WITHDRAWN
WRIGHT STATE UNIVERSITY LIBRARIES

Medical Management of HIV and AIDS

Springer
*London
Berlin
Heidelberg
New York
Barcelona
Budapest
Hong Kong
Milan
Paris
Santa Clara
Singapore
Tokyo*

Ann Millar (Ed.)

Medical Management of HIV and AIDS

With 31 Figures

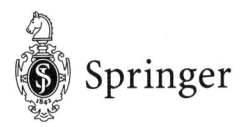

Springer

Ann Millar, MBChB, MRCP, MD
University of Bristol, Southmead Hospital, Bristol BS10 5NB, UK

ISBN 3-540-19958-6 Springer-Verlag Berlin Heidelberg New York

British Library Cataloguing in Publication Data
Medical Management of HIV and AIDS
I. Millar, Ann
616.9792
ISBN 3-540-19958-6

Library of Congress Cataloging-in-Publication Data
Medical management of HIV and AIDS/Ann Millar (ed.).
    p.   cm.
  Includes bibliographical references and index.
  ISBN 3-540-19958-6 (hardcover: alk. paper)
  1. AIDS (Disease)—Treatment. I. Millar, Ann, 1995-   .
  [DNLM: 1. HIV Infections—therapy. 2. Acquired Immunodeficiency
Syndrome—therapy.   WC 503.2 M489 1996]
RC607.A26M435   1996
616.97'9206—dc20
DNLM/DLC   95-40049
for Library of Congress

Apart from any fair dealing for the purposes of research or private study, or criticism or review, as permitted under the Copyright, Designs and Patents Act 1988, this publication may only be reproduced, stored or transmitted, in any form or by any means, with the prior permission in writing of the publishers, or in the case of reprographic reproduction in accordance with the terms of licences issued by the Copyright Licensing Agency. Enquiries concerning reproduction outside those terms should be sent to the publishers.

© Springer-Verlag London Limited 1996
Printed in Great Britain

The use of registered names, trademarks, etc. in this publication does not imply, even in the absence of a specific statement, that such names are exempt from the relevant laws and regulations and therefore free for general use

Product liability: The publisher can give no guarantee for information about drug dosage and application thereof contained in this book. In every individual case the respective user must check its accuracy by consulting other pharmaceutical literature.

Typeset by EXPO Holdings, Malaysia
Printed by Bell & Bain Ltd., Glasgow. Bound by Green Street Bindery, Oxford
28/3830-543210 Printed on acid-free paper

Preface

In the decade since AIDS was first recognised the enormous and worldwide social and medical implications of this disease have been increasingly recognised. The exponential increase in the number of people infected with HIV has been paralleled by the written literature on the subject. When this book was initially conceived the question was why another book? It seemed to me at that time and since, that as HIV presented ever more complex problems, they were best solved when considered within a wider context, using basic principles of individual medical specialties and applying them. For this reason, all the chapter authors were experienced in a particular field and applied that knowledge to HIV. All the authors were working at the Middlesex Hospital in London when the AIDS services there were expanding to fill a need, from 2 beds in 1986 to two wards today. The authors were frontline staff looking after all aspects of HIV infection within a wider general medical context. Many are now consultants or senior lecturers. It is the aim of the book to provide an insight into HIV and AIDS as a overview for someone starting to work in this field or who sees such patients occasionally and requires some basic guidelines. For this reason the chapters are based predominantly on organ systems and are divided into sections covering the presentation, methods of investigation and treatment or action required of relevant conditions. The final section of each chapter describes some thoughts on the future directions in that aspect of HIV and AIDS. The reader will judge whether this approach is a success.

I would like to thank all those who have worked so hard on this book, particularly all the chapter authors, and many in the publishing world.

HIV infection and AIDS have rewritten not only the medical textbooks but also caused a complete rethink of the provision of health care. Almost all we know about this condition is on the basis of clinical observation of those infected with HIV. I hope this text will help benefit some of them in the future.

Contents

Contributors xi

1 The Out-patient Management of HIV Infection
Patrick French 1
   Introduction 1
   Acute HIV Seroconversion Illness (CDC I) 1
   The Management of Asymptomatic HIV-positive
      Patients (CDC II and III) 3
   Constitutional Disease (CDC IVA) 14
   Sexually Transmitted Diseases and HIV-positive
      Patients 14
   References 16

**2 Counselling and Clinical Psychology in HIV
Infection and AIDS**
Alison Harris and Shamil Wanigaratne 19
   Introduction 19
   Definitions of Psychotherapy and Counselling 19
   The Role of Clinical Psychologists 20
   Prevention of HIV Infection 23
   HIV Antibody Test Counselling 24
   Psychological Assessment, Treatment Approaches and
      Psychological Techniques 26
   Psychological Treatment Approaches and Techniques . . 30
   Psychological Reactions and Problems 30
   The Worried Well 39
   Haemophiliacs 40
   Children and HIV 41
   Relapse Prevention: A New Approach 42
   The Developing Area of Health Psychology 43
   Research Issues in Psychotherapy and HIV 45
   References 45

**3 Psychological and Psychiatric Aspects of HIV
and AIDS**
Stanton Newman and Mary Fell 49
   Introduction 49

Forms and Incidence of Psychological and Psychiatric
   Disturbance 50
Suicide 53
Assessment of Mood State and Psychiatric Status 54
Psychiatric Assessments 55
Neuropsychological Assessment 56
Other Management Issues 56
Conclusion 57
References 57

4 Respiratory Problems of HIV Infection and AIDS
Ann Millar 60
Introduction 60
Clinical Presentation 60
Investigations 62
Management 69
References 79

5 Gastroenterological Problems of HIV Infection and AIDS
Ian McGowan and Duncan Churchill 86
Introduction 86
Presentation of Gastroenterological Problems 86
Investigation of Gastroenterological Problems 93
Management of Specific Problems 97
Future Developments 111
References 111

6 Neurological Complications of HIV Infection and AIDS
*Hadi Manji, Ruth McAllister, Sean Connolly and
Alan Thompson* 117
Introduction 117
Common Neurological Presentations 118
Investigation of Neurological Problems 124
Pathophysiology and Management 132
Neurological Complications due to HIV 143
The Future 155
References 156

7 Dermatological Problems in HIV Infection and AIDS
Chris Bunker 162
Introduction 162
Clinical Features 162
Diagnostic Investigations 175
Management 178
Science and Research 182
References 185

8 Haematological Complications of HIV Infection, AIDS and HIV-associated Lymphoma
Sally E. Kinsey 190
Introduction 190
Peripheral Blood Presentation 190
Peripheral Blood Features 191
Effect of Drugs Used in the Management of
  HIV Infection 198
Lupus Anticoagulant 200
Protein S Deficiency 200
HIV-related Immune Thrombocytopenia 201
HIV-related Lymphoma 202
Conclusions 207
References 208

9 Clinical Manifestations of HIV Infection and AIDS in Injecting Drug Users
Christopher Sonnex 213
Introduction 213
Symptoms 213
Investigations 217
Clinical Management 218
Other Issues 219
Conclusion 219
References 219

10 AIDS in Africa
Adam Malin and Anton Pozniak 225
The Size of the Problem 225
Transmission Modes 227
Origins 229
HIV-2 230
The Natural History of HIV Infection in Africa 231
WHO Case Clinical Definition for AIDS 232
Gastrointestinal Disease 233
Pulmonary Disease 234
Tumours 238
Skin Diseases 240
Sexually Transmitted Diseases 241
Rheumatological Problems 245
Neurological Disease 246
Paediatric Problems 247
Other Tropical Problems 248
The Future 250
References 250

Subject Index 256

Contributors

Chris Bunker
Consultant Dermatologist, Chelsea and Westminster Hospital, Fulham Road, London SW10 9NH

Duncan Churchill
Lecturer, Honorary Senior Registrar, Department of GU Medicine and Communicable Diseases, St Mary's Hospital Medical School, Jefferiss Trust Laboratories, Praed Street, London W2 1NY

Sean Connolly
Clinical and Research Fellow in Neurophysiology, Harvard Medical School and Massachusetts General Hospital, Massachusetts, USA

Mary Fell
Psychologist in Clinical Training, Department of Psychology, Eastern Health Board, Dublin 2

Patrick French
Consultant in Genitourinary Medicine, James Pringle House, The Middlesex Hospital, Mortimer Street, London W1N 8AA

Alison Harris
Clinical Psychologist, Primary Care Team, Clinical Psychology Department, Stockport Healthcare, Stepping Hill Hospital, Poplar Grove, Stockport SK2 7JE

Sally E Kinsey
Consultant Haematologist, St. James's University Hospital, Leeds LS9 7TF

Ruth McAllister
Senior Registrar in Psychiatry, Maudsley Hospital, Denmark Hill, London SE5 8AF

Ian McGowan
Blinder Research Fellow, UCLA Department of Medicine, Digestive Diseases Center, 1240 MRL, Los Angeles, CA 90095-7019, USA

Adam Malin
Clinical Lecturer, Department of Clinical Sciences, London School of Hygiene and Tropical Medicine, Keppel Street, London WC1E 7HT

Hadi Manji
Senior Registrar and Lecturer in Neurology, Royal Free Hospital, Pond Street, Hampstead, London NW3

Ann Millar
Consultant Senior Lecturer in Respiratory Medicine, Department of Respiratory Medicine, Southmead Hospital, Westbury on Trym, Bristol BS10 5NB

Stanton Newman
Head of Department and Chairman of the Board of Psychiatry, University College London Medical School Department of Psychiatry, Wolfson Building, Riding House Street, London W1N 8AA

Anton Pozniak
Senior Lecturer in Genitourinary Medicine, Kings Healthcare, 15–22 Caldecott Road, London SE5 9RS

Christopher Sonnex
Consultant Physician, Department of Genitourinary Medicine, Addenbrooke's NHS Trust, Hills Road, Cambridge CB2 2QQ

Alan Thompson
Consultant Neurologist, National Hospital for Neurology and Neurosurgery, Queen Square, London WC1

Shamil Wanigaratne
Clinical Psychologist, Drug Dependency Unit, 112, Hampstead Road, London W1N 8AA

1 The Out-patient Management of HIV Infection

Patrick French

Introduction

The human immunodeficiency virus (HIV) produces a chronic infection in which patients are asymptomatic or mildly symptomatic for the majority of its duration and are managed as out-patients. As the HIV epidemic progresses, more physicians will come into contact with this group of patients and this chapter outlines the management options available.

These options are constantly changing and as time has gone on there has been a trend for prophylactic and antiretroviral therapy to be introduced at earlier stages of HIV disease. Early in the AIDS epidemic the importance of both secondary prophylaxis for opportunistic infections and the use of antiretroviral therapy in patients with Centre for Disease Control (CDC) IV disease were realised (Fischl et al. 1987; Richman et al. 1987). Shortly after this the benefits of zidovudine in patients with early symptomatic HIV infection and primary prophylaxis for *Pneumocystis carinii* pneumonia (PCP) in patients with CDC IV disease were noted (Fischl et al. 1988, 1990a).

More recently, it has been recognised that asymptomatic patients (CDC II and III) with evidence of immunosuppression may benefit from PCP prophylaxis (CDC 1989). Although several studies of zidovudine in this group of patients have been published, the role of antiretrovirals remains uncertain (Gazzard 1993). Because of these medical interventions it is crucial to monitor asymptomatic patients, both clinically for signs of HIV disease progression and, with laboratory parameters, for evidence of immunosuppression.

This chapter also outlines the management of the HIV seroconversion illness (CDC I) which can usually be managed in the out-patient department. Finally the role of sexually transmitted diseases (STDs) and screening HIV-positive patients for STDs is discussed. Patients may have co-infection with other STDs at presentation with HIV and many patients with HIV continue to put themselves at risk of STDs.

Acute HIV Seroconversion Illness (CDC I)

Although there is no clear definition of what constitutes an HIV seroconversion illness, it appears that most patients (between 53% and 93%) are symptomatic at the time of HIV seroconversion (Tindall et al. 1991). The onset of symptoms is usually between 14 and 28 days after acquiring the virus although it can occur a great deal later (Ranki et al. 1987). It was first described as having glandular fever-like features (Cooper et al. 1985) but in fact it may have widely varying symtomatology from a mild febrile disease to a severe meningo-encephalitis (Carne et al. 1985). The hallmarks of this syndrome are a self-limiting febrile illness of acute onset often associated with a truncal macular rash (Fig. 1.1), generalised lymphadenopathy and sore throat. The clinical features of the 139 patients with symptomatic HIV seroconversion reported in the medical literature up to 1991 were summarised by Clark et al. (see Table 1.1). Although this condition is self limiting there is evidence that patients with a symptomatic seroconversion (particularly a severe prolonged illness) progress more rapidly to CDC IV (late symptomatic HIV infection) disease (Pedersen et al. 1990; Schechter et al. 1990).

This syndrome has a wide differential diagnosis (see Table 1.2) and there are also difficulties in interpreting HIV serology. Patients may not produce detectable levels of HIV antibody until the end, or after, the clinical illness and so repeat serology is mandatory for confirmation of the diagnosis. Most patients will produce detectable antibody 2–6 weeks after the onset of symptoms. There is often a transient HIV antigenaemia during seroconversion and it is useful to test for HIV p24 antigen if this diagnosis is suspected.

Because this condition is self limiting its medical management is mainly that of symptom relief. The pyrexia, myalgia and arthralgia may be controlled by non-steroidal anti-inflammatory drugs (e.g. ibuprofen 400 mg three times daily)

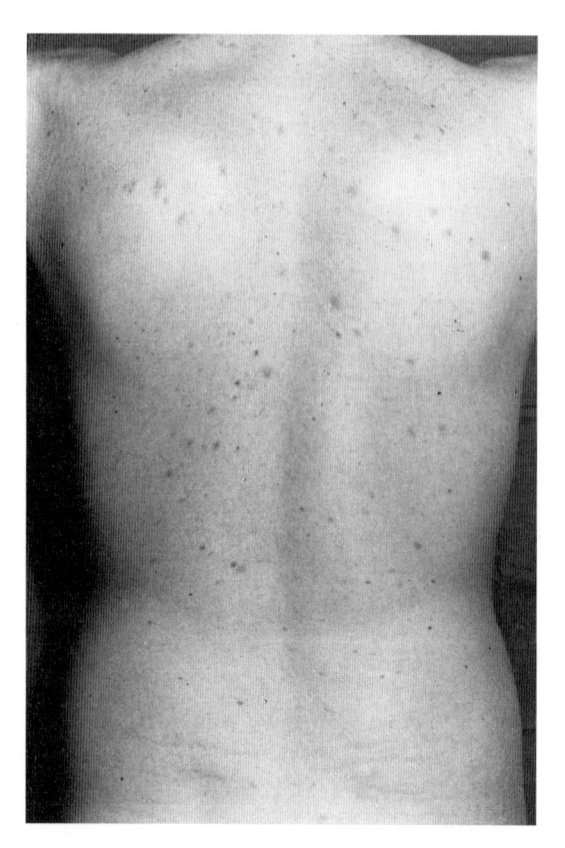

Fig. 1.1. A macular truncal rash in a man with HIV seroconversion illness.

Table 1.1. Signs and symptoms of acute HIV-1 infection (Clark et al. 1991)

Sign or symptom	Frequency (%)
Fever	97
Lymphadenopathy	77
Pharyngitis	73
Rash	70
Myalgia or arthralgia	58
Thrombocytopenia	51
Leukopenia	38
Headache	30
Diarrhoea	33
Nausea or vomiting	20
Hepatosplenomegaly	17
Oral thrush	10
Encephalopathy	8
Neuropathy	8

Table 1.2. The differential diagnosis of HIV seroconversion illness (Tindall et al. 1991)

Epstein–Barr virus mononucleosis
Cytomegalovirus mononucleosis
Toxoplasma gondii
Rubella
Secondary syphilis
Viral hepatitis
Disseminated gonococcal infection
Herpes simplex

or aspirin, and discomfort from mouth ulceration and sore throat may be eased by anaesthetic mouthwashes such as benzydamine 0.15% (Difflam) or aspirin gargles. The important exception to this symptomatic approach to management is the treatment of opportunistic infections which can present during this phase of infection. Some patients at seroconversion have transient but profound depletion of circulating lymphocytes and may need short courses of therapy for opportunistic infections, particularly oral (Fig. 1.2) and oesophageal candidiasis (Cilla et al. 1988). Oral candidiasis may be controlled with local antifungal therapy such as nystatin pastilles but oesophageal candidiasis requires systemic therapy with imidazoles (e.g. fluconazole 50 mg per day).

The role of antiretrovirals in the management of patients with acute seroconversion is uncertain. Although zidovudine (AZT) has been reported to reduce HIV antigenaemia in animal models of HIV seroconversion there are as yet no studies suggesting its efficacy in humans although some centres offer short courses of zidovudine to patients with acute HIV seroconversion (Tindall et al. 1991).

The Management of Asymptomatic HIV-positive Patients (CDC II and III)

Most patients with HIV infection are physically well for the majority of their illness. During this time care is entirely out-patient based (whether hospital out-patient, general practitioner (GP) or shared care).

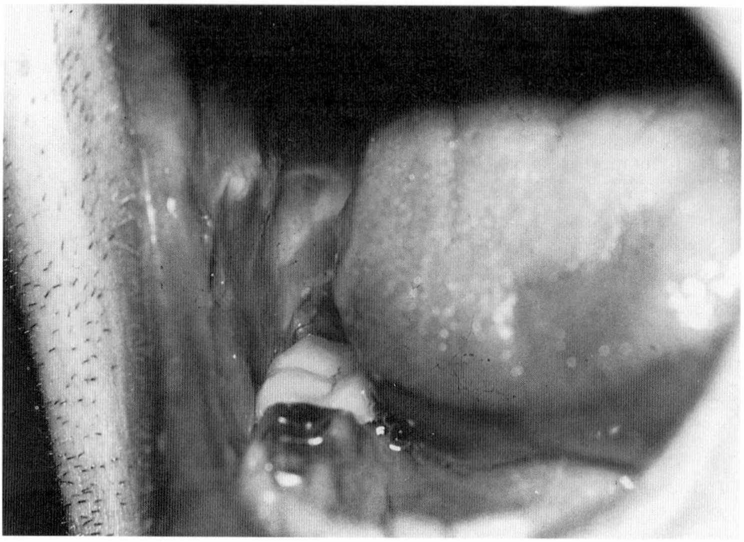

Fig. 1.2. Oral candidiasis in a man with HIV seroconversion illness.

At the Mortimer Market Centre, London we suggest review of asymptomatic patients at least tri-monthly with either visits to the out-patient clinic or alternating assessments between the GP and out-patients with the use of a shared care card. During this visit a clinical and laboratory assessment for evidence of immunosuppression can be made. This regular review also allows patients the opportunity to discuss concerns which they may feel do not warrant an appointment.

In addition HIV-infected individuals often have minor ailments which may not constitute symptomatic HIV infection but are nevertheless troublesome.

Clinical Assessment

Clinical assessment should include a full "review of systems" questionnaire to exclude the presence of constitutional symptoms (see Table 1.3). A social history establishes the level of support available to the patient and identifies any housing or employment problems. At each visit it is useful to enquire about drugs including "complementary" medicines and food supplements (which are often expensive and unnecessary). An alcohol and "recreational" drug history should be elicited as these may be important factors in patients who continue to have "unsafe" sexual intercourse.

A history of sexual behaviour should always be taken. This is the essential starting point in discussing "safer sex" practices and determines whether screening for sexually transmitted diseases is required (see below). As well as being at risk of sexually transmitted diseases women with HIV are often of child-bearing age and should therefore be counselled and advised about contraception.

Injecting drug users should be asked about the type of drug injected, needle sharing and injecting technique. Patients should be encouraged to convert to non-parenteral drug taking. If this is not possible they should be advised to use

The Out-patient Management of HIV Infection

Table 1.3. Definition of CDC IVA disease (CDC 1987)

One or more of the following must be present in the absence of a concurrent illness or condition other than HIV to explain the findings:
1. Fever persisting for more than 1 month
2. Involuntary weight loss of more than 10% from baseline
3. Diarrhoea for more than 1 month

clean needles, not to inject "street" drugs and not to share needles. These aspects of care are best managed by a drug dependency unit or needle exchange.

Examination concentrates on determining whether there is any disease progression. It is important to remember that secondary tumours such as Kaposi's sarcoma and non-Hodgkin's lymphoma may occur when the T4 lymphocyte count is relatively high (Crowe et al. 1990), in contrast to opportunistic infection.

General Examination

Weight and temperature should be measured, as weight loss and persistent pyrexia may fulfil the criteria for constitutional symptoms (see Table 1.3).

Skin (See Chapter 7)

Although skin conditions such as psoriasis, facial molluscum contagiosum and seborrhoeic dermatitis may first present, or deteriorate, as HIV disease progresses their presence in itself does not indicate progression. Careful examination may reveal lesions of Kaposi's sarcoma not seen or recognised by the patient.

Seborrhoeic dermatitis is a common complaint in this group of patients with the typical scaling greasy plaques affecting naso-labial folds, eyebrows, scalp and chest. Also many patients complain of generalised dry skin with associated pruritus.

Herpes zoster (shingles) may be an indicator of immunosuppression in HIV infection especially if it affects more than one dermatome. Herpes zoster may take a more aggressive course in HIV-infected patients but usually responds well to high dose acyclovir therapy.

The frequency and severity of ano-genital herpes simplex virus (HSV) infection may be increased by worsening immune function, and continuous mucocutaneous HSV for more than 1 month in the presence of HIV constitutes an AIDS defining diagnosis (CDC 1987). Patients with troublesome recurrences may benefit from acyclovir prophylaxis.

Lymph Nodes

At each routine visit cervical, axillary and inguinal lymph nodes should be examined. Persistent generalised lymphadenopathy (PGL), defined as palpable lymphadenopathy (nodes >1 cm) at two or more extrainguinal sites for more than 3 months, constitutes CDC Group III disease. Before this diagnosis can be made it is important to exclude other causes of generalised lymphadenopathy (see Table 1.4). In cases of doubt a lymph node biopsy should be considered (see Table 1.5). The

Table 1.4. The differential diagnosis of persistent generalised lymphadenopathy (CDC III)

1. Acute viral infections
    Epstein–Barr
    Cytomegalovirus
    Rubella
2. Secondary syphilis
3. HIV-related conditions
    a. Opportunistic infections
        Mycobacterium avium intracellulare
        Mycobacterium tuberculosis
        Histoplasmosis capsulatum
    b. Secondary tumours
        Lymphoma
        Kaposi's sarcoma

Table 1.5. Indications for lymph node biopsy (Voetberg and Lucas 1991)

Constitutional symptoms
Tender/painful lymphadenopathy
Asymmetrical lymphadenopathy
Patients from developing countries

characteristic histological feature of PGL is follicular hyperplasia which, as disease progresses, changes to germinal centre atrophy and fibrosis with regression of lymphadenopathy. The presence of lymphadenopathy is not a prognostic indicator as there is no difference between CDC II (asymptomatic HIV infection without PGL) and CDC III patients in the rates of progression to CDC IV disease (Moss et al. 1988).

Mouth

Examination of the mouth is a vital part of the assessment of asymptomatic HIV-positive patients. Periodontal disease is common and patients should be regularly assessed by a dentist on at least a 6-monthly basis. Gingivitis leading to bleeding, gum recession and caries is a frequent complication (Fig. 1.3).

Oral ulceration is another common problem and may be a manifestation of a wide variety of diseases. In patients with ulceration secondary to candidiasis or Kaposi's sarcoma the diagnosis is usually clinically obvious. In many cases, however, the aetiology of the ulceration is obscure and further investigations are required. The two most common diagnoses are herpes simplex and aphthous ulceration. Both present a history of recurrent painful mouth ulceration and have similar clinical appearances of ulcers with clearly demarcated borders, sloughed bases and local tenderness.

The palate should be carefully examined as it is a common site for Kaposi's sarcoma and may be the first site of presentation (Stafford et al. 1989).

Oral candidiasis is an important sign of immunosuppression in the absence of any other predisposing factors (see Table 1.6) and may have differing clinical appearance. However, it typically appears as white plaques on the palate and buccal mucosa. These plaques can be scraped off using a tongue depressor reveal-

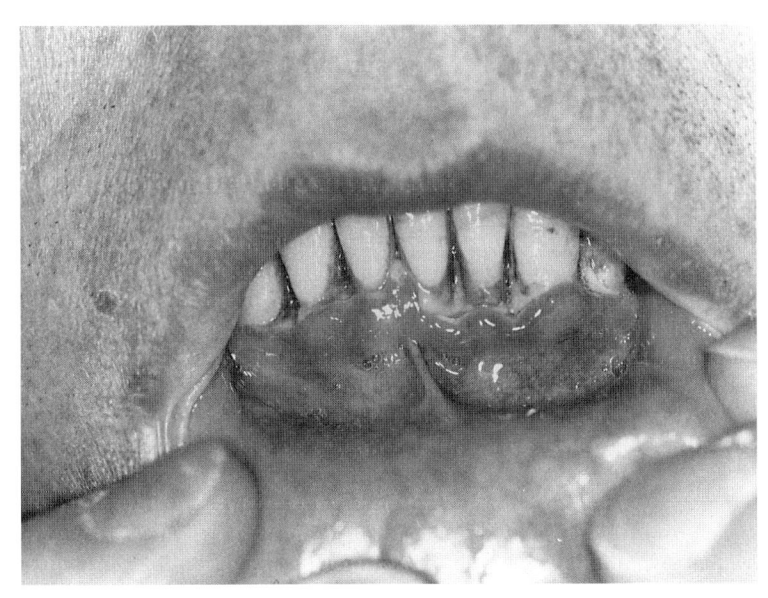

Fig. 1.3. Gingivitis and severe gum recession in an otherwise asymptomatic man with HIV infection.

Table 1.6. Predisposing causes of oral candidiasis

1. Systemic immunosuppression
    e.g. Acute HIV seroconversion
    HIV CDC IV disease
    Immunosuppressive therapy (corticosteroids, transplant recipients, cancer chemotherapy)
2. Local immunosuppression
    e.g. Steroid inhaler
3. Local disturbance in mouth microflora and maceration
    e.g. Dental plates
    Persistent sweet sucking

ing an erythematous base. In cases of doubt a wet mount of lesion scrapings should be prepared with 10% KOH to attempt to identify fungal hyphae. A positive oral culture for *Candida* sp. is of no significance as it may merely indicate fungal colonisation. Oral candidiasis is common in symptomatic HIV infection with up to 70% suffering from an attack at some point during the course of the disease.

Oral hairy leukoplakia (OHL, see Chapter 7) presents as adherent (i.e. not scraped off by a tongue depressor), grey/white linear lesions affecting the lateral border of the tongue (Fig. 1.4) and occasionally the buccal mucosa. It is a benign condition previously considered to be pathognomonic of HIV infection and associated with increased risk of progression to CDC IV disease (Greenspan et al. 1984, 1987). More recently it has been noted that OHL can occur in the absence of HIV infection (Epstein et al. 1990). Although it is found more commonly as disease progresses it is not in itself closely associated with an increased risk of disease progression (Feigel et al. 1990). It is clear that the presence of OHL alone does not represent disease progression but indicates that further examination and investigation of immune status is required (Lau et al. 1991).

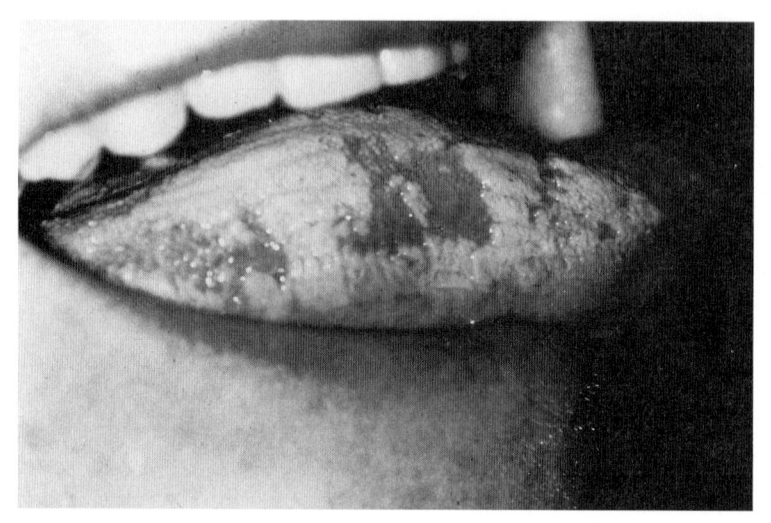

Fig. 1.4. Oral hairy leukoplakia on the lateral border of the tongue.

Although OHL is a benign condition, "OHL-like" lesions have been reported to cause oesophageal ulceration (Kitchen et al. 1990). Those with apparently symptomatic OHL should be investigated for concomitant candidiasis and treated if necessary.

Abdomen

Examination should include palpation for hepatomegaly and splenomegaly. Although splenomegaly may be associated with PGL other causes should be excluded particularly mycobacterial disease and lymphoma.

Respiratory System

All patients should have a careful respiratory examination and chest x-ray. This is particularly important in patients from the developing world and injecting drug users who may be at particular risk of *Mycobacterium tuberculosis* (see Chapter 4).

Musculoskeletal System

A relapsing, non-erosive, asymmetrical, seronegative arthritis has been described in association with HIV infection (Forster et al. 1988). The cases described occurred in HIV-positive men without AIDS and were in the main associated with psoriasis or urethritis (with or without conjunctivitis) and all patients who had HLA typing performed were HLA B27 positive. The arthritis was poorly responsive to NSAIDs and followed a relapsing progressive course. HIV-positive patients with arthritis should be referred to a rheumatologist for assessment.

Nervous System (Chapter 6)

The first clinical manifestation of HIV may be cognitive impairment and some workers have found a high prevalence of progressive subclinical neurological deficits in asymptomatic patients (Koralink et al. 1990) although others have disagreed with these findings (Janssen et al. 1989; McArthur et al. 1989). The significance and natural history of patients with subclinical neurological deficits (particularly whether these patients develop HIV-related dementia) is not yet known (Koralink et al. 1990). Where early AIDS-related dementia is suspected it is often useful to refer the patient to a clinical psychologist for serial psychometric testing.

The examination of the central nervous system should include fundoscopy for cytomegalovirus retinitis and cotton wool spots (see Chapter 6). It is probable that fundoscopy for cytomegalovirus retinitis should be reserved for patients with evidence of immunosuppression.

Cardiovascular System

Asymptomatic patients may have subclinical autonomic neuropathy or adrenocortical insufficiency and it may be worthwhile assessing the patient for postural hypotension (Membrano et al. 1987; Villa et al. 1987). Auscultation for heart murmurs should also be performed; this is particularly important if the patient is an intravenous drug user and therefore at risk of bacterial endocarditis.

Laboratory Assessments/Investigations

At the first visit to clinic it is useful to perform some baseline investigations (Table 1.7).

Several different serum markers of disease activity have been used alone and in combination to predict disease progression in HIV infection. T-Cell lymphocyte subsets (particularly absolute CD4 lymphocyte numbers and CD4 lymphocyte %) are probably the most reliable single index available. However other

Table 1.7. Baseline investigations

Full blood count (n.b. thrombocytopenia)
Liver function tests
Urea and electrolytes
Toxoplasma gondii serology
Hepatitis B serology
Syphilis serology

P-A Chest x-ray
+/− Lung function tests (including CO transfer factor) (Shaw et al. 1988)

Immunological tests
T-lymphocyte subsets
+/− p24 antigen
+/− beta 2 microglobulin
+/− neopterin

markers such as beta 2 microglobulin, neopterin and p24 antigenaemia also have a role in the monitoring of HIV disease.

T-Lymphocyte Subsets

Abnormalities in peripheral blood T-cell numbers may occur at seroconversion and persist throughout the course of HIV infection (Pedersen et al. 1990). However in most patients there is a variable period in which infection appears to be "latent" (marked HIV replication continues in lymphatic tissue) and T-cell subsets remain normal (the T4 count is usually within normal range but lower than before infection). The earliest abnormality is often a raised CD8 count leading to a decreased or inverted CD4 : CD8 ratio. In the majority of patients this is followed by a progressive fall in the CD4 count and later a fall in the CD8 count.

Although some workers have found the CD4% and CD4 : CD8 ratio to be more reliable indicators of disease progression risk than CD4 counts (possibly because of inaccurate total lymphocyte counts) (Taylor et al. 1989), most studies have related CD4 counts alone to the development of CDC IV disease. As lymphocyte subsets are increasingly used as prognostic markers and in deciding on therapy, it has become more evident that single results in individual patients should be treated with caution. Patients should have their blood samples taken at the same time of day and transported to the laboratory and processed promptly. It is important to interpret any result as part of a trend and to repeat abnormal or unexpected results. It is vital to look at results only in the context of the clinical status of the patient and to realise that factors other than from HIV infection can alter CD4 counts (Table 1.8). Patients who are having their lymphocyte subsets monitored should be assessed to exclude other causes of T-cell fluctuation.

At the Mortimer Market Centre, T-cell subsets are monitored in asymptomatic patients at 3-monthly intervals or more frequently if CD4 counts are falling rapidly. Low levels are repeated once or twice for confirmation.

Beta 2 Microglobulin

This is a low molecular weight protein that forms the light chain of the class 1 major histocompatibility complex which is present on the surface of most somatic cells. Raised levels of beta 2 microglobulin have been found to correlate

Table 1.8. Factors influencing T-lymphocyte counts (Bird 1990; Landay 1989)

Biological
    Acute intercurrent infection
    Drug therapy (e.g. cephalosporin, danarubicin)
    Diurnal variation (low at 1100, high at 2300)
    Stress and exertion (decrease with exertion)
Procedural
    Temperature of specimen in transit
    Delay in analysis
    Changes in laboratory anilites (antibiotics)
    Changes in laboratory procedure/methodology

well with disease progression in HIV infection (Jacobsen et al. 1991) and are probably related to HIV-induced activation of lymphocytes and macrophages. However this rise can be seen with other vital infections and malignancies.

It has been suggested (in treatment trials) that beta 2 microglobulin may be a more accurate marker of disease activity than T4 counts alone because it also reflects macrophage infection (Jacobsen et al. 1989). One additional advantage beta 2 microglobulin has over T-cell counts is that it can be measured in stored serum and can therefore be used in retrospective studies.

Neopterin

This is a metabolite of guanosine triphosphate and is released by macrophages when they are stimulated by activated T-lymphocytes. Although it is not often measured in routine practice some workers have found it a more accurate predictor of disease progression when used in combination with CD4 counts than CD4 counts alone (Fahey et al. 1990).

HIV Antigen

HIV p24 antigen is often transiently detected in the serum of patients during HIV seroconversion. It then usually becomes undetectable for most of the period of asymptomatic infection only to reappear as disease progresses. If present it tends to be suppressed at the initiation of antiretroviral therapy and can be measured in stored serum. However, up to 20% of asymptomatic patients may have p24 antigen while other patients may develop CDC IV disease without producing detectable p24 antigen. Therefore although p24 antigen has a role in diagnosing HIV seroconversion and monitoring response to antiretroviral therapy it has only a limited place in the assessment of the individual asymptomatic HIV-positive patient.

Treatment 1: Clinical Problems

Skin

For seborrhoeic dermatitis local applications of combined hydrocortisone 1%/antifungal creams (such as Daktacort or Canestan HC) and shampoos based on coaltar (Polytar), selenium (Selsun) or antifungal agents (Ketoconazole) are often beneficial.

Dry skin may be controlled by using aqueous cream as a soap substitute and using emollients either as bath additives (e.g. Aveenos sachets or Oilatum Emollient) or after showering (e.g. Diprobase). Patients who fail to respond to these simple medications should be referred to a dermatologist.

Shingles can be treated with acyclovir 800 mg × 5/day for 5–10 days if the patient is treated within the first few days of symptoms.

Herpes simplex prophylaxis with acyclovir at a dose of 200 mg 6-hourly appears to be effective as suppressive therapy in these patients, although some may require a higher dose. There have been reports of acyclovir-resistant strains of HSV developing in patients with CDC stage IV disease on suppressive therapy (Erlich et al. 1989) but there is no evidence of subsequent sexual transmission or latency of these strains. Acyclovir-resistant herpes simplex can be adequately treated with alternative medications such as foscarnet until the HSV reverts to the wild, acyclovir-sensitive strains (Chatis et al. 1989).

Mouth

Acute episodes of gingivitis can be managed with metronidazole 400 mg twice daily for 3 days and chlorhexidine (Corsodyl) mouth wash gargled twice daily for 10 days. Good oral hygiene and regular dental care reduce the chance of attacks.

In the management of oral ulceration empirical treatment for herpes simplex with acyclovir 200 mg × 5/day for 5 days and anaesthetic gargles (e.g. Difflam) is often justified while awaiting herpes simplex cultures. "Aphthous" ulceration is a diagnosis of exclusion and symptom relief with anaesthetic gargles and mouth toilet (installation of Corsodyl via a soft-tipped syringe) is often all that is required until spontaneous healing occurs. If the site is favourable corticosteroid pellets (hydrocortisone 2.5 mg × 4/day) applied to the ulcer may encourage healing. In patients with ulceration that fails to respond to this simple non-toxic medication ulcer biopsy should be performed to exclude tumours such as lymphoma and opportunistic infections (e.g. cytomegalovirus) (French et al. 1991). In cases of aphthous ulceration poorly responsive to this therapy more toxic systemic medication such as corticosteroids or thalidomide may be necessary.

In the first instance oral candidiasis can be treated with topical antifungal agents (miconazole gel, amphotericin lozenges, nystatin pastilles etc.) although in later disease systemic therapy such as the imidazoles (ketoconazole 200 mg twice daily or fluconazole 50 mg once daily) may be necessary for adequate control. Two-week courses of antifungal therapy may be sufficient to treat candidiasis initially but continuous systemic prophylaxis with imidazoles may be needed in recurrent disease and is advisable in all patients with oesophageal involvement.

Patients concerned about the appearance of OHL may get some cosmetic benefit from local acyclovir cream.

Treatment 2: Primary Prophylaxis for Opportunistic Infections

The risk of *Pneumocystis carinii* pneumonia (PCP) developing in patients with CD4 counts of less than $200 \times 10^6/l$ when followed up over a period of 12 months has been estimated as 18.4%. The 12-month risk of developing PCP if a patient has a CD4 count of $200–350 \times 10^6/l$ is 4% and between 351 and $500 \times 10^6/l$ is 1.4% (Phair et al. 1990). This observation has led to the recommendation that primary PCP prophylaxis should be offered to all patients with CD4 counts below $200 \times 10^6/l$ (CDC 1989). Daily oral cotrimoxazole (960 mg once daily) is more effective than monthly nebulised pentamidine (300 mg monthly) as primary PCP prophylaxis (Schneider et al. 1992) and daily dapsone (50 or 100 mg once daily) also seems effective and well tolerated (Kemper et al. 1990; Martin et al. 1992).

It has been estimated that up to 28% of patients with AIDS and positive *T. gondii* serology will develop cerebral toxoplasmosis (Grant et al. 1990) and there is increasing evidence that primary prophylaxis is effective in these patients (Clotet et al. 1991). It is advisable to screen all asymptomatic patients for serological evidence of previous toxoplasmosis as there can be a lower index of suspicion of toxoplasma encephalitis in patients with evidence of previous infection, while patients with negative *T. gondii* serology can be counselled on how to avoid future infection (Durack et al. 1984). Advice should include eating well cooked meat, thoroughly cleaning vegetables and if they own a cat disposing of cat litter daily (to prevent oocysts maturing to the infective form). Systemic PCP prophylaxis regimes such as daily cotrimoxazole or dapsone appear effective as primary cerebral toxoplasmosis prophylaxis (Girard et al. 1992). Prophylaxis should be offered to all *T. gondii* antibody-positive patients with CD4 counts <200 × 10^6/l.

Immunocompromised HIV-positive patients with a past history of *Mycobacterium tuberculosis* infection are at high risk of disease reactivation (Markowitz et al. 1991). It has recently been reported that primary prophylaxis with isoniazid 300 mg daily with pyridoxine 10 mg daily may be effective in these patients (Wadhawan et al. 1991; Pape et al. 1992). The British Thoracic Society have recommended that all HIV antibody positive patients in the UK with evidence of previous tuberculosis and a CD4 count below 200 × 10^6/l should receive prophylaxis with isoniazid 300 mg and pyridoxine 10 mg (BTS 1992). Patients attending clinic with HIV infection should therefore have a P-A chest x-ray. This may reveal previous tuberculosis and serves as a baseline film to compare with future films should the patient develop chest disease later in the course of the illness (see Chapter 4).

Treatment 3: Antiretroviral Therapy

There have been several placebo-controlled double-blind studies investigating the role of the thymidine analogue zidovudine (AZT) in reducing the risk of disease progression. Although two of these studies (Volberding et al. 1990; Cooper et al. 1993) showed a small decrease in the progression rate to symptomatic disease the clinical significance of this finding and its bearing on survival were uncertain. The preliminary data of a larger study with far greater number of end-points (severe ARC, AIDS, death) suggest that there is no significant progression or survival benefit of zidovudine in this population (Aboulker and Swart 1993). Two open studies examined the suggestion that zidovudine may increase the length of survival. Both found an initial benefit of reduced progression which persisted in one study to prolonged survival (Graham et al. 1992) although the other study did not find this (Hamilton et al. 1992). It is likely that monotherapy with zidovudine produces a small and short-lived benefit to asymptomatic patients. It therefore only has a limited role in the management of this group although some authorities believe zidovudine should be offered to patients with CD4 counts below 200 × 10^6/l (NIAID 1993). In the future other nucleoside analogues (didanosine (ddI) and dideoxycytosine (ddC)) and non-nucleoside (i.e. protease inhibitors) antiretrovirals may be used in combinations with zidovudine in an attempt to reduce the problems of viral resistance, which appears to be the fundamental cause of the limited benefit of zidovudine. These studies are currently under way.

Inosine pranobex has been noted to enhance proliferative responses of T lymphocytes and the activity of natural killer cells in vivo. A single trial suggests it may reduce the risk of progression to CDC IV disease (Pedersen et al. 1990). However these findings remain unconfirmed.

Ditiocarb sodium (imuthiol) has also been shown to be beneficial in reducing disease progression (Lang et al. 1988). Its mechanism of action is obscure and further European studies are in progress to confirm these findings.

Constitutional Disease (CDC IV A)

It was noted early in the AIDS epidemic that patients at risk of AIDS suffered from symptoms for which no cause apart from HIV infection itself could be found. These non-specific constitutional symptoms and signs were later included in the CDC classification as CDC IVA disease (Table 1.3). However before symptoms can be attributed to HIV infection alone other causes of these symptoms must be excluded (see Table 1.9).

If symptoms persist and CDC IVA disease is diagnosed the patient should be offered both primary PCP prophylaxis and zidovudine (Fischl et al. 1988; Fischl et al. 1990). It is probably best to stagger the onset of these two therapies in order to elucidate the cause of any adverse drug reactions. The choice of starting dose of zidovudine is controversial. There is now good evidence that lower dose regimes (500–600 mg/day) compared to standard zidovudine doses (1000–1500 mg), both regimes in 2–4 divided doses, are as effective and produce less toxicity, especially myelosuppression (Fischl et al. 1990; Collier et al. 1990). There are worries, however, about the central nervous system penetration of lower zidovudine doses. Constitutional symptoms usually respond well to zidovudine and if the symptomatic response is poor alternative or additional causes should be sought.

Sexually Transmitted Diseases and HIV-positive Patients

World-wide, the major route of HIV transmission is sexual and the presence of HIV is often associated with other sexually transmitted diseases (STDs) (Kell

Table 1.9. The differential diagnosis of constitutional symptoms

1. HIV-associated conditions
  a. Opportunistic infections
    Fungal e.g. cryptococcosis
    Protozoal e.g. *Pneumocystis carinii*
    Viral e.g. cytomegalovirus
    Mycobacterial e.g. *M. tuberculosis, M. avium-intracellulare*
    Bacterial e.g. *Salmonella spp.*
  b. Lymphoma with B (constitutional) symptoms
2. Infections not related to HIV
    Bacterial endocarditis (in intravenous drug users)
    Pulmonary tuberculosis
    Other chronic/relapsing infections e.g. brucellosis, syphilis, Epstein–Barr virus

et al. 1991). It is advisable therefore to offer all patients with HIV a screen for STDs at their first visit and to re-screen patients who continue to put themselves at risk of infection.

The relationship between HIV and other STDs is complex. It is probable that there is an increased risk of HIV transmission in patients with ulcerative STDs (Stamm et al. 1988; Simonsen et al. 1988). It is also possible that non-ulcerative STDs may facilitate the transmission of HIV (Laga et al. 1990).

The natural history of some STDs can be affected by concomitant HIV infection. There is anecdotal evidence that infectious syphilis may progress more rapidly to late stage disease (Johns et al. 1987) in the presence of HIV infection although this remains to be confirmed in a large study. Hepatitis B virus (HBV) can reactivate in the presence of HIV-associated immunosuppression (Vento et al. 1989) and it is possible for HIV infected patients with natural immunity to HBV to acquire infection with different strains of HBV (Maeland et al. 1989). HIV infected individuals who subsequently develop HBV are at greater risk of becoming chronic carriers. It is therefore important that HIV-positive patients who are found to be susceptible to HBV are offered vaccination.

It has been noted that women with HIV are at increased risk of cervical intra-epithelial neoplasia (CIN) and are also more likely to develop invasive disease (Agarossi et al. 1991). Invasive cervical carcinoma has recently been included in the revised CDC AIDS definition (1992) in the USA. The minimum STD screen must therefore include HBV and syphilis serology and, for women, yearly cervical cytology with or without colposcopy.

It should be borne in mind that patients with sexually transmitted diseases (particularly women) are often asymptomatic. In addition to the serological tests for hepatitis B and syphilis, screening should include tests for *Chlamydia trachomatis*, *Neisseria gonorrhoeae* and *Trichomonas vaginalis* (see Table 1.10). But it should be remembered that patients with STDs are best managed in genito-urinary medicine clinics where there is expertise in counselling, tests of cure and contact tracing. Drug regimes used at this centre for the common STDs are shown in Table 1.11. If a patient is at risk of, or has symptoms suggesting, an STD they should be referred to a genitourinary medicine physician for assessment.

Table 1.10. Screening tests for sexually transmitted diseases

Site of test	N. gonorrhoeae	C. trachomatis	Other
Pharynx	Culture	–	–
Male urethra	Gram stain and culture	ELISA +/- culture	–
Female urethra	Gram stain and culture	–	–
Vaginal	–	–	*T. vaginalis*: dark ground microscopy and culture
Cervical	Gram stain and culture	ELISA +/- culture	Herpes simplex if suspected
Rectal (if clinically indicated or N. gonorrhoeae suspected)	Gram stain and culture	Culture (if proctitis present)	Herpes simplex (if proctitis present)

Table 1.11. Treatment for selected sexually transmitted diseases

N. gonorrhoeae
Amoxycillin 3 g + probenecid 1 g both orally* *or* ciprofloxacin 250–500 mg orally (for penicillin-resistant *N. gonorrhoeae*, pharyngeal gonorrhoea, patients allergic to penicillin)

C. trachomatis
Doxycycline 100 mg twice daily for 7 days orally *or* erythromycin stearate 500 mg twice daily for 14 days*

T. vaginalis
Metronidazole 400 mg twice daily orally for 5 days *or* metronidazole 2 g orally as a single dose

Syphilis (T. pallidum)
Procaine penicillin 600,000 units i.m. daily for 10 days plus probenecid 1 g orally daily (for primary, secondary and early latent infection)* *or* doxycycline 100 mg twice daily orally for 15 days
Procaine penicillin 900,000 units i.m. daily for 21 days plus probenecid 1 g orally daily (for late latent and tertiary syphilis)* *or* doxycycline 100 mg twice daily for 30 days orally

* Safe in pregnancy and lactation.

References

Aboulker J-P, Swart AM (1993) Preliminary analysis of the Concorde trial. Lancet i: 889–890
Agarossi A, Casolati E, Muggiasca L, Ravasi L, Brammbilla T, Conti M (1991) Natural history of cervical HPV i and CIN in HIV positive women. VII International Conference on AIDS, Florence MB 2425 (Abs)
Bird AG (1990) Monitoring of lymphocyte subpopulation changes in the assessment of HIV infection. Genitourin Med 66: 133–137
British Thoracic Society (1992) Guidelines on the management of tuberculosis and HIV infection in the United Kingdom. Br Med J 304; 1231–1233
Carne CA, Tedder RS, Smith A, et al. (1985) Acute encephalopathy coincident with seroconversion for anti-HTLV-III. Lancet ii: 1206–1208
CDC (1986) Classification system for human T-lymphotropic virus type III/lymphadenopathy-associated virus infection. MMWR 35: 334
CDC (1987) Revision of the CDC surveillance case definition for acquired immunodeficiency syndrome. MMWR 36: suppl 15, 35–145
CDC (1989) Guidelines for prophylaxis against *Pneumocystis carinii* pneumonia for persons with human immunodeficiency virus. MMWR 38: suppl 5
CDC (1992) Revised classification systems for HIV infection and expanded surveillance case definitions for AIDS among adolescents and adults. MMWR 41: (no RR-17)
Chatis PA, Miller CH, Schrager LE, Crumpacker CS (1989) Successful treatment with foscarnet of an acyclovir-resistant mucocutaneous infection with herpes simplex virus in a patient with acquired immunodeficiency syndrome. N Engl J Med 320: 297–300
Cilla G, Trallero EP, Furundarena JR, Cuadrado E, Iribarren JA, Neira F (1988) Esophogeal candidiasis and immunodeficiency associated with acute HIV infection. AIDS 2: 399–400.
Clark SJ, Saag MS, Decker WD, et al. (1991) High titres of cytopathic virus in plasma of patients with symptomatic primary HIV 1 infection. N Engl J Med 324: 954–960
Clotet B, Sirera G, Romeu J et al. (1991) Twice-weekly dapsone-pyrimethamine for preventing PCP and cerebral toxoplasmosis. AIDS 5: 601–602
Collier AC, Bozzette S, Coombs RW et al. (1990) A pilot study of low-dose zidovudine in human immunodeficiency virus infection. N Engl J Med 323: 1015–1021
Cooper DA, Gold J, Maclean P et al. (1985) Acute AIDS retrovirus infection. Definition of a clinical illness associated with seroconversion. Lancet i: 537
Cooper DA, Gatell JM, Kroon S et al. (1993) Zidovudine in persons with asymptomatic HIV infection and CD4[+] cell counts greater than 400 per cubic millimetre. N Engl J Med 329: 297–303
Crowe S, Stewart K, Carlin J, Hoy JF (1990) The relationship between opportunistic infections (OI) and malignancy in HIV patients and CD4 lymphocyte number. VI International Conference on AIDS, San Francisco: SB 526 (abstr)
Durack DT (1984) Prevention of central nervous system infection in patients at risk. Am J Med 231–237
Epstein JB, Sherlock CS, Greenspan JS (1990) Hairy leukoplakia like lesions in patients without HIV infection. VI International Conference on AIDS, San Francisco: Th.B.377 (abstr)

Erlich KS, Mills J, Chatis P et al. (1989) Acyclovir-resistant herpes simplex virus infections in patients with the acquired immunodeficiency syndrome. N Engl J Med 320: 293–296
Fahey JL, Taylor JMG, Detels R et al. (1990) The prognostic value of cellular and serologic markers in infection with human immunodeficiency virus type 1. N Engl J Med 322: 166–172
Feigel DW, Greenspan D, Winkelstein W et al. (1990) Prevalence of hairy leukoplakia by CD4 count level. VI International conference on AIDS, San Francisco: Th.B.376 (abstr)
Fischl MA, Richman DD, Grieco MH et al. (1987) The efficacy of azidothymidine (AZT) in the treatment of patients with AIDS and AIDS-related complex. N Engl J Med 317: 185–191
Fischl MA, Dickinson GM, La Voie L (1988) Safety and efficacy of sulphamethoxazole and trimethoprim chemoprophylaxis for *Pneumocystis carinii* pneumonia in AIDS. JAMA 259: 1185–1189
Fischl MA, Richman DD, Hansen N et al. (1990a) The safety and efficacy of zidovudine (AZT) in the treatment of subjects with mildly symptomatic Human immunodeficiency virus infection type 1 (HIV) infection. A double blind placebo controlled trial. Ann Intern Med 112: 727–737
Fischl MA, Parker CB, Pettinelli C et al. (1990b) A randomised trial of a reduced daily dose of zidovudine in patients with the acquired immunodeficiency syndrome. N Engl J Med 323: 1009–1014
Forster SM, Seifert MH, Keat AC et al. (1988) Inflammatory joint disease and human immunodeficiency virus infection. Br Med J 296: 1625–1627
French PD, Birchall MA, Harris JRW (1991) Cytomegalovirus ulceration of the oropharynx. J Oto Laryng 105: 739–742
Gazzard BG (1993) After Concorde. Br Med J 306: 1016–1017
Girard P-M, Landman R, Gaudebout C et al. (1992) Dapsone-pyramethamine vs aerosolized pentamidine for primary prophylaxis of pneumocystosis and neurotoxoplasmosis. VIII International Conference on AIDS, Florence. WeB 1017 (Abs)
Graham NMH, Zeger SL, Park LP et al. (1992) The effects on survival of early treatment of human immunodeficiency virus infection. N Engl J Med 326: 1037–1042
Grant IH, Gold JWM, Rosenblum M et al. (1990) *Toxoplasma gondii* serology in HIV-infected patients: the development of central nervous system toxoplasmosis in AIDS. AIDS 4: 519–521
Greenspan D, Greenspan JS, Conant M et al. (1984) Oral "hairy" leucoplakia in male homosexuals: evidence of association with both papilloma virus and a herpes-group virus. Lancet ii: 831–834
Greenspan D, Greenspan JS, Hearst NG et al. (1987) Relation of oral hairy leukoplakia to infection with the human immunodeficiency virus and the risk of developing AIDS. J Infect Dis 155: 475–481
Hamilton JD, Hartigan PM, Simberkoff MS et al. (1992) A controlled trial of early versus late treatment with zidovudine in symptomatic human immunodeficiency virus infection. N Engl J Med 326: 437–443
Jacobsen MA, Abrams DI, Volberding PA et al. (1989) Serum beta 2-microglobulin decreases in patients with AIDS or ARC treated with azidothymidine. J Inf Dis 159: 1029–1036
Jacobsen MA, Bachetti P, Kolokathis A et al. (1991) Surrogate markers for survival in patients with AIDS and AIDS related complex treated with zidovudine. Br Med J 302: 73–78
Janssen RS, Saykin AJ, Cannon L et al. (1989) Neurological and neuropsychological manifestations of HIV1 infection: association with AIDS-related complex but not asymptomatic HIV1 infection. Ann Neurol 26: 592–600
Johns DR, Tierney M, Felsenstein D (1987) Alteration in the natural history of neurosyphilis by concurrent infection with the human immunodeficiency virus. N Engl J Med 316: 1573–1577
Kell PD, Barton SE, Summerbel CD, Lawrence AG (1991) Sexually transmitted diseases in HIV-1 seropositive women at presentation. Int J STD AIDS 2: 204–206
Kemper CA, Tucker RM, Lang OS et al. (1990) Low-dose dapsone prophylaxis of *Pneumocystis carinii* pneumonia in AIDS and AIDS-related complex. AIDS 4: 1145–1148
Koralink IJ, Beaumanoir A, Hausler R et al. (1990) A controlled study of early neurologic abnormalities in men infected with asymptomatic human immunodeficiency virus infection. N Engl J Med 323: 864–870
Laga M, Nzila N, Manoka AT et al. (1990) Non ulcerative sexually transmitted disease (STD) as risk factors for HIV infection. VI International Conference on AIDS, San Francisco. Th.C.97 (abstr)
Landay AL, Muirhead KA (1989) Procedural guidelines for performing immunophenotyping by flow cytometry. Clin Immunol Immunopath 52: 48–60
Lang J-M, Touraine J-L, Trepo C et al. (1988) Randomised double-blind, placebo controlled trial of ditiocarb sodium ("imuthiol") in human immunodeficiency virus infection. Lancet ii: 702–706
Kitchen VS, Helbert M, Logan R et al. (1990) EBV associated oesophageal ulcer in AIDS. Gut 31: 1223–1225
Lau RKW, Jenkins P, Pinching AJ (1991) The natural history of human immunodeficiency virus infection. Genitourin Med 67: 71–72

McArthur JC, Cohen BA, Selnes OA et al. (1989) Low prevalence of neurological and neuropsychological abnormalities in otherwise healthy HIV1 infected individuals: results from the multicentre AIDS cohort study. Ann Neurol 26: 601–611

Maeland A, Skaug K, Storvold G, Kittlesen P (1989) Reactivation of hepatitis B. Lancet i: 1083

Martin MA, Cox PH, Beck K, Styer CM, Beall GN (1992) A comparison of the effectiveness of three regimens in the prevention of *Pneumocystis carinii* pneumonia in human immunodeficiency virus-infected patients. Arch Intern Med 152: 523–528

Marcowitz N, Reichman L, Kvala P et al. (1991) *Mycobacterium tuberculosis* (TB) in HIV +/HIV- homo/bisexual men, intravenous drug users and women with heterosexually acquired HIV. VIIth International Conference on AIDS, Florence MB 2166 (Abs)

Membrano L, Irony I, Were W et al. (1987) Adrenocortical function in acquired immunodeficiency syndrome. J Clin Endocrinol Metab 65: 482–487

Moss AR, Bacchetti P, Osmond D et al. (1988) Seropositivity for HIV and the development of AIDS or AIDS related condition: three year follow up of the San Francisco cohort. Br Med J: 745–750

National Institute of Allergy and Infectious diseases (1993) HIV therapy guidelines.

Pape JW, Jean S, Ho J, Haffner A, Johnson WD (1992) Effect of isoniazid on the natural history of HIV infection in Haiti. VIII International Conference on AIDS, Florence. PoB 3091 (Abs)

Pedersen C, Lindhardt BO, Jensen BL et al. (1989) Clinical course of primary HIV infection: consequences for subsequent course of infection. Br Med J 299: 154–157

Pedersen C, Dickmeiss E, Gaub J et al. (1990) T-cell alterations and lymphocytes responsiveness to mitogens and antigen during severe primary infection with HIV: a case series of seven consecutive seroconverters. AIDS 4: 523–526

Pedersen C, Sandstrom E, Petersen G et al. (1990) The efficacy of inosine prabonex in preventing the acquired immunodeficiency syndrome in patients with human immunodeficiency virus infection. N Engl J Med 322: 1757–1763

Phair J, Munoz A, Detels R et al. (1990) The risk of *Pneumocystis carinii* pneumonia among men infected with human immunodeficiency virus type 1. N Engl J Med 322: 161–165

Ranki A, Valle S-L, Krohn M et al. (1987) Long latency period precedes overt seroconversion in sexually transmitted human immunodeficiency virus infection. Lancet ii: 589–593

Richman DD, Fischl MA, Grieco MH et al. (1987) The toxicity of azidothymidine (AZT) in the treatment of patients with AIDS and AIDS-related complex. N Engl J Med 317: 192–197

Schechter MT, Craib KJP, Le TN et al. (1990) Susceptibility to AIDS appears early in HIV infection. AIDS 4: 185–190

Shaw RJ, Roussak C, Forster SM, Harris JRW, Pinching AJ, Mitchell DM (1988) Lung function abnormalities in HIV-infected patients, with and without overt pneumonitis. Thorax 43: 436–440

Schneider MME, Hoepelman AIM, Schattenkerk JKME et al. (1992) A controlled trial of aerosolized pentamidine or trimethoprim-sulphamethoxazole as primary prophylaxis against *Pneumocystis carinii* pneumonia in patients with human immunodeficiency virus infection. N Engl J Med 327: 1836–1841

Simonsen JN, Cameron W, Gayinka MN et al. (1988) Human immunodeficiency virus infection among men with sexually transmitted diseases. N Engl J Med 319: 274–278

Stafford ND, Herdman RCD, Forster S, Munro AJ (1989) Kaposi's sarcoma of the head and neck in patients with AIDS. J Laryn Oto 103: 379–382

Stamm WE, Handsfield HH, Rampalo AM, Ashley RL, Roberts PL, Corey L (1988) The association between genital ulcer disease and acquisition of HIV infection in homosexual men. JAMA 260: 1429–1433

Swart A-M, Weller I, Darbyshire J H (1990) Early HIV infection: to treat or not to treat? Br Med J 301: 825–826

Taylor JMG, Fahey JL, Detels R, Giogi JV (1989) CD4 percentage, CD4 number, and CD4: CD8 ratio in HIV infection: which to choose and how to use. J AIDS 2: 114–124

Tindall B, Cooper DA (1991) Primary HIV infection: host responses and intervention strategies. AIDS 5: 1–14

Vento S, Di Perri G, Garofano T, Concia E, Bassetti (1989) Reactivation of hepatitis B. Lancet ii: 108–109

Villa A, Foresti V, Confalonieri F (1987) Autonomic neuropathy and HIV infection. Lancet ii: 915

Voetberg A, Lucas SB (1991) Tuberculosis or persistent generalised lymphadenopathy in HIV disease. Lancet I: 56–57

Volberding PA, Lagakos SW, Koch MA, et al. (1990) Zidovudine in asymptomatic human immunodeficiency virus infection. N Engl J Med 322: 941–949

Wadhawan D, Hira S, Mwansa N, Tembo G, Perine P (1991) Preventative tuberculosis chemotherapy with isoniazid among persons infected with human immunodeficiency virus. VIIth International Conference on AIDS, Florence WB 2261 (Abs)

2 Counselling and Clinical Psychology in HIV Infection and AIDS

Alison Harris and Shamil Wanigaratne

Introduction

Counselling and psychological interventions are major components in the care of people with HIV infection or AIDS, their partners and family. These may be crucial in containing any further spread of infection, preventing or ameliorating severe psychological distress or psychiatric illness, enabling patients to cope with aversive medical and surgical procedures or improving the quality of life for those who are affected by HIV and AIDS.

Many health care workers are mystified by psychological problems and are unaware of the potential benefits to the patient from psychological therapy. This inhibits their ability to make useful referrals to psychologists and counsellors.

As well as reviewing widely recognised problems and corresponding counselling and psychological techniques, this chapter will describe medical aspects of HIV which are amenable to psychological intervention. These adjuncts to medical care are still rarely taken up by those caring for such patients, in part due to psychologists' neglect in promoting them. In particular, psychological approaches developed under the rubric of "health psychology" such as the management of pain and nausea, and helping a patient to cope with invasive procedures are already in use in other medical settings, but still rarely considered in the specialised AIDS ward or out-patient clinic.

Medical practitioners working in non-specialised settings, in general practice, or in areas where there are few resources may find that great demands are placed on them to care for the mental health needs of their HIV and AIDS patients. This may be a daunting prospect. By outlining the range of potential psychological and emotional problems faced by people with HIV and AIDS and the range of psychological interventions available, this chapter aims to provide a framework for these issues and to facilitate appropriate referral.

Definitions of Psychotherapy and Counselling

Counselling people with HIV infection has been widely written about but rarely defined, so confusion reigns about what it is and who should be doing it. It has sometimes been prescribed as a block treatment: "please see for counselling".

Conversely, many health care workers feel they have the skills for it without any proper training. Both situations are potentially harmful to the patient and are to be avoided.

The British Association for Counselling produced the following definition of counselling in 1985:

> People become engaged in counselling when a person, occupying regularly or temporarily the role of counsellor offers or agrees explicitly to offer time, attention and respect to another person or persons temporarily in the role of client.
>
> The task of counselling is to give the client an opportunity to explore, discover and clarify ways of living more resourcefully and toward greater well-being. The term "counselling" includes work with individuals and with relationships which may be developmental, crisis support, psychotherapeutic, guiding or problem solving.

There is controversy about the distinction between the terms psychotherapy and counselling and how similar the two activities are. Counselling is often seen as focusing on experiences and feelings in the here and now while psychotherapy deals with past experiences and how they might be related to current emotions, experiences and behaviour. Counselling may be a specific, goal-orientated, problem-solving, short-term activity with psychotherapy aimed at more global and deep-rooted change.

Psychotherapy has been described in terms of a "wide" and a "narrow" definition. The wide definition proposed by the Clinical Psychology Division of the British Psychological Society is "the practice of all psychological therapies". This potentially encompasses a wide range of procedures, including behavioural, cognitive and psychodynamic approaches (Nitsun et al. 1989). The narrow definition of the term "psychotherapy" is usually associated with psychoanalytic or psychodynamic therapy. Nitsun, Wood and Bolton propose categories of psychotherapy which encompass the wide range of activities referred to so far:

Category 1: Counselling: emphasising basic skills such as listening, reflection, empathy

Category 2: Psychotherapy: this includes the broad range of specific psychotherapeutic skills ranging from behaviour therapy to alternative approaches such as Gestalt therapy. It could also include group methods and family and couple therapy

Category 3: Psychoanalytic psychotherapy: referring to the range of dynamic approaches, including Jungian, Freudian, Kleinian and object relations schools

The Role of Clinical Psychologists

Clinical psychologists provide a range of psychological therapies following a thorough psychological assessment, in addition to using basic counselling skills.

Clinical psychology may be defined as the application of the principles, procedures and concepts of experimental psychology to health care and is a specific profession within the National Health Service. Nearly all the District Health Authorities in Great Britain have a psychology department. The theoretical underpinnings of clinical psychology and the consequently widely applicable skills of the profession mean that most clinical psychologists have the potential expertise to work with people with HIV and AIDS.

Who To Refer To

With the proliferation of HIV counsellors, health advisers, therapists and psychologists, other workers in the field may be at a loss to know who to refer patients to.

In many departments, specialist clinical psychology posts have been created. But, even in districts with no HIV specialist psychologists, referral is nearly always possible to the District Psychology Department.

A recent review of clinical psychology services commissioned by the Department of Health described three levels of psychological skills:

Level 1

Both clinical staff and managers need and use certain psychological skills. These may be regarded as rudimentary, but are nevertheless extremely important in enabling them to apply their vocational skills. Basic "psychological" methods include:

Developing a relationship with the patient and relatives (establishing rapport, communicating empathy)

Maintaining a supportive relationship (advising and supporting)

Interviewing technique (ability to listen, draw out and challenge)

Recognising, interpreting and using verbal and non-verbal cues relating to problems

The use of basic psychological interventions which are not necessarily consciously acknowledged as such and can be or are carried out with basic training such as: counselling, stress/anxiety management (only in the form of "off the shelf" packages, relaxation techniques, supportive group work, simple behavioural techniques

At this level, the application of psychological skill is the lubricant of good professional practice.

Health advisers, counsellors, social workers, occupational therapists and psychiatric nurses have most of the above skills.

Level 2

Skills required to undertake *circumscribed* activities entailing psychological interventions for which one is qualified and/or has had specific training (such as behaviour modification, or behavioural psychotherapy).

Within certain mental health disciplines such as occupational therapy or social work, some practitioners choose to develop a special interest either in a psychological intervention, specialising in family or marital therapy for example, or in treating a particular disorder, for example psycho-sexual or eating disorders.

At levels 1 and 2 there should be an awareness of the criteria for referral to a clinical psychologist.

Level 3

Activities which require specialist psychological intervention skills in circumstances where there are deep-rooted underlying influences, or which call for the capacity to draw on a multiple theoretical base to devise an individually tailored strategy for a complicated presenting problem. Flexibility is the key to competence at this level, which comes from a broad and sophisticated understanding of the various psychological theories. It necessitates the ability to select and adapt more complex approaches and to combine approaches if appropriate. (Adapted from the Management Advisory Service Review of Clinical Psychology, 1989).

For level 1 and level 2 skills, referrals will be made to the appropriate professional according to local arrangements. Criteria for referrals to a psychologist are listed in Table 2.1.

Further referral may be made to a clinical psychologist for a number of reasons. A recent review of clinical psychology described what a wide range of associated professions (such as psychiatrists) said they used clinical psychology for:

Particularly severe or complex problems

Where a patient needs to be seen by the clinical psychologist to devise a care programme, which may be carried out by other professionals

Where emotional or cognitive problems are regarded as primary to a physical condition

Where some aspect of a patient's psychological state is interfering with the effectiveness of other (for example, medical) treatments

Other disciplines will often consult a clinical psychologist for advice, rather than make a direct referral

Table 2.1. Presenting problems for which referral to a psychologist is recommended

1. Severe difficulty adjusting to a diagnosis of HIV infection or AIDS.
2. Beliefs about being infected with HIV despite negative HIV antibody tests and clinical tests.
3. Problem drinking or drug use.
4. Chronic depression associated with functional withdrawal or decline.*
5. Suicidal planning or activity.*
6. Acute or chronic anxiety (including panic attacks).
7. Thought disorders or cognitive impairment.
8. Obsessions and compulsions, including compulsive risky sex, of concern to the patient.
9. Sexual problems.
10. Relationship problems.
11. Any other psychological or emotional problem that is disrupting a patient's everyday functioning.

* With severe depression, suicidal planning or activity, referral to a psychiatrist should always be considered.

Prevention of HIV Infection

At the present time the only way of containing the spread of HIV infection in Britain is by means of voluntary changes in people's behaviour. It has been cogently argued that the greatest potential contribution of behavioural scientists to curtailing the HIV epidemic is by helping people to change their behaviour through avenues such as counselling, health education and health promotion (Baum and Temoshok 1990). Once behaviour change has taken place, helping people "maintain" the change (preventing relapse) is a crucial challenge for behavioural scientists.

These "primary prevention" activities of behavioural scientists can be classified in terms of three elements. An appreciation by health care workers of all three elements is important if preventive efforts are to be effective.

Information

Public health communications providing factual information about HIV infection and AIDS are the main feature at this level. Effective communication involves a choice of medium, target group and appropriate message. Constant evaluation and modification of these communications are key factors in their effectiveness. Many public health campaigns on HIV and AIDS would be greatly enhanced if they exploited psychological knowledge and expertise. For example, recent surveys of injecting drug users show that in general whilst there are marked changes in needle sharing practices this group continues to have unsafe sex (Higgins et al. 1991).

Counselling on HIV Antibody Testing

Counselling on HIV antibody testing is an opportunity for behaviour change. The decision to have a test for most people is usually due to the perception of having been at risk of exposure to the HIV virus and is an emotionally stressful event. Hence, in theory, counselling may be used to motivate reduction in high risk behaviour.

Pre-test counselling, apart from helping the individual arrive at an informed decision to be tested or not, should always include information on and discussion of safer sex practices and changes in high risk sexual behaviour. Post-test counselling should also include the above components regardless of whether the person tests positive or negative. (See section on pre-test and post-test counselling.)

Behaviour Change

Efforts to promote behaviour change are targeted at individuals in three broad categories. These are:

1. Those who are experiencing difficulties in making the decision to change
2. Individuals requiring additional help or skills to make changes

3. Those who are having difficulty in maintaining the changes in behaviour they have already made (Baum and Temoshok 1990)

Producing change is a challenge and requires innovative techniques. Needle exchange schemes for intravenous drug users aimed at harm minimisation and more accessible health care are an example of preventitive work influenced by behavioural scientists in this area.

There are also examples of community-based AIDS risk-reduction programmes for gay men aimed at providing information and skills for behaviour change (Kelly et al. 1989; Kelly and St Lawrence 1990). Such group programmes provide a social environment that supports engagement in lower-risk behaviour. These programmes aim to change subcultural norms and include workshops on eroticising safer sex and giving information in real-life settings such as bath-houses in San Francisco. Unfortunately the vast majority of such efforts have little scientific basis and are not based on the evidence available of what makes for an effective intervention (Fisher and Fisher 1992). There is now compelling evidence that interventions aimed at maintenance of behaviour change are as important as those aimed at initiation of change (Coates et al. 1990; O'Reilly et al. 1990). Programmes based on relapse prevention, a therapeutic model derived from treatment of addictive behaviours, have been shown to have a significant effect on maintenance of behaviour change in gay men (Wanigaratne et al. 1992a). The holistic nature of the model enables health education (for example safer sex) and health promotion (for example coping with anxiety and depression, lifestyle balance and exercise) techniques to be incorporated into these programmes. There is a need to extend this type of approach to other groups with high-risk behaviour. (See section on Relapse Prevention.)

HIV Antibody Test Counselling

Pre-test Counselling

In the large specialist centres, the practice has grown up whereby pre-test and post-test counselling are carried out by health advisers who are usually based in departments of genito-urinary medicine. In these settings, health advisers have the specialised skills to carry out good quality counselling and have the expertise to refer patients on to other professionals such as clinical psychologists, where appropriate.

A range of helping professionals and individuals, including physicians, may be involved in counselling patients with HIV. At a minimum it should be expected that these individuals have undergone training in basic counselling skills and have a good working knowledge of HIV infection and AIDS. Such counselling is most effective when there is enough time available. A range of professionals are involved in this "front-line" counselling activity. The basic aims and key features of pre-test counselling are outlined below. The reader is referred to Green and McCreaner (1988) and Miller and Bor (1991) for more detailed descriptions.

Reassuring patients of confidentiality is an essential pre-requisite to effective pre-test counselling.

Aims of Pre-test Counselling

The aims of pre-test counselling can be summarised as follows:

To ensure that any decision to take a test is fully informed and based on an understanding of the personal, medical, legal and social implications of a positive result

To provide necessary preparation for those who are likely to face the trauma of a positive result

To provide necessary information on reducing the risk of acquiring or passing on HIV, whether or not a person elects to have a test (McCreaner 1988)

Patients presenting for pre-test counselling will have varying perceptions of their risk of infection. A key task in preventive work is to provide information and to encourage changes in behaviour which will reduce the risk of HIV being contracted or transmitted at this stage. Advice on safe sex is a minimum requirement at this stage (Glover and Miller 1990).

Pre-test counselling can be effective in reducing risky behaviour. In a review of 45 studies examining the effectiveness of HIV antibody test pre-test counselling Higgins et al. (1991) found different effects according to the target group. In gay men (26 studies) a majority of the studies report a decrease in the number of sexual partners and frequency of anal intercourse and an increase in condom use for both seropositive and seronegative men, with greater percentage reduction in seropositive men. All studies on intravenous drug users (9 studies) showed a decrease in risky injection practices but only a small proportion (3 studies) showed a decline in risky sexual behaviour. The studies on heterosexuals (10 studies) provided mixed results. These differential effects must be taken into account so that counselling is tailored to the needs and interests of the individual.

The counsellor should neither encourage nor discourage a patient to have a test, but should help the patient weigh up for themselves the pros and cons of testing. However the clinical advantages of early medical intervention should be fully discussed.

For many individuals pre-test counselling is their first experience of counselling. This provides for many an opportunity to seek help for other medical, psychological and social problems. Hence those carrying out pre-test counselling should be sensitive to this and be prepared to deal with such problems and have access to other professionals (doctors, psychologists, psychiatrists, social workers and so on) for more specialised work if required.

Post-test Counselling

The content of post-test counselling depends largely on whether the result is positive or negative. To carry out post-test counselling the counsellor must meet the following basic requirements:

1. Have basic counselling skills
2. Have skills and experience in breaking bad news
3. Have up-to-date factual information about HIV and AIDS, including current treatment and infection control options

4. Have access to adequate medical and psychological back-up services
5. Have a working knowledge about voluntary and statutory services available for people with HIV and AIDS

The basic aims of post-test counselling are:

1. Giving information
2. Providing emotional support
3. Assessing coping resources (e.g. social support networks)
4. Reiterating safer sex information

Following a positive result it is important that the patient is seen at least twice for post-test counselling (Glover and Miller 1990) and in many cases may need further sessions. The amount of information a patient takes in after the shock of a positive result can be very limited. Hence it is important not to overload the patient with information at this stage but to invite them back as soon as possible for a follow-up appointment.

Poor handling of breaking bad news or a lack of post-test counselling can have damaging consequences. Patients may feel unable to return to the clinic and may lose confidence in the staff. This may then result in increased morbidity and poor information about HIV infection. Keeping this in mind, utmost consideration must be given to ensure that all criteria involved in post-test counselling are adequately met. Readers requiring more detailed descriptions of post-test counselling are referred to Green (1988).

Psychological Assessment, Treatment Approaches and Psychological Techniques

Learning one is seropositive is associated with significantly higher levels of depression, anxiety, obsessive-compulsive behaviour and general levels of distress (Ostrow et al. 1989), although the degree of psychological distress reported is similar to that of patients with other medical conditions. It is vital to take into account an individual's psychosocial functioning and history prior to acquiring HIV as this appears to be the most important risk factor in coping with HIV infection (King 1989).

A patient referred to a clinical psychologist undergoes a thorough psychological assessment. This assessment is made at several levels and is aimed at arriving at a comprehensive picture of the patient's problems. The assessment process in general (except neuropsychological assessment (see later)) does not follow the discrete pattern of most medical investigations. It may take place over one or more sessions. Psychological assessment is continuous and integral to the treatment process.

There are many areas of overlap between a psychological assessment and a psychiatric assessment. Background information such as developmental milestones, personal history and family history are common to both types of assessment. At a fundamental level psychological assessment involves a dialogue between the patient and the psychologist about the patient's problems. There may not always be congruence between the patient's assessment of their problems and that of the psychologist.

A patient may come to the initial assessment without a clear perception of their problems and/or views about the impact of those problems on different aspects of their lives, such as relationships, family, friends, employment or health. The dialogue with the psychologist can help the patient arrive at a more focused picture of their problems. This alone is enough for some patients to begin the process of problem-solving using their own resources. In this way the boundary between assessment and therapy is often blurred.

The dialogue from a psychologist's perspective is aimed at gathering information on different areas of a patient's life, history and functioning. Much of this could take place in interview format (loose or structured such as the Present State Examination) and by the use of standardised questionnaires, such as the Beck Depression Inventory (BDI), or Spielberger State–Trait Anxiety Inventory (STAI). For a more detailed description of these please see Chapter 3 (Newman and Fell).

Psychological assessment typically covers the following areas: a detailed description of the presenting problem, the mental state of the patient, personal history, family history, physical problems, social support, past contact with mental health services and other agencies involved. These are described in more detail below.

Presenting Problem

A detailed description of the problem includes the nature of the problem, time of onset, triggers, duration and frequency of occurrence.

A psychologist working within a behavioural framework may assess the presenting problem using functional analysis according to different schemata. All of these schemata are based on an analysis of the antecedents, consequences and the nature of the problem behaviour. An example of such a schema has the acronym "SORC" and measures the following elements of behaviour:

1. Stimuli (the environmental situation that precede the problem – triggers)
2. Organismic (physiological and psychological factors within the individual)
3. Responses (the problem, its frequency, intensity and form)
4. Consequences (events that appear to reinforce the behaviour in question (Goldfried and Sprafkin 1976; Hersen and Bellack, 1982)).

Self-report instruments, such as drink diaries or anxiety diaries, are often used in this type of assessment (see Table 2.2).

The description of presenting problems often involves a rating of the severity of the problem by the patient and the therapist. This together with other standardised measures such as the BDI can be used to evaluate the success of psychological interventions.

The Mental State of the Patient

Mental state includes the basic *behaviour* of the patient during the interview, such as posture, gestures, eye contact, level of arousal and level of activity. A mental state examination of a patient also includes an assessment of the following:

Table 2.2. My drink diary

Day	Time of drinking	Number of units*	Type of alcohol	In company or alone	Where drinking took place	Feeling before and afterwards	Effects of drinking	Money spent on alcohol
Monday								
Tuesday								
Wednesday								
Thursday								
Friday								
Saturday								
Sunday								
Totals	–	–	–	–	–	–	–	£

* Name ....Completion Date ..../..../.... 1 Unit = half pint ordinary beer, single measure vermouth or spirits, 1 glass wine or small sherry; 1 + units = 1 standard can lager; 2 + units = 1 strong can lager, 4 units = 1 extra stong can lager

speech, mood, evidence of depersonalisation or derealisation, obsessional problems, delusions, hallucinations and illusions, orientation in time and place, attention and concentration, memory and insight.

A psychiatric assessment would also involve detailed examination of the above areas (Gelder et al. 1983; Leff and Isaacs 1990).

Personal History

Personal history includes birth and early development, childhood health, education, occupational history, sexual history, orientation, functioning and home situation and finances.

Family History and Contact

Family history and contact includes parent's relationship, separations between and from parents, illness in the family, recent events in the family and quality of current relationships.

Physical Problems

Physical problems include the history of any past or current physical illnesses.

Social Support

Social support includes groups, family, friends and partners.

Past Contact with Mental Health Services and Other Agencies

Problem, dates, duration and type of past contact with mental health services are included in the psychological assessment. Involvement with social services, probation service, voluntary organisations and so on should also be discussed with the patient.

In practice, the emphasis of a psychological assessment would vary according to the theoretical orientation or the treatment model of choice of the psychologist. For example a psychologist working within a psychodynamic model would place a greater emphasis on childhood experiences and relationships. Similarly a cognitive or behavioural psychologist would concentrate more on the behaviour, feelings and patterns of thinking associated with the problem. The main purpose of assessment is to determine the best therapeutic help for the patient, tailored to their individual history and current needs. The experience and skill of the psychologist would be used to match treatment options to the patient's particular problem. Measures have also been developed to aid this process by taking into account patients' opinions about their problems and expectations of treatment (Pistrang and Barker 1992).

Psychological Treatment Approaches and Techniques

Psychologists have at their disposal an extensive battery of techniques based on broader theoretical approaches, which can be applied to a range of problems. Table 2.3 outlines the types of services available from clinical psychologists working with people with HIV.

Effectiveness of Psychological Therapies

In the world of general medicine the evaluation of a treatment or a drug may be fairly straightforward. Because of the complexities of an individual's psychosocial world and the multiple factors involved in psychological therapy evaluation psychological therapies is a much harder task. Outcome criteria may be numerous and difficult to define.

Over 30 years ago a paper by Hans Eysenck, claiming that patients receiving psychotherapy did no better than patients receiving no treatment, led to an explosion of psychotherapy evaluation research. Major reviews of these studies (Vandenbos and Pino 1980; Rachman and Wilson 1980; Smith et al. 1980; Lambert et al. 1986) all conclude that in the majority of cases, psychotherapy does indeed produce more positive changes in individuals with psychological problems than no treatment.

The most substantial support for the effectiveness of psychotherapy has come from studies using meta-analysis. This is a statistical technique which enables the averaging of results of a large number of outcome studies. In a pioneering study using this technique, which included 400 outcome studies, Smith and Glass (1977) found that, on average, individuals receiving psychotherapy fared better than 75% of untreated individuals. This finding has been supported by subsequent meta-analytic studies (Shapiro and Shapiro 1982, 1983; Brown 1987).

Although research indicates that a majority of people clearly benefit from psychotherapy, when the different therapies are compared for their differential effectiveness the picture is less clear. Studies that have compared the major categories of therapy described above have failed to show a clear superiority of one type of therapy to another (Sloane et al. 1975; Luborsky et al. 1975; Shapiro 1983). This is an area of much controversy and there is much more to be discovered about how psychotherapy works.

In recent years many therapists have adopted an eclectic approach and the "matching" of type of therapy to the patient and the problem has become of major interest to both practitioners and researchers.

Psychological Reactions and Problems

At all stages from a seropositive result through asymptomatic infection to AIDS and finally death, a patient may experience a range of psychological reactions which will require continuous support and counselling. Some reactions will of course be understandable, healthy responses to a life-threatening situation. On

Table 2.3. Types of services available from a clinical psychology department

Levels of intervention
1. *Individual assessment and therapy* (includes individuals, carers, couples and groups)
2. *Team/Departmental* (such as staff support, organisational consultancy)
3. *District* (planning and policy making, interventions at the level of whole communities)

Psychological models used
Cognitive
Behavioural
Psychodynamic
Systemic

Services offered
Psychological assessment (including cognitive assessment)
Psychological therapies
Clinical supervision
Consultation
Staff support
Research (including service evaluation)
Teaching
Training
Policy-making
Planning

Examples of target problems
Anxiety
Depression
Preparation for dying
Complex grief reactions
Sexual problems
Sexual abuse
Eating problems
Obsessional–compulsive problems including the "worried well"
Relationship problems
Psychological adjustment to chronic illness
Coping with pain
Alcohol/drug use
Stress
Staff "burn-out"
Anger control

Some common psychological approaches and techniques
Counselling (including Pre-HIV antibody testing and Post-HIV antibody testing)
Cognitive therapy
Behaviour therapy
Psychodynamic therapy
Hypnotherapy
Family therapy
Couple therapy
Group therapy
Neuropsychological rehabilitation

Specific packages
Anxiety management
Stress management
Pain management
Problem solving
Anger control
Guided mourning
Relapse prevention
Sex therapy

these occasions, talking to a psychologist, health adviser or other counsellor (depending on the division of labour in a particular team) can be of considerable benefit in adjusting to changed expectations or circumstances and in coping with illness.

At other times, patients may develop more severe psychological problems requiring specific referral to a clinical psychologist. A range of psychological problems which may be experienced by people with HIV and AIDS and which are appropriately treated by clinical psychologists, are discussed in some detail below.

Anxiety Problems

The person with HIV or AIDS has many legitimate sources of worry. Some patients, in common with the general population, may have been prone to anxiety problems in the past. They and others may develop more specific or severe, but nevertheless treatable problems. These may include simple phobias, social phobia, agoraphobia, panic attacks and generalised anxiety.

Symptoms of anxiety are likely to be physical (cardiovascular, respiratory, muscular, gastro-intestinal or sexual), cognitive and behavioural. Unfortunately many of them are similar to symptoms of HIV disease and it is often tricky to differentiate them. Close collaboration between the medical practitioner and the psychologist is crucial in such cases.

Intervention

A major and avoidable contributor to patients' anxiety is a reluctance on the part of health care workers to provide frank and clear information about the patient's present condition, chances of recovery and how long they can expect to live for. Time and again, doctors believe they have fully informed the patient, but the patient remains confused.

However, in addition to information-giving, successful psychological treatments are available for the anxiety problems listed above. Psychological therapy (using a cognitive–behavioural approach) is now the treatment of choice for a wide range of anxiety problems. Benzodiazepines should be regarded as a short term palliative only and preferably avoided altogether in view of withdrawal problems.

A key element of a behavioural approach is exposure to whatever stimulus arouses anxiety, although this needs to be structured in a particular way for maximum effect. This is where the specialist knowledge of the clinical psychologist or nurse behaviour therapist is indispensable.

In many cases, for example with panic attacks, cognitive therapy for the anxiety-provoking thoughts associated with somatic symptoms is an essential component of therapy. Cognitive strategies include identifying irrational, anxiety-provoking thoughts, devising rational substitutes and coping statements, learning to appraise the situation more rationally and challenging negative "automatic thoughts".

Other important components may be behavioural techniques such as relaxation training or meditation in order to reduce physiological arousal; the planning of lifestyle changes and of distracting, pleasurable activities as alternative behaviours.

Depression

Most people experience mild, transient depression on occasions. But depression becomes a problem when it occurs frequently, is particularly intense or intractable and begins to disrupt everyday life. An important minority of people with HIV experience significant depression. Again, somatic symptoms of depression may mimic those of HIV disease progression and so the medical practitioner must take care not to overlook or mistake these signs in someone who is physically unwell. Symptoms may be somatic, cognitive or behavioural.

Intervention

Cognitive therapy has been shown to be highly effective and reduces initial symptoms comparably to anti-depressant medication although with a greatly reduced relapse rate (Teasdale 1988). Psychological interventions can be used in isolation, or in combination with drug treatments in the treatment of depression.

As well as identifying negative "automatic" thoughts and errors of thinking in order to learn more rational ways of analysing experiences, cognitive therapy is usually conducted as a package including important behavioural techniques such as increasing activity levels, planning and doing pleasurable activities.

Long-term psychodynamic psychotherapy may be valuable where an individual's depression is thought to be closely linked to their early experiences. Unfortunately, resources for this tend to be limited in the National Health Service.

Obsessions and Compulsions

An obsession is defined as an intrusive, repetitive thought, image or impulse that is unacceptable and/or unwanted and gives rise to subjective resistance (Rachman and Hodgson 1980). Obsessions are to be distinguished from compulsions, which are stereotyped and compulsive activities or rituals which are recognised by the person to be excessive or senseless. Like obsessions, compulsions cause distress and provoke subjective resistance.

Obsessive behaviour associated with fear of HIV infection may include obsessional checking for physical symptoms, obsessional washing of self and home, and obsessional avoidance of any source of infection, however slight. This may disrupt the patient's life considerably, resulting in an inability to carry out work or social activities.

Obsessional thoughts or ruminations may include thoughts of death or dying, persistent fear of infection or guilt concerning past sexual activities.

Intervention

Obsessive-compulsive problems are treated most successfully by behavioural methods based on techniques such as exposure and response prevention (Rachman and Hodgson 1980). Information is gathered on the triggers, frequency, content and consequences of the obsession or compulsion, including patterns of avoidance behaviour. In vivo or imaginal prolonged exposure is arranged to a range of stimuli in ascending order of discomfort and the patient is required to refrain from their usual obsessional response.

With obsessional problems thorough assessment is vital to a successful outcome; for example depression is often a major factor and needs to be treated otherwise the intervention may fail (Foa and Emmelkamp 1983).

Sexual Problems

Sexual problems and relationship difficulties are often found in people with AIDS, those who are HIV positive, and the worried well. As with the rest of the population, these might arise because of depression, anxiety, fear of infecting a loved one, fear of being infected, or poor body image because of the physical manifestations of AIDS, amongst other reasons.

Safer sex techniques are advocated for everybody in order to reduce the risk of HIV transmission. This can lead to sexual problems as individuals may find it difficult to change their established sexual practices. Psychological techniques, for example, relapse prevention, can assist with managing these changes (see below).

Intervention

Psychological intervention can facilitate improvements in sexual relationships where there is no physical impairment. This may take the form of behavioural treatments such as Masters and Johnson couple therapy. Couple therapy can also be effective in resolving relationship difficulties which are associated with the virus, or difficulties which have been present for some time and are exacerbated by living with HIV and AIDS. Couple therapy can be based on a wide range of theoretical approaches from practical behavioural techniques to more exploratory psychodynamic methods.

Chronic Pain

Chronic pain is most usefully defined as any pain lasting 6 months or more. At least 40% of terminally ill people suffer severe pain (Twycross 1975). It is important to separate physical from psychological aspects of pain, although the two may be closely interrelated.

Pain in terminal illness may be particularly difficult to tolerate because it is meaningless and unrelenting. Chronic exhaustion and debility as a result of the deterioration of other bodily functions can only exacerbate the experience of pain in patients with AIDS.

Intervention

Psychological methods of pain management are relatively well developed. The best results appear to be obtained by a multi-faceted package of psychological interventions rather than by one technique used alone.

Again, research findings have lead to the emergence of the cognitive-behavioural approach as the treatment of choice. This approach has four main aims:

1. To re-orient the patient away from helplessness towards a greater sense of control
2. To enable patients to monitor and identify the relationships between thoughts, feelings, behaviours, their environment and symptoms
3. To teach the skills needed to solve problems
4. To develop more effective ways of thinking, feeling and responding (Erskine and Williams 1989). This includes education and the acquisition of new skills (such as goal setting, relaxation techniques) and cognitive coping strategies (such as distraction and the use of imagery) (Turk and Rennert 1981).

Hypnotherapy (in groups as well as individually) also appears to be effective in alleviating pain for some patients. The strength of hypnotherapy is that patients learn self-hypnosis and so have a tool for coping with pain which is under their own control.

Neuropsychological Problems

Neuropsychological problems in HIV are far less common than was believed in the early years of treatment of HIV infection. The risk of developing symptoms of dementia among healthy, HIV-infected patients is very low (Selnes et al. 1990). The risk grows with increasing degrees of immunosuppression and progression of the illness to symptomatic stages. Indeed there remains a worrying enthusiasm, particularly on in-patient AIDS wards, for overdiagnosing dementia in the absence of any evidence from relevant neurological and psychological investigations. This tendency runs the risk of overlooking other causes of apparent cognitive or behavioural changes, such as depression, and of thereby failing to take remedial action. In any case, minor degrees of cognitive impairment are more common in AIDS than is a full-blown dementia. Slowed information-processing appears to be most typical as an early sign. Nevertheless a small percentage of people with ARC or AIDS will develop neuropsychological problems. These changes and their assessment are outlined elsewhere in this book (see Chapter 3).

The early term "AIDS dementia complex" (ADC) is now outmoded and has been replaced by the World Health Organization proposed term of "HIV-1 associated cognitive/motor complex" (HACC) (Egan 1992). HACC is divided into severe and mild forms, the severe forms being "HIV-1 associated dementia complex" (HDC). A milder form of HACC is "HIV-1 associated minor cognitive/motor disorder" (HMCD).

Neuropsychological assessment has the following aims:

1. To provide an objective measurement of current cognitive functions for use as a baseline against which to assess future changes

2. To determine to what extent apparent problems result from (i) neurological abnormalities, (ii) other physical factors, or (iii) depression and anxiety
3. To develop a plan of management and rehabilitation

Intervention

Psychological assessments seldom settle diagnostic questions decisively although the information gained may contribute to an emerging diagnostic picture in tandem with other investigations. Some investigations, such as MRI scans, need clinical confirmation as abnormal findings can exist in the absence of clinical symptoms and, indeed, in a normal population.

Psychologists can use this neuropsychological assessment to develop a plan of management and rehabilitation. This may include providing advice on strategies for overcoming problems associated with deficits or individual therapeutic help for those who are coming to terms with cognitive difficulties in themselves or significant others. The assessment may also be used to judge whether a patient is able to cope at home or is competent to make crucial decisions on their medical treatment.

Addictive Behaviours

There is mounting evidence of the need for psychological techniques in the reduction of addictive behaviour related to HIV.

There is frequently an apparent increase in addictive behaviours such as problem drinking, smoking, intravenous drug use, eating and compulsive risky sex as a reaction to the knowledge of being infected with HIV. Drinking and drug taking have been linked to unsafe sex and relapse from safer sex (Stall et al. 1990; O'Reilly et al. 1990).

Interventions

The emphasis of treatment of addictions has shifted markedly from a medical to a psychosocial perspective over the last decade. Today, there exists a more holistic approach termed the biopsychosocial model (Engel 1960; Schwartz 1982).

Counselling forms the basis of any modern approach in the treatment of addictions. Interventions focus on the decision to change (Prochaska and Diclementi 1983; Miller 1985) and the maintenance of change (Marlatt and Gordon 1985). The holistic approach to addictions also means that treatment goals have become much broader and flexible in comparison to the traditional abstinence-only goal.

Injecting Drug Users (IDUs)

There are two aspects to interventions with this group, direct interventions with drug users and the prevention of transmission of HIV.

Direct Interventions with Drug Users

The aim of psychological interventions with IDUs is the same as with any other person with HIV infection or AIDS. Nevertheless this group of individuals may have special needs associated with their addictive behaviour. Their pattern of uptake and use of services (such as primary health care or counselling) may also differ markedly from other groups of patients.

Health care workers often find that to work effectively with IDUs in general they have to adopt a more flexible approach within clear boundaries, giving a non-judgemental and caring message. There is also a clear need to move towards a much broader philosophy of treatment than the traditional abstinence orientated approach.

Intervention for HIV infection or for Drug Addiction? HIV is a much greater threat to life than injecting drug use per se. Although the management of AIDS and HIV in this group is inseparable from the management and treatment of drug abuse itself, it must be clear that these must not be seen as the same thing (Robertson 1990). For example, the option of help to change the addictive behaviour can always be made available to the patient who is receiving medical treatment or counselling for HIV-related problems. It must be made clear that the decision is entirely the patient's own and the help they are receiving should in no way be contingent upon their decision.

Some counsellors use the counselling approach termed "motivational interviewing" (Miller 1985) to encourage changes in the addictive behaviour. Since the relationship between the patient and the counsellor is the pivotal factor in this approach and the aim of the approach is to facilitate behaviour change, caution must be exercised not to force the patient in the "right" direction. Further research is needed to look at the outcome of this approach with patients with HIV and AIDS.

Relapse Prevention (Marlatt and Gordon 1985; Wanigaratne et al. 1990) (see later), a new development in psychological therapy for addictions, has particular relevance here. This approach is aimed at maintenance of behaviour change and includes interventions aimed at changing lifestyles.

Opiate substitute therapy (e.g. methadone maintenance) in many cases may be an essential "anchor" for psychological work with this patient group.

Prevention of Transmission of HIV

In Europe, the total number of cases of AIDS among drug users is increasing rapidly and in some centres is likely to overtake those cases acquired by sexual intercourse or blood product transfusion in the next few years (Robertson 1990). The need for effective prevention strategies targeted at this group is an urgent priority. Prevention strategies are aimed at three distinct groups. These are chronic injectors, those on the periphery of drug use, and potential drug users.

The success of preventive work in this area depends on a multidisciplinary approach carried out at different levels. Because the fundamental requirement here is self directed change in an individual's behaviour and maintenance of that change, psychologists have an obvious contribution to make. Changing attitudes and perceptions, learning new skills and increasing confidence in the ability to use those skills are basic elements of most psychological interventions.

Chronic Injectors. With this group "needle exchange schemes" aimed at preventing the spread of HIV through sharing of needles is at present the foremost intervention (Stimson et al. 1988). Needle exchanges with user-friendly, non-judgemental working philosophies and a flexible, innovative and progressive approach appear to hold much promise. Not only do they appear to attract this difficult-to-read group but they also succeed in providing a much-needed funnel into other services such as primary health care, counselling and drug treatment. The effectiveness of needle exchanges in the prevention of spread is still being evaluated. The data on compliance from popular needle exchange schemes show a great deal of promise (Hart et al. 1989).

Those on the Periphery of Drug Use. Work on the practice of safer sex which includes counselling, education and provision of condoms are the main intervention with this group.

Potential Drug Users and New Users. Preventive work with new drug users and potential drug users is the major challenge for multidisciplinary work in the future. Education programmes for young people, innovative schemes operating at street level (for example the CLASH team in Camden and Islington Health District) and treatment centres with broad, flexible and user friendly operational philosophies are some of the responses to this challenge.

Preparing for Dying and Death

Many challenges, both practical and emotional, have to be faced by the person facing death and their loved ones. Healthcare workers who avoid assisting the patient in this work, whether consciously or not, are likely to increase rather than reduce, the distress of patients in the long run.

Lovers and family members may experience grief reactions and may withdraw emotionally, prior to the death of the person with AIDS. Psychological intervention at this point can alleviate distress, and preparation for bereavement can reduce serious grief reactions or abnormal grieving following the death. Abnormal grief reactions may take the form of inhibited mourning, uncontrolled grieving for a prolonged period, withdrawal from friends or work, or severe depression.

Intervention

Intervention is necessary and appropriate with both the person who is facing death and their significant others. Studies show that 70%–90% of terminally ill patients would like to be told if they are dying yet 60%–90% of physicians are opposed to telling them (Wilson 1989)!

The best way a doctor can emotionally support a patient is to answer questions honestly, frankly and fully, without embarrassment and avoiding all euphemisms. Euphemisms include phrases such as "things don't look good" without a specific explanation.

A common misunderstanding arises between the doctor and the patient with AIDS at the point where curative treatment becomes palliative care. It is important to make this crystal clear to the patient who may interpret phrases such as "we're going to give you something to make your symptoms go away" as meaning they will be cured.

All expressions of psychological and emotional distress by the person who is facing terminal illness warrant an offer of professional support, even just time to talk, and should not be dismissed as an inevitable part of dying. Conversely, a wish for privacy or for no intrusion by professionals should be respected. For the person who is dying, psychological intervention can facilitate a life review, reduce fear and achieve some form of emotional resolution.

There is a common belief that individuals progress through certain stages during the normal grieving process (Kubler-Ross 1970). However, individual reactions vary greatly and not everyone goes through every stage nor in the prescribed order.

Many carers express profound concern, particularly following confirmation of their loved one's impending death, that they are not reacting appropriately since their behaviour does not accord with popular images of grief. This seems often to be the case when carers are extremely busy, assuming responsibility for practical affairs as well as providing nursing care and emotional support to the patient. They simply do not have the time for preparatory grieving or do not dare to add to the burdens of the dying person. Reassurance should be given that they are not "abnormal" or callous and that they are likely to experience the emotions they presently feel cut off from, when the time is right.

Counselling on practical issues such as funeral arrangements, financial affairs and information to be provided about cause of death, may need to be done with the person who is seriously ill and their family or partner.

Behavioural techniques, such as guided mourning (Mawson et al. 1981) can benefit those experiencing abnormal grief reactions. It is worth remembering that many people with HIV have already experienced multiple bereavements, if many friends have died of AIDS, and they may require longer-term bereavement work.

The Worried Well

This term refers to people with an obsessional fear of HIV infection. Many have a strong belief that they are infected which they know to be irrational. The so-called "worried well" usually have a low risk sexual history and have tested negatively for HIV antibodies in repeated tests (Miller, et al. 1988). Their fears may be so strong as to disrupt their work-life and lead to extreme social withdrawal.

This relatively common problem may be the modern expression of latter-day "syphilophobia" or "venereophobia". More than 50% of a sample of GPs in London described attenders who constantly visited their surgery with a fear of AIDS (King, 1989). These patients usually exhaust the patience and available time of their doctors in a fruitless search either for reassurance or for confirmation of their worst fears.

Such people should be referred to the psychologist (with their agreement) when it becomes apparent that repeated negative tests for HIV antibody plus the fullest information about viral transmission are not enough to allay their fears.

Intervention

Fortunately, such fears are amenable to psychological intervention using cognitive and behavioural techniques according to the specific details of the problem. Attention must be paid to depression and social withdrawal, which are often major factors in the development and maintenance of such obsessional fears.

Reassurance is not a solution for people with obsessional anxieties and may, in fact, help to maintain the problem.

Haemophiliacs

Haemophiliacs infected with HIV face particular challenges which result from their life-long underlying disorder. Since haemophilia is an inherited disorder, the whole biological family is drawn into and affected by the threat of haemophilia and what have been the fatal consequences, for many, of its treatment.

Many carrier mothers suffer life-long feelings of guilt at having passed on the genetic defect to their sons. This guilt has been compounded for some mothers who know their children have also become infected with HIV as a direct result of their actions in giving them treatment for bleeding episodes. Screening of donors and heat treatment of blood products since 1985 is presumed to have stopped any further infection with HIV.

Those infected with HIV as a result of contaminated blood product transfusions may be of any age. For example at the Royal Free Hospital, London, seroconversion occurred in patients aged from 2 years to 70 years. In the UK, the highest prevalence of infection through this route is in adolescents. This creates many dilemmas for counsellors. There may be a conflict between the counselling needs of the parents and of the adolescent. Parents may not wish to burden their son with a new life-threatening diagnosis. At the same time the adolescent will be going through many life changes, developing his sexuality, trying to establish an identity as an adult, and in need of information about safer sex. Furthermore, the logistics of prophylactic treatment and antiviral therapy mean that youngsters cannot be denied knowledge of being infected with HIV. He is likely to be highly reluctant to disclose his HIV status to new partners. Counselling should include advice about contraception and safer sex, and should give informal access to free condoms.

Many older haemophiliacs were already socially and physically disadvantaged before being infected with HIV, as a result of regular hospital admissions in earlier life affecting their education and employment prospects.

The death of a person with haemophilia from AIDS will not usually mean the end of a family's involvement with services as brothers, children and female partners may also be infected. School teachers, peers and other members of the local community usually know about a boy's haemophilia. Confidentiality about HIV infection is, therefore, almost impossible to maintain since assumptions are made, even when false. In this way, youngsters with haemophilia have become stigmatised at school, with serious consequences for all aspects of their well-being.

Haemophiliacs and other family members infected with HIV are often said to be very angry. They are angry at having been infected with HIV when this might have been prevented. Their anger and grief has been exacerbated by having to pursue lengthy litigation procedures. In addition, many haemophiliacs with HIV feel bitter about the poor or non-existent advice on safer sex they received following infection. This has led to a good deal of sexual unhappiness and also to the infection of their sexual partners.

Many haemophilia treatment centres now offer substantial counselling and support to patients with HIV in making decisions about whether or not and how best to conceive a baby. In addition large haemophilia centres have long run an open-door type of medical service which is empowering to patients and offers benefits in the treatment of HIV infection.

Staff Support

Some staff in haemophilia centres are involved with an individual patient from birth to marriage and now, more frequently, until their death. HIV has had a devastating affect on some members of staff, particularly in centres where haemophilia treatment was aggressively pursued leading to a higher rate of HIV infection in patients. Regular, intensive staff support is essential to rebuild confidence, reduce stress and ensure a healthy staff team. For a fuller discussion of the complex relationship between counselling and the medical problems of HIV antibody positive haemophiliacs see Jones (1988).

Children and HIV

Children can be affected by HIV and AIDS in two broad ways; directly by being affected themselves in utero or at birth, or indirectly by their parents' illness and death. The recent finding that in Western Europe vertical transmission occurs in only about 20% of births to HIV positive women, is overshadowed by the realisation that those babies who escape HIV infections are nevertheless going to lose at least one, if not both of their parents, in childhood.

The social and emotional consequences for children with HIV are enormous. These may include social stigma at school, separation from parents due to their own illness, parent's illness or death, fostering, adoption and being cared for by elderly grandparents.

Breaking bad news to children is a crucial task. The way in which children find out about their own or their parent's illness plays a major part in their adjustment (Forrest 1989). The child's level of understanding and the emotional context in which the child is given the news are key factors in the process. An understanding of the developmental stages of children's ability to conceptualise serious illness (Bluebond Langer 1978; Lansdown 1980) and death (Kane 1979) should be of help to the professional involved in such a task. Breaking bad news to children if it is done in a skilful and considerate way may help reduce later emotional disturbances in these children.

Caring for children affected by HIV requires substantial proactive and reactive interventions with complex co-ordination of many health service and social service agencies.

Parents of children with HIV disease have to cope with depression, anxiety and multiple losses. Professionally-run support groups can assist parents in coping with this, reducing their isolation and providing an opportunity for anticipatory mourning (Crandles et al. 1992).

For a comprehensive source of information on HIV infection and babies and children the reader is referred to Sherr (1991).

Relapse Prevention: A New Approach

This is a new development in psychological interventions in the field of addictions. Relapse Prevention is a cognitive–behavioural approach aimed at maintenance of "self-directed" change. It is a holistic approach in that it consists of assessment procedures, cognitive and behavioural strategies, skills training and lifestyle change procedures.

Relapse Prevention is based on a process model of relapse developed from over a decade of psychological research into relapse in addictive behaviours (Marlatt and Gordon 1985).

Self directed change and its maintenance are the most crucial human factors in the prevention of spread of HIV. So the potential utility of an approach such as Relapse Prevention in the field of HIV and AIDS is immense. There are three key areas of application of this approach: with those who have problems in maintaining self directed change in practising safer sex; with injecting drug users; and with problem drinkers.

Maintaining Self-directed Change in High Risk Sexual Behaviours

Many individuals experience difficulty in maintaining self directed change in long-standing and highly reinforced behaviours such as sexual practices. The problem has been particularly highlighted in the gay community of AIDS epicentres where a vast majority of people have dramatically changed their sexual behaviours. A small section in this population reportedly find it difficult to change their behaviour or maintain safer sex practices such as always using condoms and lubricants for anal intercourse (Kelly et al. 1989). Individuals belonging to this group are at high risk in terms of both acquiring and spreading HIV infection.

Studies of Relapse Prevention interventions with gay men who have requested help with their compulsive high risk sexual behaviours show both a significant reduction in risk behaviour and long term maintenance of change (Marlatt and Gordon 1989; Wanigaratne et al. 1992a).

Wider application of such approaches is clearly needed at present with both gay and heterosexual individuals. This can be ensured by making such interventions widely available and easily accessible to individuals who need it and by vigilance of clinicians in discovering difficulties in this area for their patients.

Relapse Prevention with Injecting Drug Users

With injecting drug users relapse prevention has applications at three levels: interventions directed towards changing and maintaining change in drug use itself; interventions directed towards changing injecting practices; changing to and maintaining safer sex. The full potential of relapse prevention techniques with IDUs is yet to be exploited. Its inclusion as part of the total range of treatment and service options available to users of "needle exchanges" would be a valuable step.

Problem Drinkers

Problem drinking can be linked to HIV and AIDS in two ways: as a co-factor leading to unsafe sexual behaviour (Wanigaratne et al. 1992b); as a maladaptive coping mechanism by those with HIV and AIDS. For those seeking help with their problem drinking, relapse prevention offers a flexible and holistic approach to both changing drinking habits and maintaining those changes.

The Developing Area of Health Psychology

The importance of psychological processes in the experience of health and illness is being increasingly recognised. Health psychology focuses on three processes: the aetiology of health problems; the concurrence of psychological processes and medical problems; and the development and refinement of specific psychological techniques for medical problems (Broome 1989). It is already clear that the application of psychology can make a significant contribution to medical care. In addition the potential contribution of psychology to medical disorders in children is as great as in adults, although this area has been slow to develop due to a lack of resources.

There are several specific medical specialities where psychology has been shown to make an important and broad-ranging contribution to patient management. Obstetrics and gynaecology is probably the best developed example (e.g. Reading 1982; Broome and Wallace 1984), although rheumatology, dermatology, gastroenterology, haematology and cardiology are amongst the others.

The psychological contribution to medical disorders can be subdivided into (a) that relating to specific disease processes, whether at the stage of prevention, interruption of disease processes or symptom reduction, and (b) general contributions to the effective management of medical or surgical patients, including advice on improving overall service delivery and clinical audit-type research.

Symptom Reduction

Psychological interventions have been developed for the reduction of a wide range of medical symptoms (Ferguson and Taylor 1980; Pinkerton et al. 1982). Two common problems where psychological methods work well and provide an alternative to medication are pain (see p. 34) and insomnia.

Preparation for Medical and Surgical Procedures

One of the most successful areas of health psychology has been in the preparation of patients for medical and surgical procedures. Patients differ in their psychological responses to minor and major surgery, depending on personality, coping skills and available social support. Pre-operative psychological interventions including information-giving (on both surgical procedures and on psychophysiological and cognitive reactions to be expected) and teaching of behavioural, cognitive or psychological and physical stress management procedures. These interventions have been shown to reduce post-operative distress and lead to earlier discharge from hospital and reduced use of analgesia.

Attention has now moved on to a consideration of which aspects of special preparation are most helpful. The general conclusion is that the most successful preparation procedures do not merely provide additional information about what will happen, but also use cognitive therapy to help patients deal with their worries about surgery, and teach them psychological and physical coping techniques for dealing with their post-operative state.

Though all patients receive some kind of preparation for surgery, the benefits of special psychological preparation compare well with standard procedures. Such interventions are not time-consuming and are cost-effective in terms of earlier discharge and reductions in medication.

Communication and Compliance

Patients do not always understand what doctors tell them, and often cannot remember what they have been told. Many have a poor understanding of their illness. Often this lack of understanding militates against adherence to medical advice and ultimately leads to low satisfaction with treatment. Doctors have a responsibility to improve this situation and various remedies are recommended, based on extensive research (Ley 1989). These include improving oral communications and providing written information. Guidelines for improving oral communications with patients include the following:

1. Present the most important information first
2. Stress importance
3. Use simpler words and shorter sentences
4. Categorise the information, listing and then repeating category names before each category of information is presented
5. Use repetition
6. Use specific, rather than general, statements
7. Use additional interviews to see that information has been understood

Written information can maximise understanding and recall. It can be used for reference and should be simple and readable. A variety of psychological interventions have been developed to improve compliance (Meichenbaum and Turk 1987), although the whole concept of "compliance" is fraught with assumptions of authority, power and superior knowledge. In general, measures to improve so-called treatment compliance will clearly have to be achieved largely by encouraging greater awareness and skill within the health care team as a whole.

Research Issues in Psychotherapy and HIV

Although the effectiveness of psychological therapies has been demonstrated in general use, there have been precious few evaluation studies of therapy with people with HIV and AIDS in particular. Outcome measures should take into consideration the biological, psychological and social spheres, but are difficult to operationalise in practice. Outcome criteria could range from markers of disease progression to various measures of psychological and social adjustment.

Counselling is in widespread use as discussed earlier, but again relatively little work has been done to evaluate such interventions. The assumptions regarding the effectiveness of counselling in this area are so widely accepted that withholding such interventions for research purposes could raise considerable ethical difficulties.

There are inherent methodological difficulties in evaluating psychological interventions. The heterogeneity of therapy content and delivery, and the diversity of outcome criteria are the common problems of psychotherapy evaluation (Garfield and Bergin 1986). Outcome criteria may also be specific to the type of intervention. Furthermore there are problems that are specific to the evaluation of counselling people with HIV and AIDS. Disease progression (for physical health), mood states, quality of life, level of functioning, self esteem, family and other relationships, sexual functioning and vocational functioning are some of the outcome criteria that have been used (Christ and Weiner 1985; Fornstein 1984). HIV has raised the profiile of the emerging field of psychoneuroimmunology (Solomon and Temoshok 1990). The study of the effects of psychological interventions on the immune systems of those infected with HIV and those with AIDS is now an urgent priority.

Today, HIV counselling services provide for an unprecedented number of counselling clients. This offers a unique opportunity for research which could not only improve the efficacy of psychological assessment and therapy in HIV services, but in the wider field of psychotherapy as a whole.

References

Baum A, Temoshok L (1990) Psychosocial aspects of acquired immunodeficiency syndrome. In: Temoshok L, Baum A (eds) Psychosocial perspectives on AIDS: etiology, prevention, and treatment. Laurence Erlbaum, New Jersey
Bluebond Langer M (1978) The private worlds of dying children. Princeton University Press, New Jersey
British Association for Counselling (1985) Counselling – Definition of Terms. Information sheet available from BAC, Rugby, Warwickshire CV21 3BX
Broome AK, Wallace L (eds) (1984) Psychology and gynaecological problems. Tavistock, London
Broome AK (1989) (ed) Health psychology: processes and applications. Chapman and Hall, London
Brown J (1987) A review of meta-analysis conducted on psychotherapy outcome research. Clin Psychol Rev 7: 1–23
Christ GH, Weiner LS (1985) Psychosocial issues in AIDS. In: De Vita VT, Hellman S, Rosenburg SA (eds) AIDS: etiology, diagnosis, treatment and prevention. JB Lippincott, Philadelphia
Coates TJ, Stall RD, Hoff CC (1990) Changes in sexual behaviour among gay and bisexual men since the beginning of the AIDS epidemic. In: Temoshok L, Baum A (eds) Psychosocial perspectives on AIDS: etiology, prevention and treatment. Lawrence Erlbaum, New Jersey
Crandles S, Sussman A, Berthaud M, Sunderland A (1992) Development of a weekly support group for caregivers of children with HIV disease. AIDS care 4: 325–351
Egan V (1992) Neuropsychological aspects of HIV infection. AIDScare 4: 3–10

Engel G (1960) A unified concept of health and disease. Perspectives Med Biol 3: 459-485
Erskine A, William AC (1989) Chronic pain. In: Broome AK (eds) Health psychology: processes and applications. Chapman and Hall, London
Ferguson JM, Tayldor CB (1980) The comprehensive handbook of behavioural medicine. MTP Press, Lancaster
Fisher JD, Fisher WA (1992) Changing AIDS-risk behaviour. Psychol Bull 111: 455-474
Foa EB, Emmelkamp PMG (1983) Failures in behaviour therapy. John Wiley and Sons, New York, Chichester
Fornstein M (1984) The psychosocial impact of the acquired immunodeficiency syndrome. Semin Oncol 11: 77-82
Forrest G (1989) Breaking bad news to children in paediatric care. In: Couriel J, Hull R, Harten-Ash VJ (eds) Breaking bad news: current approaches. Duphar Medical Relations, Southampton
Garfield SL, Bergin AE (1986) (eds) Handbook of psychotherapy and behaviour change. Wiley, New York
Gelder M, Gath D, Mayou R (1983) Oxford textbook of psychiatry. Oxford University Press, Oxford
Glover L, Miller D (1990) Counselling in the context of HIV infection and disease. In: Mindel A (ed) AIDS: A pocket book of diagnosis and management. Edward Arnold, London
Goldfried MR, Sprafkin JN (1976) Behavioural personality assessment. In: Spence JT, Carson RC, Thibaut JW (eds) Behavioural approaches to therapy. GLP, New Jersey
Green J (1988) Post-test counselling. In: Green J, McCreaner A (eds) Counselling in HIV infection and AIDS. Blackwell, Oxford
Green J, McCreaner A (1988) (eds) Counselling in HIV infection and AIDS. Blackwell, Oxford
Hart G, Woodward N, Carvell A (1989) Needle exchange in central London: operating philosophy and communication strategies. AIDS care 1: 125-134
Hersen M, Bellack AS (1982) Behavioural assessment. Pergamon, New York
Higgins DL, Galarotti C, O'Reilly KR, Schnell DJ, Moore M, Rugg DL, Johnson R (1991) Evidence for the effects of HIV antibody counselling and testing on risk behaviours. JAMA 226: 2419-2429
Jones P (1988) The counselling of HIV antibody positive haemophiliacs. In: Green J, McCreaner A (eds) Counselling in HIV infection and AIDS. Blackwell, Oxford
Kane B (1979) Children's concepts of death. J Gen Psychol 134: 141-153
Kelly JA, St. Lawrence JS (1990) The impact of community-based groups to help persons reduce HIV infection risk behaviours. AIDS care 2: 25-36
Kelly JA, St Lawrence JS, Hood HV, Brasfield TL (1989) Behavioural interventions to reduce AIDS risk activities. J Consult Clin Psychol 57: 60-67
King MB (1989) Psychosocial status of 192 out-patients with HIV infection and AIDS. Br J Psychiat 154: 237-242
Kubler-Ross E (1970) On death and dying. Tavistock, London
Lambert MJ, Shapiro DA, Bergin AE (1986) Evaluation of therapeutic outcomes. In: Garfield SL, Bergin AE (eds) Handbook of psychotherapy and behaviour change. Wiley, New York
Lansdown R (1980) More than sympathy. Tavistock, London
Leff JP, Isaacs AD (1990) Psychiatric examination in clinical practice. Blackwell, Oxford
Ley P (1989) Improving patient's understanding, recall, satisfaction and compliance. In Broome AK (ed) Health psychology: processes and applications. Chapman and Hall, London
Luborsky L, Singer B, Luborsky L (1975) Comparative studies of psychotherapy. Arch Gen Psychiat 32: 495-1008
McCreaner A (1988) Pre-test counselling. In: Green J, McCreaner A (eds) Counselling in HIV infection and AIDS. Blackwell, Oxford
Management Advisory Service (MAS) Report to the NHS (1989): Review of Clinical Psychology Services
Marlatt GA, Gordon JR (1985) Relapse prevention. Guildford, New York
Marlatt GA, Gordon JR (1989) Relapse prevention: future directions. In: Gossop M (ed) Relapse and addictive behaviour. Tavistock/Routledge, London
Mawson D, Marks IM, Ramm L, Sterns (1981) Guided mourning for morbid grief: a controlled study. Br J Psychiat 138: 185-193
Meichenbaum D, Turk DC (1987) Facilitating treatment adherence: a practitioner's guidebook. Plenum Press, New York
Miller D, Acton TMG, Hedge B (1988) The worried well: their identification and management. J R Coll Physicians Lond 22: 158-165
Miller R, Bor R (1991) AIDS: A guide to clinical counselling. 2nd edn. Science Press, London

Miller WR (1985) Motivation for treatment: a review with special emphasis on alcoholism. Psychol Bull 98: 84–107

Nitsun M, Wood H, Bolton W (1989) The organisation of psychotherapy services: a clinical psychology perspective. Clinical Psychology Forum, no. 23, British Psychological Society, Leicester

O'Reilly KR, Higgins DL, Galavotti C, Sheridan J (1990) Relapse from safer sex among homosexual men: evidence from four cohorts in the AIDS community demonstration projects. Paper no FC. 717, presented at Sixth International Conference on AIDS, San Francisco, USA

Ostrow DG, Joseph JG, Kessler R, Soucy J, Tal M, Eller M, Chmiel J, Phair J (1989) Disclosure of HIV antibody status: behavioural and mental health correlates. AIDS Education and Prevention, Guildford, New York

Park LP, Munoz A, Armenian H, Margolick J, Giorgi JV, Ferbas J, Bauer K, Kaslow RA, Fahey JL (1990) Interaction between HIV-1 infection and smoking on CD4 lymphocyte count. Paper no. 675, presented at Sixth International Conference on AIDS, San Francisco, USA

Paul GL (1967) Strategy for outcome research in psychotherapy. J Consult Psychol 31: 109–118

Pinkerton SS, Hughes H, Weinrich WW (1982) Behavioural medicine: clinical applications. Wiley, New York

Pistrang N, Barker C (1992) Clients' beliefs about psychological problems. Counselling Psychology Quarterly 5: 325–335

Prochaska DO, DiClementi CC (1983) Stages and processes of self-change of smoking: towards an integrative model of change. J Consult Clin Psychol 51: 390–395

Rachman S, Hodgson R (1980) Obsessions and compulsions. Prentice-Hall, Century Series, Englewood Cliffs, NJ

Rachman S, Wilson GT (1980) The effects of psychological therapy (2nd edn). Pergamon, New York

Reading A (1982) Psychological aspects of pregnancy. Longmans, London

Robertson R (1990) AIDS and drug misuse. In: Mindel A (ed) AIDS – a pocket book of diagnosis and management. Edward Arnold, London

Schwartz GE (1982) Testing the biopsychosocial model: The ultimate challenge facing behavioural medicine. J Consult Clin Psychol 50: 1040–1053

Selnes OA, Miller E, McArthur J et al. (1990) HIV Infection: no evidence of cognitive decline during the asymptomatic stages. Neurology 40: 204–208

Shapiro DA, Shapiro D (1982) Meta-analysis of comparative therapy outcome research: a critical appraisal. Behavioural Psychotherapy 10: 4–25

Shapiro DA, Shapiro D (1983) Comparative therapy outcome research: methodological implications of meta-analysis. J Consult Clin Psychol 51: 42–53

Sherr L (1991) HIV and AIDS in mothers and babies. Blackwell, Oxford

Sloane RB, Staples FR, Cristos AH, Yorkston NJ, Whipple K (1975) Psychotherapy versus behaviour therapy. Harvard University Press, Cambridge, MA

Smith ML, Glass GV (1977) Meta-analysis of psychotherapy outcome studies. Am Psychol 32: 752–760

Smith ML, Glass GV, Miller TI (1980) The benefits of psychotherapy. John Hopkins University Press, Baltimore, Maryland

Solomon GF, Temoshok L (1990) A psychoneuroimmunologic perspective on AIDS research: questions, preliminary findings and suggestions. In: Temoshok L, Baum A (eds) Psychosocial perspective on AIDS. Lawrence Erlbaum, New Jersey

Stall R, Ekstrand M, Pollack L, Coates TJ (1990) Relapse from safer sex: the AIDS behavioural research project. Paper no. Th C. 108 presented at Sixth International Conference on AIDS, San Francisco, USA

Stiles WB, Shapiro DA, Elliot RK (1986) Are all psychotherapies equivalent? Am Psychol 41: 165–180

Stimson GV, Alldritt L, Dolan K, Donoghoe M (1988) HIV transmission risk behaviour of clients attending syringe exchange schemes in England and Scotland. Br J Addict 83: 1449–1455

Teasdale JD (1988) Cognitive vulnerability to persistent depression. Cognition and Emotion 2:247–274

Turk D, Rennert K (1981) Pain and the terminally ill cancer patient: a cognitive social learning perspective. In Sobel H (ed) Behaviour therapy in terminal care. Ballinger, USA

Twycross RG (1975) Disease of the central nervous system: relief of terminal pain. Br Med J 4: 212–214

Vandenbos GR, Pino CD (1980) Research on outcome of psychotherapy. In: Vandenbos GR (ed) Psychotherapy practice, research and policy. Sage, California

Wanigaratne S, Wallace W, Pullin J, Keaney F, Farmer R (1990) Relapse prevention for addictive behaviours: a manual for therapists. Blackwell, Oxford

Wanigaratne S, Aroney R, Williams M (1992a) Initiating and maintaining safer sex: description and evaluation of group work with gay men in London, UK. Poster presentation at VIII International Conference on AIDS/III STD World Congress, Amsterdam, Netherlands

Wanigaratne S, Clone H, Evan J (1992b) Alcohol consumption and safer sex: a survey of sexually transmitted disease clinic attenders. Royal College of Psychiatrists Conference "Addiction Problems and Responses" – A European perspective, Birmingham, UK

Wilson C (1989) Terminal care: using psychological skills with the terminally ill. In Broome AK (ed) Health psychology: processes and applications. Chapman and Hall, London

3 Psychological and Psychiatric Aspects of HIV and AIDS

Stanton Newman and Mary Fell

Introduction

In any chronic life-threatening illness, the difficulties of coping with the physical, social and emotional aspects are considerable. The impact of HIV and AIDS on the psychological state of the individual covers a range of areas of functioning, including mood and cognition.

Mood states are commonly examined using self-report questionnaires. These produce a score on a continuous scale from normal through ranges of mood change to mood disturbance. In this way they are able to examine both minor fluctuations in mood and also to give an indication of clinically severe mood disturbance. Self-report questionnaires are useful, therefore, to plot changes in mood at different stages of the disease and treatment, and also to compare the mood of those with HIV to that of other groups. While individuals who are HIV-seropositive report a range of concerns such as uncertainty about the disease and treatment, anxiety about any new physical symptoms, sadness, helplessness, lowered self esteem, guilt, worthlessness, suicidal thoughts, social withdrawal and anticipatory grief, sense of isolation and reduced support, anger (Holland and Tross 1985; Maj 1990a), the most commonly assessed mood states are those of depression and anxiety.

A different but related approach comes from psychiatry which also considers disturbances of mood state as well as psychoses. Self-report measures of mood state, as described above, produce results highly correlated with psychiatric assessments. Psychiatric assessments may take the form of a clinical psychiatric interview with traditional diagnostic categories (DSM IIIR) or by means of standardised assessments. The value of standardised instruments is that they are less likely to show variations from examiner to examiner and more likely to offer an accurate picture of the incidence of psychiatric disturbance.

Neuropsychology stems from two parent disciplines, neurology and psychology (Walsh 1978). While there has always been an interest in the relationship between brain and behaviour, this has been especially evident in the last few decades, with neuropsychology becoming a discipline in its own right. A neuropsychologist assesses nervous system functions associated with cognitive abilities such as memory, attention, language etc. Many of these assessments rely on already established correlations between localised brain damage and deficits on psychological tests designed to assess specific psychological functions

(Beaumont 1983). Because neuropsychological assessment is complex, training is required to properly perform and evaluate the results.

HIV is now known to be capable of causing neurological disease (Ho et al. 1985; McAllister et al. 1988; see Chapter 6), with CSF abnormalities identified soon after seroconversion (McArthur et al. 1988). This suggests that the nervous system is an early target for HIV and emphasises the importance of neuropsychological evaluation. Within the context of HIV/AIDS, neuropsychology has a number of functions: (a) to obtain early identification of cognitive changes in HIV-seropositive individuals, (b) to identify the areas of functioning most affected, (c) to examine changes in cognitive functioning by serial examination of neuropsychological performance and (d) to examine the effects of treatment on cognitive functions.

Forms and Incidence of Psychological and Psychiatric Disturbance

Depression

Raised levels of depressed mood and an increased incidence of depression have been found to occur in many chronic illnesses such as rheumatoid arthritis and multiple sclerosis (Stewart and Sullivan 1983; Newman et al. 1989). It might be expected that an increased incidence of depression would occur in HIV/AIDS. A WHO report (World Health Organization 1988) claims that a depressive episode may occur at any point of HIV infection, but generally these episodes cluster (a) in the period following an HIV diagnosis as a reactive state linked to the realisation of the health threat, loss of self esteem and guilt, and (b) in the initial stage of HIV-1 associated cognitive/motor complex (see below), where affective disturbance may precede the onset of cognitive abnormalities.

McAllister et al. (1992) compared depressed mood at various stages of infection and found that, on a self-report measure, the CDC IV group were more depressed than the CDC II/III group who, in turn, were more depressed than the seronegative group. These findings imply an increase in levels of depressed mood with disease progression. Reports on such self-report measures may be confounded by the inclusion of somatic items, the removal of which may eliminate group differences (Fell et al. 1993).

A number of factors have been found to influence levels of depressed mood in other chronic illnesses and these have also been reported in HIV and AIDS. Ostrow et al. (1989) examined depressed mood in 4954 gay men and found that self-reported HIV-related symptoms, such as swollen glands and weight loss, are associated with higher psychological symptom scores regardless of HIV status. Grant and Atkinson (1990) suggest that distress may be more evident at transitional points of HIV infection; these transitions often involve physical symptoms. Ostrow also reports that the individuals who perceived themselves to have more social supports, in particular people to confide in, had lower depression scores. Moulton et al. (1987) found that individuals who feel personally responsible for becoming HIV seropositive are more depressed than those who feel that they were not to blame. These findings, along with others, suggest that the level of depressed mood observed in HIV and AIDS is susceptible to influence from other psychological and social variables.

The question has arisen as to whether there is an increased incidence of psychiatric disturbance in asymptomatic HIV-positive individuals compared to those who are seronegative. King (1989) interviewed 192 HIV seropositive outpatients attending two London hospitals and found an incidence of psychiatric disorder in 31% of the sample. Psychiatric problems were generally mild and characterised as depression or prolonged adjustment reactions. Almost half of those with a psychiatric diagnosis reported emotional problems before HIV diagnosis; later studies support this to some extent (Rundell et al. 1990; Misrachi et al. 1991). King claims that this level of psychiatric disorder is similar to that seen in other patient groups. As the known cases of HIV infection do not distribute normally through the population and tend to be currently concentrated in specific groups, the incidence of any form of disturbance in these groups needs to be considered before the HIV virus can be implicated in the aetiology.

Anxiety

The time of testing for the presence of the HIV virus may be expected to be a time of particular anxiety for many individuals. Jadresic et al. (1990) examined anxiety in two groups of subjects around time of testing; those later found to be HIV seropositive and those found to be seronegative. Assessments were made prior to the notification of results and 6 months later. No differences were found between the two groups prior to the notification of results. It is interesting in this study that there was a significant drop in anxiety at 6 months after testing in those who were seropositive; this was maintained when they were repeatedly assessed 1 year after testing (Pugh et al. 1991). The authors conclude that knowledge of HIV seropositivity does not have a long-term adverse effect on mood. These findings parallel other studies of screening (e.g. Perry et al. 1990a) and suggest that the reduction of uncertainty in those found positive may be the important underlying reason for the fall in their levels of anxiety following screening. These findings must, however, be considered in relation to the increased risk of suicide in the short term, around the time of testing for seroconversion (see below).

Levels of anxiety reported by a homo/bisexual male population at different stages of infection have been investigated at the Middlesex Hospital, London (Fell et al. 1993). Significant increases in levels of anxiety were only apparent in the symptomatic stages of disease. Group differences disappeared once past psychiatric history had been controlled for, again highlighting the importance of considering this factor. Atkinson et al. (1988), using a psychiatric assessment procedure, found a greater lifetime prevalence of anxiety disorder among homosexual men compared to heterosexual men, thus emphasising the need for a comparable control group in any examination of mood and psychiatric disturbance in HIV.

Psychosis

Psychotic states are rarely reported in the early stages of infection. For example, Naber (1990) reviewed the records of a large cohort and found no incidence of psychotic illness in asymptomatic patients.

Early research, mainly in the form of case studies, suggested that many AIDS patients may present initially with a psychiatric syndrome (see Detmer and Lu 1986-1987, for a review). More recent research suggests that this is not as common as was first believed. The incidence of psychoses has been investigated by Naber et al. (1990) in Munich. In a study which combined subjects who were formally assessed and others whose case notes were reviewed, he found psychotic symptoms in 9 of 720 patients. Four patients had paranoid hallucinatory syndrome, 4 a delirious state, 1 a manic syndrome. The psychiatric diagnoses were exogenous or organic psychosis in 7, schizophrenia in 1 and a manic depressive illness in 1. These patients were in late stages of infection (ARC or AIDS). He concluded that the incidence of psychotic symptoms was not markedly elevated in HIV-infected patients with advanced disease. Naber, along with Maj (1990a), cautions that various diagnoses e.g., endogenous psychoses, drug-induced or psychogenic psychosis need to be considered before HIV-induced psychosis is diagnosed.

Neuropsychological Changes

Where individuals at CDC stages II/III and IV, and seronegative control groups have received formal neuropsychological assessment, significant differences have been found on some tests. For example, McAllister et al. (1992) found that performance of the CDC IV group was significantly poorer than that of the seronegative and the CDC II/III groups on three tests of attention and concentration and one test of visuo-spatial ability. These findings, along with those of other studies, indicate that neuropsychological changes are apparent when the disease has reached an advanced stage (Janssen et al. 1989; Miller et al. 1990).

One of the most controversial of CNS manifestations of HIV is what has been referred to as the AIDS Dementia Complex (ADC; Price and Brew 1988), and is now generally referred to as HIV-1 associated cognitive/motor complex (WHO 1990).

ADC has been so named because (a) it occurs in the context of advanced HIV infection and immunological compromise when an AIDS diagnosis is appropriate, (b) dementia refers to the cognitive decline which is the most obvious aspect of the disorder, and (c) the cognitive decline is generally accompanied by disturbed motor functions and sometimes behavioural change, justifying the term "complex" (Price and Brew 1988; Sidtis and Price 1990). Attributing any cognitive, motor or behavioural slowing to ADC is potentially problematic, as the symptoms may be those of a secondary dementia, that is, a dementia which is secondary to systemic problems associated with HIV infection (Navia et al. 1986). Differentiating between this and a primary dementia is important, as many of the problems of the former are both treatable and reversible (Woo 1985). Poor nutrition, including alcohol consumption and drug use, may cause metabolic encephalopathy with very similar symptoms (McAllister et al. 1988). The potentially negative effect of an AIDS diagnosis on the patient's cognitive functioning should be borne in mind (Bruhn et al. 1987). As regards frequency, the progression from a minor impairment to dementia appears to be rarer than originally believed (Goodwin et al. 1991).

Because of these manifestations and difficulties it has recently been proposed that a new term, HIV-1 associated cognitive-motor complex, be used (WHO 1990). For HIV-1 associated cognitive/motor complex to be judged as present, it has been suggested that the following guidelines be adopted: (a) laboratory evidence of sustained HIV-1 infection, (b) an acquired abnormality in at least two cognitive abilities, present for at least 1 month, verified by reliable history and neuropsychological assessment, and causing impairment in work or in activities of daily living, (c) an absence of clouding of consciousness allowing one to check the above, (d) exclusion of other aetiologies, (e) an acquired abnormality of motor function, and (f) a decline of motivation or of emotional control, or a change in social behaviour. It is generally felt that this cognitive/motor complex does not appear until the symptomatic stages of infection, if then (Maj 1992).

While HIV-1 associated cognitive/motor complex has been established as a clinical entity, the problem lies in identifying its actual onset. An abundance of studies have attempted to do this with varying results. One of the initial studies in this area was that of Grant et al. (1987), claiming that neuropsychological deficits existed in HIV-positive asymptomatic individuals, and suggesting that a progression of brain involvement occurs in persons with HIV infection that can begin with rather subtle cognitive changes early in the natural history of this viral disease. Other small studies have reported similar findings (e.g. Saykin et al. 1988).

Several larger prospective studies have been conducted, controlling for the many extraneous variables such as mood state, drug use and alcohol consumption. The Multicentre AIDS Collaborative Study investigation has reported on the prevalence of neurological abnormalities in seropositive men in CDC II/III and HIV seronegative homosexual men (Miller et al. 1990; McArthur et al. 1989). No significant differences were detected between the asymptomatic seropositive men and the seronegative men on neuropsychological test batteries. Similar findings have been reported from other study centres (Jannsen et al. 1989; Selnes et al. 1990; McAllister et al. 1992). In general, the larger studies, in contrast to those involving fewer than 70 subjects, have failed to demonstrate any group differences in neuropsychological performance between asymptomatic seropositive and seronegative individuals (Newman et al. in press).

Suicide

Suicide is a major concern for the carers of those who are HIV seropositive. Perry et al. (1990b) have examined the frequency of suicidal ideation among seropositive individuals, showing that 28.6% reported suicidal ideation 2 weeks before testing and 27.1% 1 week after testing. At a 2-month follow up, the percentage of individuals reporting suicidal ideation had dropped to 16.3%. This suggests that the period around testing is a particularly difficult time for those subsequently diagnosed as seropositive (Maj 1990a).

Considering more advanced infection, Glass (1988) suggests that there may be two periods of particularly high risk for suicide during the course of HIV/AIDS. Shortly after an AIDS diagnosis the patient may experience feelings of panic, depression or hopelessness. The second high risk period occurs later in the illness and is related to biological factors as CNS complications arise. Naber et al. (1990), in a retrospective study of case notes in the USA, concluded that 1% of individuals made a suicide attempt on learning their diagnosis. Using suicide notes from New York, 1985, Marzuk et al. (1988) reported that the relative risk for suicide in men with AIDS aged 20–59 years was 36.3 times that of men aged 20–59 years without this diagnosis, and 66.15 times that of the general population. Numbers of suicides might have been underestimated as an AIDS diagnosis may not have been reported to the medical examiner or suicide cases may have been concealed in other death classifications. Insufficient information, lack of treatment facilities and psychological support at that stage of the AIDS epidemic could perhaps account for these high rates. There is evidence that some of these cases of suicide reported depression and chronic anxiety. While some have argued that suicide in AIDS patients occurs as a manifestation of a psychiatric disorder (Glass 1988), others have suggested it may be considered to be a rational choice for some individuals with a terminal illness such as AIDS. Whatever the explanation offered, these findings emphasise the importance of counselling around the time of testing for the presence of the virus and for continuing contact with support and counselling services over the course of infection.

Assessment of Mood State and Psychiatric Status

The following gives an account of various procedures which may be used in attempting to assess mood state and psychiatric status.

Self-report Measures of Mood

Self-report measures of mood can be divided into general evaluations of mood and more specific mood inventories.

General Measures of Mood

(a). The Profile of Mood States (POMS) assesses transient, distinct mood states (McNair et al. 1971). It consists of a checklist of 65 adjectives rated on a 5-point scale ranging from "not at all" to "extremely". Six factors are measured: tension-anxiety (9 items), depression-dejection (15), anger-hostility (12), fatigue-inertia (7), vigour-activity (8), and confusion-bewilderment (7). With a healthy population, administration takes about 3–7 minutes; with very ill patients, it may take up to 15–20 minutes (Shacham 1983).

(b). The Hospital Anxiety and Depression scale (HAD) is a self-report measure designed to look at the severity of anxiety and depression in a hospital setting (Zigmond and Snaith 1983). It consists of 14 statements, 7 measuring depression, 7 measuring anxiety, with 4 possible responses to each. The individual is asked to note the reply which comes closest to how s/he has been feeling in the last week. Responses are scored on a 4-point scale with higher scores indicating more severe anxiety/depression. On both the anxiety and depression subscales, scores of 7 or less indicate non-cases, 8–10 doubtful cases, with 11 or more for definite cases.

Depressed Mood

(a). The Beck Depression Inventory (BDI) examines the extent of depressed mood in the last week, including the day of testing (Beck et al. 1961). There are

21 questions, each with 4 statements. Each question relates to a particular state e.g. feeling sad, and the statements allow the individual to rate the degree of severity of such a feeling. Answers are then rated on a 4-point scale, with the higher ratings being given to the more extreme/severe statements. The final score may be used as continuous measure but cut-off scores are also provided. Scores below 9 are taken as an indication of no or minimal depression, 10 to 14 borderline depression, 15 to 20 mild depression, 21 to 30 moderate depression, 31 to 40 severe depression and 41 to 63 very severe depression.

(b). The Zung is a 20-item questionnaire with 10 items worded symptomatically positive and 10 worded symptomatically negative (Zung and Durham 1965). Persons are asked to rate each on a 4-point scale, as to whether it occurred "a little of the time" through to "most of the time". The responses are then scored from 1 to 4, higher scores indicating a more depressed mood. These raw scores are then divided by 80 (maximum possible score) and expressed as a decimal. Some normative scores have been provided for a group of depressed patients (0.63–0.90) and a control group (0.25–0.43).

Anxiety

(a). The Spielberger State and Trait Anxiety Inventory (STAI) considers the level of anxiety currently experienced (state) and the general level of anxiety for the individual (trait) (Spielberger et al. 1970). Each consists of 20 statements with a 4-point scale, higher scores reflecting greater levels of anxiety.

(b). The Taylor Manifest Anxiety Scale is one of the earliest self-report measures (Taylor 1953). It consists of 50 items believed to reflect symptoms of manifest anxiety. Subjects are given the list of statements and asked to indicate how they generally feel by answering either true or false for each one.

Psychiatric Assessments

The following are three commonly used standardised psychiatric assessments:

(a). The Present State Examination (PSE) provides a structured clinical interview with the object of assessing the present mental state of adults (Wing et al. 1974). It has 107 questions and 33 observations of mood, behaviour and speech. Each question represents a symptom which is then rated as present or absent, not only on the basis of a "yes" or "no" reply, but by asking the patient to describe it in their own words ("yes") or by taking all available cues from behaviour to determine if the questioning should proceed for a particular symptom. The time period concerned is over the last month. Specific training is required in the use of this instrument.

(b). The Revised Clinical Interview Schedule (CIS–R) is designed to establish the individual's psychiatric history and current psychiatric status (Lewis and Pelosi 1990), and is based on Goldberg's et al. (1970) Clinical Interview Schedule. Increased standardisation of the revised version means that it is no longer necessary for an experienced clinician to administer it, as clinical judgements have been made in designing the questions and the rules for coding. Demographic and health queries are followed by an interview which considers fatigue, sleep problems, depression, anxiety, obsessions and compulsions, etc. Each section is scored over the past week and is rated on a 0–4 or 5 scale. The potential range of scores is 0–57. The CIS–R has also been adapted for self-administration by microcomputer (Lewis et al. 1988).

(c). The Diagnostic Interview Schedule (DIS) is a highly structured interview designed for use by lay interviewers and capable of generating computer diagnoses in terms of certain DSM III criteria (Myers et al. 1984; Regler et al. 1984). It assesses the presence, duration and severity of certain symptoms. Firstly, it determines whether or not the symptom ever occurred; then its severity, in terms of the degree to which it limits activity, if a physician or other professional has been consulted, or whether medication has been taken to treat it. It then examines whether every recurrence was explained by medical illness, alcohol or drug use. Symptoms that meet severity criteria and are not totally explained by medical conditions or substance use are grouped into patterns as designated by DSM III. The DIS does not cover all DSM III categories, inclusion being decided on the basis of expected prevalence, severity and clinical importance of the disturbances, research interest and validity of the disorder category as suggested by treatment response, family studies and follow-up studies. The DIS determines DSM III disorders with reference to several time periods, including 2 weeks prior to the interview, 1 month, 6 months and 1 year prior to interview and the entire lifetime prior to interview.

Neuropsychological Assessment

A number of established tests are available with which to assess cognitive functions. The selection of the tests to be applied depends on the requirements of the case at hand but some basic criteria need to be fulfilled (Kolb and Whishaw 1980). Thoroughness is important: if a group of tests is to be useful, a wide variety of functions should be examined. Ease of administration and scoring need to be considered, as do cost constraints. Tests should be of a reasonable length, bearing in mind that fatigue can adversely affect test scores. Constraints may also be placed on the tests used due to the testee's health: tests therefore need to be portable and adaptable. Finally, they also need to be flexible in that further alternative tests may need to be added in the light of new data. The range of neuropsychological tests is immense and the reader may consult Lezak (1983) for a comprehensive overview and description of the neuropsychological tests available, and Butters et al. (1990) for those most relevant to HIV/AIDS.

Other Management Issues

The manifestation of mood and psychiatric disturbance in those with symptomatic disease may have its origin in a number of causes which need to borne in mind when evaluating psychological or psychiatric state, particularly when determining if the psychiatric problems are organic or functional (see also Miller and Riccio 1990). Possible causes include early HIV-1 associated cognitive/motor complex (Smith 1990), previous psychiatric diagnosis (King 1989), drug-induced psychoses, reaction to an HIV diagnosis or disease progression (e.g. Atkinson et al. 1988).

Suspicion of changes in mood state and/or psychiatric disturbance will probably occur in the course of routine clinical assessment. Immediate referral to the counselling or psychiatric services should follow. This is discussed in Chapter 2. Care needs to be taken in prescribing and monitoring psychotropic drugs as there is evidence of an increased sensitivity in those with HIV infection (Maj 1990b; Miller and Riccio 1990).

Quality of life in HIV infection is now being given more serious attention, with an increasing awareness that quality as well as quantity of life is important. This is especially so with regard to treatment, many treatment evaluation studies including quality of life measures (see Burgess and Catalan 1991 for a review).

The use of neuropsychological tests to monitor the effects of pharmacological treatments is also an area of increasing importance. These tests offer a sensitive measure of the impact of treatment on level of arousal and cognitive functioning (see for example Schmitt et al. 1989).

Conclusion

The management of individuals with HIV infection is a complex and rapidly developing field. Professional help or assistance should be sought at an early stage when difficulties are first encountered. Not only should this assistance be initiated by the doctor but those who are HIV seropositive should be encouraged to request help, both from within the institution and from outside bodies.

References

Atkinson JH, Grant I, Kennedy CJ, Richman DD, Spector SA, McCutchan A (1988) Prevalence of psychiatric disorders among men infected with human immuno-deficiency virus. Arch Gen Psychiatry 45: 859–864

Beaumont JG (1983) Introduction to neuropsychology. Blackwell Scientific Publications, Oxford.

Beck AT, Ward CH, Mendelson M (1961) An inventory for measuring depression. Arch Gen Psychiatry 4: 561–571

Bruhn P and the Copenhagen Study Group of Neurological Complications in AIDS (1987) AIDS and dementia: a quantitative neuropsychological study of unselected Danish patients. Acta Psychiat Scand 76: 443–447

Burgess A, Catalan J (1991) Health related quality of life in HIV infection. Int Rev Psychiatry 3: 359–366

Butters N, Grant I, Haxby J et al. (1990) Assessment of AIDS-related cognitive changes: Recommendations of the NIMH workgroup on neuropsychological assessment approaches. J Clin Exp Neuropsychol 12: 958–963

Detmer WM, Lu FG (1986–87) Neuropsychiatric complications of AIDS: a literature review. Int J Psychiatry Med 16: 21–29

Fell M, Newman S, Herns M, Durrance P, Manji H, Connoly M, McAllister R, Weller I, Harrison M (1993) Mood and psychiatric disturbance in HIV and AIDS: changes over time. Br J Psychiatry 162: 604–610

Glass RM (1988) Aids and suicide. JAMA 259: 1369–1370

Goldberg DP, Cooper B, Eastwood MR, Kedward HB, Shepherd M (1970) A standardised psychiatric interview for use in community surveys. Br J Prevent Soc Med 24: 18–23

Goodwin GM, Egan V, Chiswick A, Brettle RP (1991) HIV and the brain: functional investigations in drug users. Int Rev Psychiatry 3: 343–356

Grant I, Atkinson JH (1990) The evolution of neurobehavioural complications of HIV infection. Psychol Med 20: 747–754

Grant I, Atkinson JH, Hesselink JR, et al. (1987) Evidence for early central nervous system involvement in the acquired immunodeficiency syndrome (AIDS) and other human immunodeficiency virus infections. Ann Intern Med 107: 828–836

Ho DD, Bredesen DE, Vinters HV, Daar ES (1985) The acquired immunodeficiency syndrome (AIDS) dementia complex. Ann Intern Med 111: 400–410

Holland JC, Tross S (1985) The psychosocial and neuropsychiatric sequelae of the acquired immunodeficiency syndrome and related disorders. Ann Intern Med 103: 760–764

Jadresic D, Riccio M, Hawkins D, Wilson B, Thompson C (1990) Long-term impact of HIV diagnosis on mood and alcohol and drug use – St. Stephen's cohort study. Paper presented at the Conference on Neurological and Neuropsychological Complications of HIV Infection, Monterey

Janssen RS, Saykin AJ, Cannon L et al. (1989) Neurological and neuropsychological manifestations of HIV-1 infection: association with AIDS-related complex but not asymptomatic HIV-1 infection. Ann Neurol 26: 592–600

King MB (1989) Psychosocial status of 192 out-patients with HIV infection and AIDS. Br J Psychiatry 154: 237–242

Kolb B, Whishaw IQ (1980) Fundamentals of human neuropsychology. Freeman & Co., San Francisco

Lewis G, Pelosi AJ (1990) Manual of the revised Clinical Interview Schedule. Institute of Psychiatry, London

Lewis G, Pelosi AJ, Glover G et al. (1988) The development of a computerised assessment for minor psychiatric disorder. Psychol Med 18: 737–745

Lezak MD (1983) Neuropsychological assessment (2nd edn). Oxford University Press, New York

McAllister RH, Harrison MJG, Johnson H (1988) HIV and the nervous system. Br J Hosp Med July: 21–26

McAllister RH, Herns M, Harrison MJG et al. (1992) Neurological and neuropsychological performance in HIV seropositive men without symptoms. J Neurol Neurosurg Psychiatry 55: 143–148

McArthur JC, Cohen BA, Farzedegan H et al. (1988) Cerebrospinal fluid abnormalities in homosexual men with and without neuropsychiatric findings. Ann Neurol 23: 534–537

McArthur JC, Cohen BA, Selves OA et al. (1989) Low prevalence of neurological and neuropsychological abnormalities in otherwise healthy HIV-1-infected individuals: Results from the multicenter AIDS cohort study. Ann Neurol 26: 602–611

McNair DM, Lorr M, Droppleman LF (1971) Profile of Mood States. Educational and Industrial Testing Service, San Diego

Maj M (1990a) Psychiatric aspects of HIV-1 infection and AIDS. Psychol Med 20: 547–563

Maj M (1990b) Organic mental disorders in HIV-1 infection. AIDS 4: 831–840

Maj M (1992) HIV-associated cognitive disorders. Paper presented at Session 150, VIII International Conference on AIDS, Amsterdam

Marzuk PM, Tierney H, Tardiff K et al. (1988) Increased risk of suicide in persons with AIDS. JAMA 259: 1333–1337

Miller D, Riccio M (1990) Non-organic psychiatric and psychosocial syndromes associated with HIV-1 infection and disease. AIDS 4: 381–388

Miller EN, Selnes OA, McArthur JC et al. (1990) Neuropsychological performance in HIV-1 infected homosexual men: the WIAC study. Neurology 40: 197–203

Misrachi A, Zulian C, DeWit S et al. (1991) Patterns of psychiatric and psychosocial hospitalisations of HIV patients. Poster presented at VII International Conference on AIDS, Florence

Moulton JM, Sweet DM, Temoshok L, Mandel JS (1987) Attributions of blame and responsibility in relation to distress and health behaviour change in people with AIDS and AIDS related complex. J Appl Soc Psychol 17: 493–506

Myers JK, Weissman MM, Tischler GL et al. (1984) Six month prevalence of psychiatric disorders in three communities. Arch Gen Psychiatry 41: 959–967

Naber D, Perro C, Schick U et al. (1990) Psychiatric symptoms in HIV-infected patients. Paper presented at a conference on Neurological and Neuropsychological Complications of HIV infection, Monterey

Navia BA, Cho E, Petito CK, Price RW (1986) The AIDS Dementia Complex: II. Neuropathology. Ann Neurol 19: 525–535

Newman SP, Fitzpatrick R, Lamb R, Shipley M (1989) The origins of depressed mood in rheumatoid arthritis. J Rheumatol 16: 740–744

Newman S, Lunn S, Harrison MJG (1993) Do asymptomatic HIV seropositive individuals show cognitive deficit–a review of 36 studies. Submitted for publication.

Ostrow DG, Monjan A, Joseph J et al. (1989) HIV related symptoms and psychological functioning in a cohort of homosexual men. Am J Psychiatry 146: 737–742

Perry S, Jacobsberg L, Fishman B et al. (1990a) Psychological responses to testing for HIV. AIDS 4: 145–152

Perry S, Jacobsberg L, Fishman B (1990b) Suicidal ideation and HIV testing. JAMA 263: 679–682

Price RW, Brew BJ (1988) AIDS Commentary: the AIDS dementia complex. J Infect Dis 158: 1049–1083

Pugh K, Riccio M, Catalan J, Jadresic D, Lovett E, Hawkins D (1991) Psychiatric findings in CDC group II gay men – one year follow-up of the St. Stephen's cohort study. Paper presented at Conference on Neuroscience of HIV Infection, Padua

Regler DA, Myers JK, Kramer M et al. (1984) The NIMH epidemiologic catchment area program: Historical context, major objectives and study population characteristics. Arch Gen Psychiatry 41: 934–941

Rundell J, Paolucci S, Beatty D et al. (1990) Psychiatric illness at all stages of HIV infection. Am J Psychiatry 145: 652–653

Saykin AJ, Janssen RS, Sprehn GC, Kaplan JE, Spira TJ, Weller P (1988) Neuropsychological dysfunction in HIV-infection: Characterisation in a lymphadenopathy cohort. Int J Clin Neuropsychol 10: 81–95

Schmitt FA, Bigley J & AZT Collaborative Work Group (1989) Neuropsychological correlates of immune system status and AZT therapy in AIDS and ARC. Paper presented at Neurological and Neuropsychological Complications of HIV Infection, Quebec City

Selnes OA, Miller E, McArthur JC et al. (1990) HIV infection: No evidence of cognitive decline during the asymptomatic stages. Neurology 40: 204–208

Shacham S (1983) A shortened version of the profile of mood states. J Pers Assess 47: 305–306

Sidtis JJ, Price RW (1990) Early HIV-1 infection and the AIDS dementia complex. Neurology 40: 323–326

Smith J (1990) Manic psychosis as a neuropsychiatric complication of HIV infection. Paper presented at the conference on Neurological and Neuropsychological complications of HIV infection, Monterey

Speilberger CD, Gorsuch RL, Luchene RE (1970) STAI: Manual for the State-Trait Anxiety Inventory. Consulting Psychologists, Palo Alto, CA

Stewart DC, Sullivan TJ (1983) Illness behaviour and the sick role in chronic disease. The case of multiple sclerosis. Soc Sci Med 16: 1397–1404

Taylor JA (1953) A personality scale of manifest anxiety. J Abnorm Soc Psychol 48: 285–290

Walsh KW (1978) Neuropsychology – a clinical approach. Churchill Livingstone, Edinburgh

Woo SKC (1985) The psychiatric and neuropsychiatric aspects of HIV disease. J Palliat Care 4: 50–53

World Health Organization (1988) Global Programme on AIDS: Report of the consultation on the neuropsychiatric aspects of HIV infection. Geneva

World Health Organization consultation on the neuropsychiatric aspects of HIV-1 infection (1990) AIDS 4: 935–936

Wing JK, Cooper JE, Sartorius N (1974) Measurement and classification on psychiatric symptoms. Cambridge University Press, Cambridge

Zigmond AS, Snaith RP (1983) The hospital anxiety and depression scale. Acta Psychiatrica Scandinavica 67: 361–370

Zung WWK, Durham NC (1965) A self-rating depression scale. Arch Gen Psychiatry 12: 63–70

4 Respiratory Problems of HIV Infection and AIDS
Ann Millar

Introduction

At present, the lungs are affected more commonly in the acquired immunodeficiency syndrome (AIDS) than any other organ system (Hope and Luce 1985; Murray et al. 1984, 1987; Murray and Mills 1990). Furthermore one respiratory illness alone, pneumocystis carinii pneumonia (PCP), will occur in 75% of patients who are antibody positive for the human immunodeficiency virus (HIV-positive) at some point in their disease without prophylactic treatment and still accounts for up to 50% of initial presentations of AIDS.

The lungs can be involved by opportunistic and conventional infectious disorders as well as non-infectious disorders such as Kaposi's sarcoma (KS), lymphocytic interstitial and non-specific pneumonitis (Murray et al. 1994, 1987; Stover et al. 1985). Many of these conditions can be life-threatening but are potentially curable, hence their diagnosis and appropriate promptly instituted treatment is essential. Primary and secondary prophylactic treatment is becoming more widely used and more effective and this will change the spectrum of disease. In this chapter, the clinical presentations of these pulmonary diseases are described, followed by the modes of investigation and subsequently some discussion of individual conditions and their management in HIV-infected patients.

Clinical Presentation

The commonest presenting symptoms of respiratory disease are breathlessness, cough, fever, haemoptysis, chest pain, constitutional disorder and malaise.

Breathlessness

Breathlessness is the most characteristic and earliest symptom of PCP and as such must be taken extremely seriously in an HIV-positive individual or someone in a high risk category for HIV (Engelberg et al. 1984). Breathlessness in this situation may be disproportionate to radiological or physiological data. It may precede physiological and radiological abdominal by up to 6 weeks

(Goodman and Tashki 1983). PCP induces hypoxaemia which is responsible for the characteristic tachypnoea and resultant hypocarbia of this condition. Pyogenic bacterial pneumonia and interstitial pneumonitis may also produce breathlessness whereas it is unusual with non-infective disorders such as Kaposi's Sarcoma (KS) until extensive disease is present. Less dramatic breathlessness may occur with pleural effusions that accompany KS or mycobacterial disease (especially *M. tuberculosis*). These conditions are often associated with additional symptoms and signs, and the breathlessness is not only less severe in intensity but also of a more gradual onset than with PCP. Upper respiratory tract infections, bronchitis and other "orthodox" chest complaints affect HIV-positive individuals and must not be forgotten (Wallace et al. 1993). Finally, the patient in the high risk group who is antibody-positive is usually very well informed about these potential illnesses and symptoms. Anxiety may produce hyperventilation and breathlessness; however, though fears must be allayed, breathlessness should not be discarded as due to anxiety alone unless the patient has been carefully reviewed for some weeks.

Cough

Cough is a non-specific symptom of many chest diseases, but is a useful pointer to the chest as the cause of non-specific symptoms of weight loss, general malaise and loss of well being, which may occur in a very indolent fashion with *M. tuberculosis* or more commonly with atypical mycobacteria. Pneumocystis carinii pneumonia is usually associated with a dry, persistent but non-productive cough but this is not a universal feature. Bacterial pneumonia may also present with cough which is more likely to be productive. Cough is more common in patients who are also smokers whatever the underlying pathology (Wallace et al. 1993).

Fever

Fever is a frequent sign, but rarely a complaint of patients with PCP. Conventional bacterial pneumonia may present with high fever in combination with other symptoms. Constitutional symptoms and intermittent fever are frequent symptoms of *M. tuberculosis* similar to those found in non-HIV-positive individuals. Atypical mycobacteria may not produce fever and lack of this sign does not exclude this infection. Absence of fever may be a useful feature to distinguish PCP from lymphocytic interstitial pneumonia (LIP), which can present with otherwise identical symptoms, signs and chest radiograph.

Chest Pain

Chest pain is an unusual symptom in PCP, though many patients complain of a difficulty in taking a deep breath in, or chest "tightness". Pleuritic chest pain would point to bacterial pneumonia as a more likely diagnosis. Non-specific but persistent chest pain may occur with intrathoracic neoplasia due to KS or B cell lymphoma. Pulmonary emboli and lung cancer are other conditions which can present with chest pain and occur with the same incidence for their age and sex as in HIV-negative patients.

Haemoptysis

Haemoptysis most commonly occurs in HIV-positive patients due to KS, which may be in the naso-oropharynx and readily visible (Meduri et al. 1986). More extensive KS in the lung parenchyma can also occasionally produce haemoptysis. Some parenchymal disease is usually present when extensive skin lesions are seen, but their mutual extent does not correlate. Haemoptysis is not a symptom of PCP but may occasionally be seen with bacterial pneumonia and tuberculosis. Pulmonary embolism and bronchogenic carcinoma may occur particularly in more elderly smokers, and such conventional diagnoses must be considered as the cause of haemoptysis.

Constitutional Disturbance and General Malaise

These symptoms may be due to chest disease such as mycobacterial infection. In any patient complaining of these symptoms, a chest x-ray must be performed and the respiratory system considered as the site of disease.

Examination

General examination of a patient may raise the possibility of AIDS-related disease when risk factors have not been elucidated in the history. Obvious weight loss, oropharyngeal candidiasis, seborrhoeic dermatitis, KS and widespread lymphadenopathy may all be present. In cases of PCP, examination is usually normal other than the tell-tale sign of tachypnoea, even with extensive disease. At most, some fine basal crepitations may be heard on auscultation. Clinically detectable signs in the chest are most commonly due to pyogenic bacterial pneumonia although classical signs of consolidation are rare. The presence of a clinically detected pleural effusion is unusual and suggestive of KS although *M. tuberculosis*, bacterial pneumonia and other malignancies can occasionally produce these physical signs. Characteristically atypical mycobacterial infection is associated with few physical signs.

Investigations

The important investigations in this condition are chest radiograph, computed tomography, oximetry (± exercise), lung function tests, nuclear medicine studies, blood tests, induced sputum, fibreoptic bronchoscopy and bronchoalveolar lavage and open lung biopsy.

Radiology

Radiological examination of the chest is the initial investigation of any patient presenting with respiratory symptoms and is a useful screening test. In HIV-positive or high-risk patients this is particularly important as radiological signs of PCP are more marked than the clinical signs. Any abnormality in the chest x-ray (CXR) of a symptomatic patient should be investigated. However, the CXR may be normal in 5%–14% of cases in the early stages of several lung diseases including PCP and MAI, and symptomatic patients require close monitoring despite the presence of a normal CXR (or arterial blood gases) (Goodman et al. 1984). The radiographic changes of pulmonary complications of AIDS are neither specific to any particular infection or neoplasm, nor to AIDS itself (Suster et al. 1986; De Lorenzo et al. 1987; Naidich et al. 1987). Characteristically, PCP presents with an initial perihilar bilateral haze which is easily overlooked, especially when the possibility of PCP is not mentioned on the request form (Fig. 4.1). This shadowing extends into a batwing distribution with peripheral sparing, this feature and the absence of Kerley's B lines differentiating this appearance from pulmonary cardiogenic oedema. These appearances can also be seen with pyogenic bacterial, mycobacterial, cytomegalovirus and fungal infection in addition to Kaposi's sarcoma and lymphoid or non-specific interstitial pneumonitis. Alveolar consolidation and resultant air bronchograms may be present in severe cases. Atypical features such as cystic changes, localised upper zone changes suggestive of tuberculosis (Milligan et al. 1985), and very rarely hilar and mediastinal lymphadenopathy (Stern et al. 1984) or pleural effusion (Naidich et al. 1987) may be present in up to 10% of cases. X-ray changes can occur rapidly in PCP so that a normal CXR may be grossly abnormal a few days later. By contrast, CXR clearing on recovery tends to be slow, reflecting the persistent lung function abnormalities often remaining on recovery (Shaw et al. 1988; Mitchell et al. 1992). The CXR has been reported to have a sensitivity as high as 85% for the diagnosis of PCP when the typical features described are present and similar specificity (Millar and Mitchell 1990). When such typical radiographic features are seen in patients with a "typical" clinical history and examination,

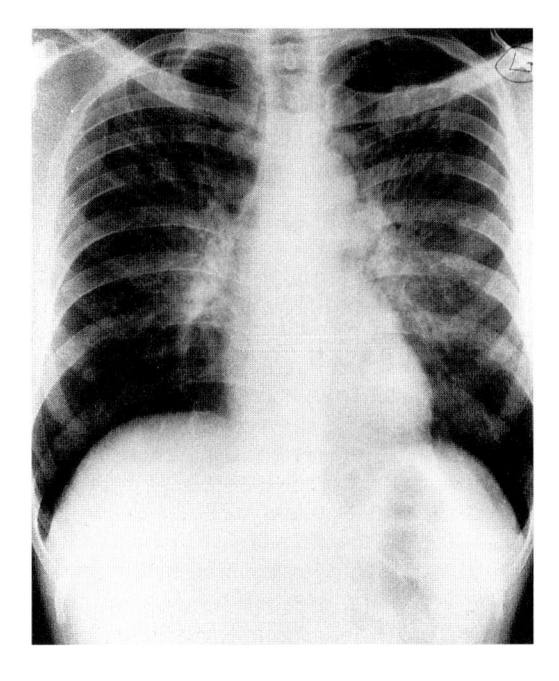

Fig. 4.1. A chest x-ray showing typical features of PCP with bilateral infiltrates and peripheral sparing.

i.e., breathlessness, dry cough, normal examination or basal crackles, and arterial hypoxaemia then the sensitivity and specificity increase to 87% and 90% respectively. The majority of pulmonary disease in AIDS is due to PCP so this is not as surprising as it may seem.

Focal radiographic changes suggest pathogens other than PCP in the lung. Localised consolidation is more likely to represent bacterial pneumonia but may occur with PCP (especially if treated with aerosolised pentamidine) or mycobacterial disease (Naidich et al. 1987). Soft upper zone shadowing, with or without cavitation or pleural effusions, is more suggestive of tuberculosis, although atypical presentations of this disease are also common. Atypical mycobacterial disease may have similar features but can have minimal radiographic signs, reflecting the lack of inflammatory response. Nodular shadowing is usually a feature of Kaposi's sarcoma. Hilar or mediastinal lymphadenopathy with or without pleural effusions on conventional CXR suggest the presence of tuberculosis, lymphoma or Kaposi's sarcoma.

More recently, computed tomography (CT) have been used to evaluate AIDS-related lung disease (Naidich and McGuiness 1991; Hartman et al. 1994). Fine section CT (2- or 3-mm cuts) may be particularly useful in cases with respiratory symptoms and normal CXR. Such patients are relatively unusual and the development of pattern recognition for PCP compared to other pulmonary pathology remains to be established. Intra-alveolar consolidation and bronchial wall thickening is highly suggestive of PCP. KS was associated with multiple diffuse masses of abnormal tissue. The diagnostic value of CT is undoubted but cannot be a panacea. Specific areas include identification of occult disease, dual pathology in patients unresponsive to treatment and CT-guided biopsies.

Oximetry

Arterial oxygenation must be assessed to determine the presence and extent of respiratory failure. There are obvious advantages for patients and staff in the use of oximetry to monitor respiratory failure in AIDS patients, as arterial puncture is avoided. It must be emphasised that high saturation levels do not ensure a well patient, due to the sigmoid shape of the oxygen dissociation curve. Exercise-induced desaturation detected by oximetry is a highly sensitive index for PCP. In the original study, of patients who were able to exercise for 10 min, 88% developed an oxygen saturation of less than 90% whereas in none of 12 healthy volunteers did this occur (Smith et al. 1988). Furthermore 20 of 24 (83%) patients with PCP and normal blood gases desaturated on exercise whereas only 2 of 19 (10%) patients with other AIDS-related respiratory problems desaturated.

Arterial puncture enables the alveolar-arterial (Aa) oxygen gradient and the level of CO_2 to be calculated, determining type II respiratory failure. Only 8% of patients with PCP have normal Aa oxygen gradients at rest and if exercise testing is added this decreases to 5% (Stover et al. 1989). The presence of hypoxaemia and an abnormal Aa gradient are therefore sensitive indices for PCP, but they are non-specific and are seen with many of the other pulmonary complications of AIDS. Severe PCP is characterised by rapidly progressive and potentially fatal hypoxaemia and therefore continuous oximetry is necessary as additional therapy may be undertaken.

Lung Function Tests

Routine pulmonary function tests are non-invasive, quick to perform and repeat and are readily available in most hospitals. Reduced values of single breath diffusing capacity (DLCO), diffusion coefficient (KCO), vital capacity (VC) and total lung capacity (TLC) have been described as reduced in HIV-related lung disease, in particular PCP, whereas simple measures of airway function (peak expiratory flow rate, forced expiratory volume in one second) are often normal (Coleman et al. 1984; Shaw et al. 1988; Mitchell et al. 1992). However the most sensitive of these investigations appears to be the DLCO which may correspond with the extent of lung involvement. This test may also be reduced in other AIDS-related lung disease and values of less than 70% predicted are found in Kaposi's sarcoma and mycobacterial infection and HIV-positive patients without overt lung disease. The decrease in DLCO which occurs in smokers or intravenous drug abusers does not seem to be the cause and the emergence of non-specific pneumonitis possibly due to HIV itself may be the explanation (Overland et al. 1980). Attempts have been made to correlate a reduction in DLCO with the HIV and/or CMV load in the lung but have not shown a direct relationship (Clarke et al. 1991; Nieman et al. 1993; Kvale et al. 1993). The DLCO remains a useful screening test, particularly when sequential measurements can be made, as a sudden fall in DLCO associated with new respiratory systems nearly always represents pulmonary disease (Shaw et al. 1988). In prospective studies Shaw et al. (1988) and Mitchell et al. (1992) found patients with acute PCP had a mean DLCO of 49% of the predicted value which improved to 71% predicted on recovery. By contrast, the mean DLCO (% predicted) for patients with AIDS-related complex was 73%, for patients with non-pulmonary Kaposi's sarcoma was 72% and for AIDS without overt lung involvement it was 73%. A progressive decline in lung function was related only to smoking and improvement did not occur with zidovudine treatment. The relatively short time scale (18 months) does not enable HIV to be excluded as a cause of changes in DLCO. Fears of cross infection both by HIV which can be present in saliva (Ho et al. 1985), and mycobacterial disease have limited the application of lung function testing. The use of disposable one-way valves for spirometry and saliva-absorbing bacteriostatic filters for gas transfer testing circumvent this problem. Simple and inexpensive modifications to conventional lung function equipment have recently been described which, if generally adopted, should remove risks of infection completely (Denison et al. 1989).

Nuclear Medicine

The use of radionucleotides in the investigation of pulmonary disease in general as well as HIV is more common in the USA than in the UK. Two agents have been used. Gallium-67 citrate is given intravenously and is taken up by inflammatory cells. Initially it was thought that diffuse uptake of gallium-67 by the lungs in an at-risk patient was both highly specific and sensitive for PCP (Coleman et al. 1984). Further studies have confirmed a high sensitivity of more than 90% for PCP but showed a low specificity of 51% (Kramer et al. 1987). This may reflect greater awareness of the possible significance of pulmonary symptoms by both physicians and patients in high-risk groups for HIV infection who therefore present earlier in the course of their disease. Gallium-67 scans may also be useful in monitoring the response of PCP to treatment. The scans may be graded 1–4 according to the intensity of gallium uptake; in one study of 12 patients with PCP and initial grade 3 or 4 scans, 10 reverted to grades 1 and 2 on recovery. Two further patients had persistent grade 4 changes following treatment of PCP and in both *Pneumocystis carinii* was still present on repeat bronchoscopy (O'Doherty et al. 1989). Another uptake pattern, with focal gallium accumulation, has been associated with the presence of *Mycobacterium avium* complex (MAC). In one small study 9 of 10 patients with MAC had such changes (Kramer et al. 1987). The main use of gallium-67 is likely to be in the patient who is not responding to treatment or with a probable inflammatory lesion, in which case it will be a guide to further investigation and/or biopsy (O'Doherty and Nunan 1993).

By contrast, ^{99m}Tc DTPA is delivered to the lung by the inhalational route and its subsequent clearance is a measurement of pulmonary epithelial permeability or "leakiness". DTPA clearance from the lung is markedly increased in patients with PCP (O'Doherty et al. 1989) and has been advocated as a screening test for this disease. Smokers also have an increased clearance, indeed this change can be seen after 3 days of smoking in a previous non-smoker (O'Doherty 1985). However, in patients with PCP a biphasic clearance curve is seen which differs from that seen in smokers but may be seen with other respiratory problems such as legionella pneumonia. On recovery from PCP, this biphasic clearance curve reverts to a monophasic curve, allowing this technique to assess response to treatment (O'Doherty et al. 1989). A small comparative study of gallium-67 and ^{99m}Tc DTPA scanning in 11 patients suggests that the latter is more specific for PCP (Rosso et al. 1986). These techniques are time-consuming, costly and require the nuclear medicine expertise. They may have little to offer over and above the more simple screening tests.

Blood Tests

The serodiagnosis of disease has obvious advantages, particularly in sick and potentially infectious patients. The possibility of using such techniques for PCP had been explored. Complement fixation tests for PCP in the epidemic childhood form of the illness have been used and initial results were encouraging: 90% of proven cases were seropositive in contrast to only 3% of a control group (Barta 1969). However immunofluorescent techniques showed that more than 75% of children were seropositive by the age of 4 years (Pifer et al. 1978) so that the presence of antibody to *Pneumocystis carinii* could not be taken to indicate active infection unless a four-fold increase in titre could be demonstrated. Conversely, AIDS patients by virtue of their immune incompetence may be unable to mount antibody responses to neoantigens and so would remain seronegative for PCP in the face of active infection. The standardization of such tests and a source of antigen have been difficult (Young 1987; Walzer et al. 1987). Further problems involve difficulty in standardising the tests and the sources of antigen. At present, both antibody and antigen detection tests are inappropriate for the diagnosis of PCP because they lack adequate reproducibility, specificity and sensitivity. The use of DNA probes to detect the presence of pneumocysts in lung tissue or bronchial washings as a diagnostic tool have resulted in very positive reports

(Tanabe et al. 1988). The diagnosis of lung disease from blood samples by such techniques remains to be explored. It is likely that application of this technology will supersede many of the more invasive investigations.

Serum lactate dehydrogenase (LDH) and peripheral lymphocyte counts may also be useful. LDL levels are substantially elevated in most cases of PCP (Zaman and White 1988; Smith et al. 1988), but also elevated to a lesser extent in HIV-positive patients with other pulmonary disease. Peripheral blood lymphopenia or reduced CD4 lymphocyte counts can be helpful indicators in that most cases of PCP occur with CD4 counts of less than 200/mm^3 (Masur et al. 1989).

Induced Sputum

Sputum production is unusual in patients with the more common HIV-related lung diseases, in particular PCP. Sputum production can be induced by inhalation of hypertonic (3%–5%) saline, the deposition of which causes airway irritation and subsequent mucus production and an osmotic influx of water into the airways. In this way the inflammatory exudate and pneumocysts pass up the conducting airways and are expectorated. Essentials for the success of this technique in producing adequate specimens are a well-fitting face mask and the co-operation of the patient, together with the encouragement of a nurse or physiotherapist for the patient to keep the mask on throughout the nebulisation. Ultrasonic nebulisers are most effective for this process.

Preliminary studies of this technique found that more than 50% of patients subsequently shown to have PCP at fibre-optic bronchoscopy or broncho-alveolar lavage are diagnosed by induced sputum (Pitchenik et al. 1986; Bigby et al. 1986). The preparation of the material obtained is also crucial. The sputum must be stained with Giemsa as well as silver stains as cystic forms predominate in the sputum and are picked up by conventional staining better than the silver staining that detects the trophozoites predominant in broncho-alveolar lavage (Fig. 4.2). At this basic level the technique requires very expert and experienced cytological examination. However, the use of Dithiothreitol to liquefy the sample and the use of specific monoclonal antibodies to pneumocystis have increased the sensitivity, reported in one series as up to 92% (Zaman et al. 1988; Kovacs et al. 1988). Conventional bacterial infection and mycobacteria may also be detected in this fashion. The use of DNA probes will undoubtedly improve the sensitivity, specificity and reproducibility of these techniques (Wakefield et al. 1991).

Fibreoptic Bronchoscopy (FOB), Broncho-Alveolar Lavage (BAL), and Transbronchial Biopsy (TBB)

Fibreoptic bronchoscopy (FOB) has been the mainstay of diagnosis for respiratory disease in HIV-positive individuals since the initial recognition of this condition (Stover et al. 1984; Orenstein et al. 1986). FOB is a readily available procedure which is safe for both the patient and operator. PCP can be diagnosed in 85% of cases by broncho-alveolar lavage (BAL) at FOB which increases to more than 90% when transbronchial biopsy (TBB) is also performed (Warren et al. 1985). TBB may add relatively little in terms of diagnosis with a marked increase in morbidity when PCP is the likely diagnosis, and BAL alone is to be

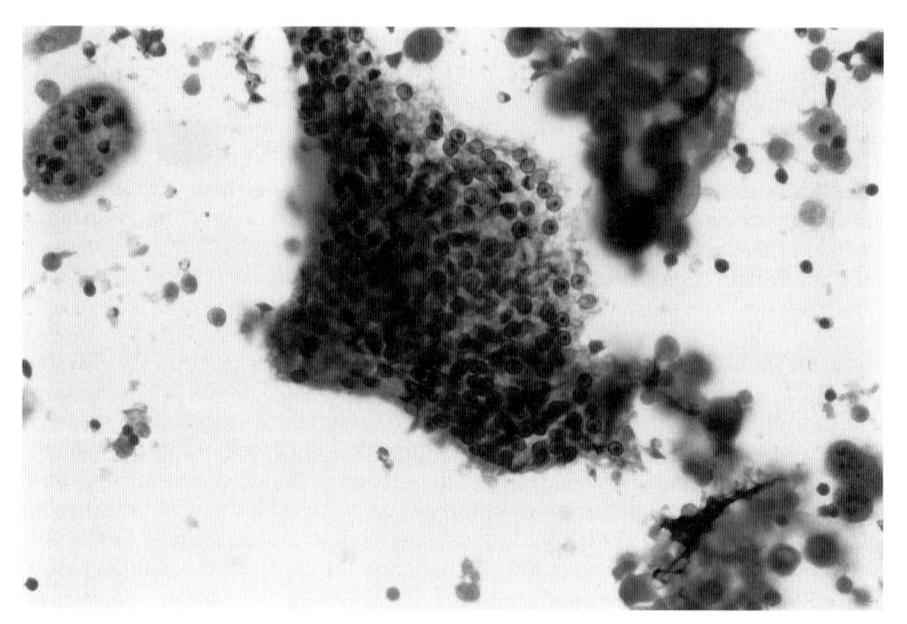

Fig. 4.2. A high power microscopic view of silver staining pneumocysts from an induced sputum sample.

recommended. TBB should be performed when atypical features are present or if a repeat bronchoscopy is performed because of failed medical therapy. Several studies have suggested that routine fluoroscopic screening is unnecessary unless changes are present on the chest radiograph.

BAL should be performed in a standard manner using warmed isotonic saline in aliquots of 60 ml unless the patient is particularly hypoxic, in which case the increased hypoxia always encountered during this procedure may be unacceptable and a smaller volume should be used (30 ml) ideally with oximetry being performed. Careful inspection of the large airways is required to identify the subtle changes of Kaposi's sarcoma which may be otherwise mistaken for the traumatic lesions of excessive suction (Hanson et al. 1987). The lavage fluid and biopsies taken are sent for histological, bacteriological and virological screening. The bronchoscopist should wear goggles, a mask and gloves, and ideally disposable clothing because a blood-laden aerosol may be formed, particularly at TBB. The risk of nosocomial infection is very low. Subsequent to the use of the bronchoscope, the apparatus should be cleaned in the conventional manner and then prior to its use in the next patient immersed in glutaraldehyde for 20 min. This means that the bronchoscope is adequately sterile for use in any patient. The length of immersion is not to eradicate HIV, which is relatively fragile, but to eradicate organisms such as atypical mycobacteria and prevent cross infection. Such precautions for both the bronchoscope and the operator should be taken in all patients as those who are potentially infective cannot be identified.

The value of bronchoscopy is undoubted, but still some cases remain undiagnosed and in most centres if a clinical diagnosis of PCP is suspected then treatment will be given on an empirical basis. However the increasing use of induced sputum and the application of molecular biological detection methods are likely to make a diagnosis in the vast majority of patients. A further importance of BAL may be to enable assessment of cellular proportions and functions to be made. The proportions in BAL can be determined by light microscopy to differ in AIDS compared to other immunocompromised patients. Methods of detecting subsets of lymphocytes and other macrophages are increasingly used and these may enable prognostic indications to be made and possible therapeutic measures to occur if abnormalities of cellular function are found and the subgroup of patients who develop respiratory failure with *Pneumocystis carinii* may be defined. Some suggestions that neutrophilia is associated with a poor prognosis have already been made.

Open Lung Biopsy

Open lung biopsy is rarely required for diagnostic purposes in these patients; however if two TBBs have failed to make a diagnosis then this may be justified (Fitzgerald et al. 1987). Kaposi's sarcoma, lymphoid interstitial pneumonia and non-specific interstitial pneumonitis may require this method for diagnosis.

Management

Pneumocystis Carinii Pneumonia

Pneumocystis carinii pneumonia (PCP) alone or in combination with co-pathogens is by far the commonest respiratory disorder seen in patients with AIDS. PCP is a ubiquitous organism which is widely distributed in the environment. Although originally considered a protozoan it is now established as a fungal organism (Edman et al. 1988; Wakefield et al. 1992). PCP causes death due to hypoxic respiratory failure and the role of frequent arterial oxygen requirements and continuous oxygen therapy is vital. These patients require management in the open ward, where they can be closely supervised.

First Line Treatment

Cotrimoxazole. Cotrimoxazole (20 mg/kg/day of the trimethoprim component) remains the treatment of choice for PCP (Fischl 1988). Cotrimoxazole is usually given intravenously for at least the first 7 days of the 21-day course. In carefully selected patients who are not hypoxic oral therapy may be considered. It is conventional to dilute the intravenous solution 1 : 250 in 0.9% saline, thus giving the patient a considerable fluid load, however a 1 : 10 dilution is the minimum necessary to keep the drug from precipitating out of solution and these more concentrated forms can be used if the treatment is given via a large central vessel. Glucose 5% can be used as the diluent. The main side effects of cotrimoxazole are nausea, skin rashes and cytopenia (Gordin et al. 1984). Nausea is usually universal and prophylactic anti-emetics should be prescribed but this symptom may be intractable. There is some evidence that keeping serum levels of trimethoprim between 5 and 8 g/ml may minimise the problem. Prophylactic folinic acid does not protect against myelotoxicity (Byberg et al. 1988).

Pentamadine. Intravenous or intramuscular pentamidine (0.4 mg/kg/day of the isethionate salt) is equally effective but the potentially serious side effects of the latter have decreased its use (Sands et al. 1985). There is no synergistic effect between pentamadine and cotrimoxazole. Comparisons of treatment with pentamidine or cotrimoxazole have been made and although serious complications are more common with the former, the choice of first line treatment did not relate to outcome (Wharton et al. 1986; Klein et al. 1992). Pentamidine may be given intravenously or intramuscularly so it is the drug of choice when venous access is difficult or fluid restriction is necessary. The main side effects are immediate hypotension or hypoglycaemia and subsequent cytopenia and nephro- and hepatotoxicity. If the therapy initially initiated is altered because of side effects then the prognosis remains unaltered, but a change of therapy because of therapeutic failure is a poor prognosis indicator.

Treatment of respiratory illness by nebulisation has obvious attractions as it is a non-invasive method for the patient and should enable high drug concentrations to be delivered to the alveoli directly and, if the capillary alveolar membrane is functioning and there is little pulmonary clearance, this may not be associated with high systemic absorption. In animal models delivery of pentamadine by such methods has been effective in the treatment of pneumocystosis. Initial trials of this therapy gave very variable responses (Montgomery et al. 1987; Girard et al. 1989; Miller et al. 1989). It became apparent that the efficacy of treatment is crucially dependent on the size of the aerosol (assessed by the mass median aerodynamic diameter (MMAD) and geometric standard deviation (GSD)) which determines particle deposition within the lungs. Side-stream nebulisers such as the System 22 Mizer (Medicaid) or the Respirgard II (Marquest) are most effective (O'Doherty et al. 1990). Nebulised pentamadine has been compared to cotrimoxazole and found to produce a slower clinical response with a greater risk of pneumothorax and extrapulmonary disease. This method of treatment is now confined to mild to moderate cases.

Second Line Treatment/Salvage Therapy

Atavaquone. Atavaquone (566C80) is a hydroxynapthoquinone which had shown considerable efficacy in both animal studies and initial human studies in the prevention and treatment of PCP (Hughes et al. 1990). Its precise mechanism of action is unknown but is suggested to be due to inhibition of the electron transport system. In a randomised double-blind study of oral therapy in 322 patients with mild to moderately severe PCP there were significantly more treatment failures with atavaquone than cotrimoxazole (20% vs 7%). However, by contrast, adverse effects requiring a change in therapy were significantly greater with cotrimoxazole (20% vs 7%). This drug is a significant advance but is still currently a second line treatment. The plasma concentration of this drug was an important determinant of outcome. It does not have the antibacterial effect of cotrimoxazole which may be a disadvantage in patients with copathogens to PCP (Hughes et al. 1993).

Dapsone/Trimethoprim. Dapsone was initially tried as a sole agent for the treatment of PCP but in this context had an unacceptable failure rate of 61% (Mills et al. 1988). The combination of oral dapsone (100 mg/kg/day) with trimethoprim (20 mg/kg/day) has been compared to oral cotrimoxazole (20 mg/kg/day trimethoprim component) in patients with first episodes of mild to moderate PCP (PaO$_2$ >60 mm Hg). The results were comparable in terms of treatment failure (10%) but major toxic side effects were commoner in the cotrimoxazole group (57% vs 30%) (Medina et al. 1990). Methaemoglobinaemia is the commonest side effect of this trimethoprim/dapsone and occurs in most patients but is usually clinically insignificant.

Clindamycin/Primaquine. The combination of clindamycin and primaquine has been used in open trials to treat mild to moderate PCP (Aa gradient <40 mm Hg) (Toma et al. 1989). It is equally effective in this patient group when given orally or intravenously with a 92% response rate with <10% serious adverse effects (Black et al. 1994). Comparative trials with first line therapy are under way.

Trimetrexate. Trimetrexate has been used as salvage therapy for patients in whom conventional therapy has been ineffective. It is an analogue of methotrexate and, as might be expected, is myelosuppressive. This drug is lipid-soluble which enables rapid penetration of the organism, within which it inhibits the dihydrofolate reductase enzyme. *Pneumocystis carinii* lacks a transport system for folate which enables folinic acid rescue to be given without reversal of the anti-pneumocyst effect. In an initial report of 16 patients who had failed treatment with or were intolerant of conventional therapy (cotrimoxazole or pentamadine), 69% responded and 69% survived when treated with trimetrexate (30 mg/m^2 (body surface area)/day) and leucovorin acid (80 mg/m^2/day) (Allegra et al. 1987). There was a high relapse rate after treatment and the side effects seen were neutropenia, liver dysfunction and skin rashes. Trimetrexate has now been compared with cotrimoxazole in moderate to severe cases of PCP (Sattler et al. 1994). The mortality rates were significantly higher with trimetrexate (31%) than cotrimoxazole (16%) but with significantly less serious and treatment terminating side effects. This drug remains a potential salvage therapy.

Eflornithine (DFMO). Eflornithine acts as an inhibitor of ornithine decarboxylase and has also been mainly used as a salvage treatment in patients unresponsive to conventional treatment. One report describes 345 such patients treated with eflornithine (400 mg/kg/day intravenously). A 23% survival was achieved in those receiving 14 days therapy and ventilated prior to treatment and 78% in those not ventilated prior to treatment (Golden et al. 1984). Anecdotal reports in the UK suggest that approximately 69% of patients respond to salvage treatment with DFMO (Smith et al. 1990). The main side effects are thrombocytopenia and diarrhoea.

Adjunctive Therapy

Steroids. The use of corticosteroids for treatment of severe cases of PCP was begun on anecdotal reports. The rationale behind their use lay in the observation that radiographic and physiological deterioration in PCP can occur so quickly that there must be a considerable inflammatory component. The precise mechanism for such activity is speculative but a reduction in chemotaxis of inflammatory cells, complement-mediated neutrophil activation, cytokine production and inhibition of phospholipase A2 have all been postulated. In practice a reduced inflammatory component buys time for conventional therapy to take effect and perhaps improves the drug delivery to the organism. It is now established that in patients presenting with a PaO_2 <8.5 kPa corticosteroids should be given as an adjunct to antibiotic therapy, usually oral prednisolone 40 mg/day (Bozzete et al. 1990; Masur et al. 1990). In mild to moderate PCP corticosteroids are not beneficial and have some adverse effects.

Continuous positive airways pressure (CPAP). Continuous positive airways pressure (CPAP) is a technique which can be used in spontaneously breathing patients to improve oxygenation and has been used in many lung disorders. The mechanism of CPAP's efficacy is unknown but it has been postulated to prevent airway collapse by being a "pneumatic splint" subsequently improving ventilation/perfusion mismatch. It has been shown to increase functional residual capacity but adverse effects on cardiac output are uncommon.

CPAP may be delivered by tight-fitting nasal or face mask. The former method also requires a chin strap and is used more commonly for sleep apnoea. In patients with PCP, CPAP circuits containing a flow generator are preferable as there is less pressure drop during peak inspiration and a reduced work of breathing in comparison with the older systems using a bag reservoir (Kesten and Rebuck 1988; Miller and Semple 1991). Some patients find this difficult to tolerate and the complications include pulmonary barotrauma, gastric aspiration, pressure necrosis and corneal ulceration. In patients with normocapnia ($PaCO_2$ <5.3 kPa) diamorphine (2.5 mg s/c prn) can be cautiously administered to relieve dyspnoea. This technique is extremely valuable in buying time for conventional therapy to be effective. It can be used on a general ward by nursing staff with no specific ICU training.

Mechanical Ventilation. At the beginning of the AIDS epidemic, patients who developed respiratory failure were commonly ventilated. However as it became evident that the outcome of such intensive care was universally appalling, both patients and their carers became reluctant to follow this route, as reflected in the falling ICU admissions in the face of increasing overall admissions. At one US centre only 14% of such patients left hospital in the period 1981–1985 and none survived a subsequent 12 months (El-Sadr and Simberkoff 1988; Luce et al. 1988). Subsequent reports have been more favourable. The use of adjunctive corticosteroids and CPAP may have reduced the number of patients developing respiratory failure from PCP. It may be that the more positive attitude to AIDS by both patients and carers, as a chronic manageable condition, leads to increased ICU referral. This is an issue that needs careful discussion between patients, carers and their physicians (Staikowsky et al. 1993).

Prophylaxis

This is the probably the most important clinical area in AIDS treatment at present. Prophylaxis may be secondary or primary. Prophylaxis is recommended for all patients with a prior history of PCP, any other AIDS related disease or a CD4 count less than $0.2 \times 10^9/l$. Conventional prophylactic therapy has been with cotrimoxazole, 2 tablets once daily (Fischl et al. 1988) and treatment failure is usually due to poor compliance. Nebulised pentamadine has been successfully used for both primary and secondary prophylaxis. There are many comparative trials to establish optimum apparatus and modes of delivery in terms of dose and frequency (Leoung et al. 1990). The current recommendations are for pentamadine 300 mg every 4 weeks through a Respirgard II or 60 mg every 2 weeks through a Fisoneb (Murphy et al. 1991; Montaner et al. 1991). If PCP occurs during this therapy it may present atypically, and is usually in the upper lobes. Improved aerosol delivery with postural manoeuvres may overcome this problem. Comparative studies of cotrimoxazole and nebulised pentamadine have established that there are significantly increased treatment failures with pentamadine for both primary (Schneider et al. 1992) and secondary prophylaxis (Hardy et al. 1992). Several studies have suggested that cotrimoxazole thrice weekly is as effective as one daily (Ruskin and LaRiviere 1991) and this may reduce intolerance.

Dapsone (100 mg/day) has been used successfully and seems to have a comparable efficacy to cotrimoxazole. Lower doses of dapsone alone or in combination with pyrimethamine are less effective than cotrimoxazole (Coker et al. 1992) but approximately equivalent to aerosolised pentamadine (Girard et al. 1993). Fansidar (Pyrimethamine/sulphadoxine) once weekly may be used but is less effective than other regimes (Gottlieb et al. 1984).

Primaquine and clindamycin in combination are currently undergoing trial for efficacy as prophylaxis.

Future Strategies

It is now established that *Pneumocystis* is a fungal agent but the precise mechanisms of its pathogenicity remain obscure. Greater understanding of these mechanisms would help the design of more specific and effective therapy. The development of effective prophylaxis gives a positive reason for patients to come forward and be HIV tested, prior to illness. However high risk groups (IV drugusers) are recalcitrant to this approach. The other problem is trials of therapy. AIDS patients are on the whole an extremely well-informed and articulate group. Some patient groups do not feel that in a terminal disease, blinded controlled trials are justified. Individual patients want what they perceive as best for them and may find unconvincing the conventional medical view of requiring data to ensure a drug is effective.

Cytomegalovirus (CMV) Pneumonitis

Cytomegalovirus is a well recognised cause of pneumonitis in patients with renal and bone marrow transplants and when the pulmonary complications of AIDS were first described, CMV was found alone and as a co-pathogen in a considerable number (Murray et al. 1984). Matching CMV donor and recipient status has drastically cut the problems of CMV pneumonitis in bone marrow transplant recipients. However when this occurs the mortality is 75%–80% and the disease is closely related to graft versus host disease in allogenic bone marrow transplants (GVHD). By contrast, CMV pneumonitis has always been rare in autologous bone marrow transplants (2%) in whom GVHD is also rare. These observations in man and others in the mouse model of CMV have led to the suggestions that pneumonitis in these patients may be due to an immune mediated mechanism. It is proposed that T-cell dependent activity may be stimulated by viral antigen which will occur in bone marrow transplants as immune recovery occurs, but by contrast will rarely occur in AIDS patients because of their persistent immunocompromise (Grundy et al. 1987). It has also become clear that in the sick, immunodeficient patient CMV replicates and will enter damaged tissue so its role as the primary pathogen has been questioned (Wallace and Hannah 1988; Pillay et al. 1993). In one review of 101 cases of pneumonitis in patients with AIDS there was evidence of CMV in 11 and despite no treatment, deaths occurred in only 2 (Millar et al. 1990). In our experience CMV detected by cytopathic change is rarely found in the lung. We have also used monoclonal antibodies which detect proteins secreted within 24 h by cells infected with CMV. However with either method of detection we have found that the treatment of co-pathogens when CMV is present has resulted in complete recovery, and in one patient with no co-pathogens recovery occurred with no specific anti-CMV therapy. However, there are some undoubted reports of CMV pneumonitis in the context of HIV (Squire et al. 1992).

In CMV retinitis where the disease seems undoubtedly due to viral replication, gancyclovir (1,3–dihydroxy-2-propodymethyl (DHPG) and foscarnet (phosphonoformate) have both been used effectively to slow the rate of disease progression. Both drugs are given intravenously. The dose regime of gancyclovir is 5 mg/kg every 12 h for 10–14 days followed by 5 mg/kg/daily maintenance with bone marrow suppression as its main side effect (Collaborative DHPG study group 1986). The dose regime of foscarnet is 60 mg/kg every 8 h for 14 days followed by 90 mg/kg/daily maintenance; the main side effects are nausea, anaemia and nephrotoxicity (Youle et al. 1990). Comparative trials suggest that these drugs are equally effective but toxicity is less of a problem with foscarnet (Meinert et al. 1992). CMV is not eradicated by these treatments and long-term maintenance therapy is required; furthermore, despite this, deterioration continues (Hirsch 1992). There have been several reported cases of viral resistance to DHPG occurring which would explain the intermittently progressive nature of the disease.

As the currently available treatment must be life-long, has considerable side effects in particular of cytopenia and requires intravenous access, it cannot be recommended unless CMV is found as a sole pathogen in a patient with severe respiratory problems. Oral formulations of gancyclovir are currently under trial but preliminary data suggest they are less effective than the intravenous route. When effective oral agents are developed it is probable that primary prophylactic regimes will be developed, with particular reference to the possibility that CMV infection may have effects on HIV progression (Webster et al. 1989).

Mycobacterial Disease

Mycobacterial disease is common in AIDS patients, affecting up to 10% of patients (Jacobson 1988) and since 1993 *M. tuberculosis* has joined atypical mycobacteria as an AIDS-defining diagnosis (CDC 1992). In both the USA and the UK the documented downward trend in *M. tuberculosis* reporting has flattened (Murray et al. 1989; Watson et al. 1991). This has been partially attributed by some authorities to tuberculosis in HIV-infected patients (CDC 1986).

Mycobacterium Tuberculosis

The incidence of tuberculosis in AIDS varies considerably with populations and the relation to the prevalence within the group, e.g. it is higher in intravenous drug abusers in the USA among non-Caucasians and Haitians (CDC 1986). Although it is not restricted to these groups, having been reported in transfusion associated with AIDS, clearly socio-economic factors associated with tuberculosis prior to AIDS are an important factor. Further evidence to support this view comes from one of the few large prospective trials of development of tuberculosis in HIV-positive individuals (Selwyn et al. 1989). This study of injecting drug users is further discussed in Chapter 9. In this study 7 out of 8 cases of tuberculosis developed in patients who were PPD positive (7/49) despite the similar incidence of PPD-positive patients in the HIV-positive (49/217) versus the HIV negative (62/303) (Selwyn et al. 1989). This implies that in this group *Mycobacterium tuberculosis* (mTB) is a result of reactivation of latent infection which would be more common in the older population and the more deprived, i.e. drug users, non-Caucasians and hispanic populations in the USA. The increasing refinement of molecular biological sequencing techniques will enable the reactivation/new infection/cross infection to be defined precisely.

In the UK the majority of the HIV-positive population are white homosexual men at present. The incidence of tuberculous infection in the UK HIV-positive population has been estimated at between 4.6% and 6% (Helbert et al. 1990; Watson et al. 1993). However, if the proportion of injecting drug users were to increase, then this may become an increasing problem. Experience in the USA where BCG vaccination is not routine, has suggested that HIV-positive individuals who are PPD positive be treated prophylactically against tuberculosis (American Thoracic Society/Centers for Disease Control 1987). This is not current practice in the UK (Joint Tuberculous Committee of the British Thoracic Society 1992).

There is a dearth of prospective data on the incidence of mTB and the relation to HIV infection. As retrospective reviews of pulmonary involvement with HIV pre-date the inclusion of mTB as a criterion for the diagnosis of AIDS and refer to it as pre-AIDS diagnosis, it is possible that from this grew the suggestion that mTB presented early in the course of HIV infection. In early HIV infection mTB presents in a conventional manner (Thuer et al. 1988). By contrast in more advanced HIV infection extra-pulmonary disease is much commoner, occurring in 60%–70% of cases (Chaisson et al. 1987; Small et al. 1991). Treatment should be given with conventional triple therapy of pyrazinamide (20–20 kg/day), rifampicin (10–15 mg/kg up to 600 mg/day) and isoniazid (10–15 mg/kg up to 300 mg/day) for 2 months followed by rifampicin and isoniazid for a minimum of 4 months. However, longer treatment has been advocated. It has been suggested that life-long treatment with at least one (usually isoniazid, up to 300 mg/day), if not two, drugs should be continued because of continued immunodeficiency (American Thoracic Society 1987; Advisory committee for the elimination of tuberculosis 1989; Joint Tuberculous Committee of the British Thoracic Society 1992).

Atypical Mycobacteria

Non-tuberculous mycobacteria present more commonly as a disseminated illness than as pulmonary disease, although the latter does occur. Two very similar forms of mycobacteria, *M. avium* and *M. intracellulare*, are referred to together as *Mycobacterium avium* complex (MAC) (Hawkins et al. 1986). Post mortem studies suggest that 25%–30% of HIV patients have MAC at post mortem. MAC is overwhelmingly the most commonly reported non-tuberculous mycobacterium although there is considerable variation between areas (e.g. 0.44% of cases in the mid-West United States compared to 0.08% elsewhere). This suggests that the "pathogenic" propensity of this organism is particularly suited to the immunosuppression caused by HIV infection. There is considerable evidence that this organism invades via the bowel wall and commonly gastrointestinal upset can be a feature of its infection. Diagnosis is usually made on the basis of blood or bone marrow detection which requires specific culture techniques in the laboratory. Some recent reports of *M. genoense* suggest that other forms of atypical mycobacteria may not have been identified because of laboratory culture techniques. The impact of MAC (and other forms of atypical mycobacteria) on symptoms and survival in AIDS patients has been controversial, with several studies suggesting that this organism was a sign of deteriorating health rather than a cause (Chaisson and Hopewell 1989). In the last few years the weight of evidence has shifted suggesting the MAC contributes to both symptoms and mortality independently of severe immunosuppression (Horsburg and Selik 1989; Chaisson et al. 1992) Chaisson studied a cohort of 1020 patients in a multicentre trial of patients treated with zidovudine and found that, stratifying for immunological differences, there was a highly significant increase in mortality associated with MAC infection. A large number of mono and combination therapies for the treatment of MAC have been tried and, to date, eradication of the MAC has not been achieved. The currently favoured combinations are rifabutin, amikacin, clarithromycin and ethambutol or rifabutin, clarithromycin and ethambutol. Rifabutin was studied in double-blind placebo-controlled trials by Cameron et al. (1992) and Gordin et al. (1992). More than 1000 patients were studied and in both studies there was a significant reduction in the development of MAC bacteraemia, although no difference in survival. In the USA these findings have led to recommendations for primary prophylaxis in patients with a CD4 count less than 200/mm^3 with rifabutin 300 mg orally once daily. There are no firm UK recommendations on prophylaxis for MAC at present but it is probable they will follow the USA guidelines.

Bacterial Pneumonia

Bacterial pneumonia is increasingly recognised as a problem (Polsky et al. 1986; Miller et al. 1994). In patients with AIDS several studies have shown an increased incidence of bacterial pneumonia with *Streptococcus pneumoniae* and *Staphylococcus aureus* being a particular problem (Miller et al. 1994). This may be the result of a relative decrease in the number of cases of PCP, perhaps due to prophylactic measures (Pitkin et al. 1993). In addition, in a cohort study of 1353 HIV-positive subjects there is an eight times greater risk for bacterial pneumonia than in seronegative control subjects, the risk increasing with a reduction in CD4 below 250 mm^3 (Wallace et al. 1993). In this and several other studies risk of bacterial pneumonia has been shown to be greater in HIV-positive injecting drug users than homosexual or bisexual subjects (Magenat et al. 1991). Ideally, treatment should be on the basis of specimen culture sensitivities. If empirical therapy is instituted after samples for culture have been taken, cover for both pneumococcal and staphylococcal disease is appropriate.

Fungal Pneumonia (other than PCP)

Fungi are relatively uncommon causes of respiratory problems in AIDS, representing 1.6% of cases in the USA (Murray and Mills 1990), where the disease is more common in general than in the UK. Treatment with intravenous amphotericin at a dose of 0.6 mg/kg/day is the first line treatment. This medication can be extremely toxic and liposomal formulations can be used as alternatives.

Non-Infective Disorders

Kaposi's Sarcoma

Kaposi's sarcoma (KS), occasionally related to the thorax, is troublesome because of oropharyngeal or endobronchial disease. This may result in haemoptysis and occasionally airways obstruction. Local radiotherapy is highly effective for such lesions (Chak et al. 1988). Whole lung irradiation has been used for more extensive disease (Meyer 1993). Most patients with cutaneous KS have some evidence of intrapulmonary disease, but the extent is not closely correlated. Pulmonary KS as a cause of marked respiratory symptoms is unusual, and when present it may be associated with minimal cutaneous manifestations (Ognibene 1985). The lesions are submucosal and although visualised at bronchoscopy, conventional forceps may not give a histological diagnosis. For this reason open lung biopsy may be useful. Chemotherapy has been used in these patients, with single agents as well as combinations of doxorubicin (adriamycin), vinblastine, vincristine, bleomycin and etoposide being reported. Doxirubicin can now be given in a liposomal formulation and several small-scale studies have suggested that this shows an improved response with fewer adverse effects (Chew et al. 1992; Dormann et al. 1992). Systemic therapy with alpha interferon has also been tried, but with variable success (partial response in 85% but major side effects in 80%). However very extensive KS is usually present in the lungs in the terminal stage of the disease and the general condition of the patient and their wishes should be considered before toxic therapy is instituted (Fig. 4.3).

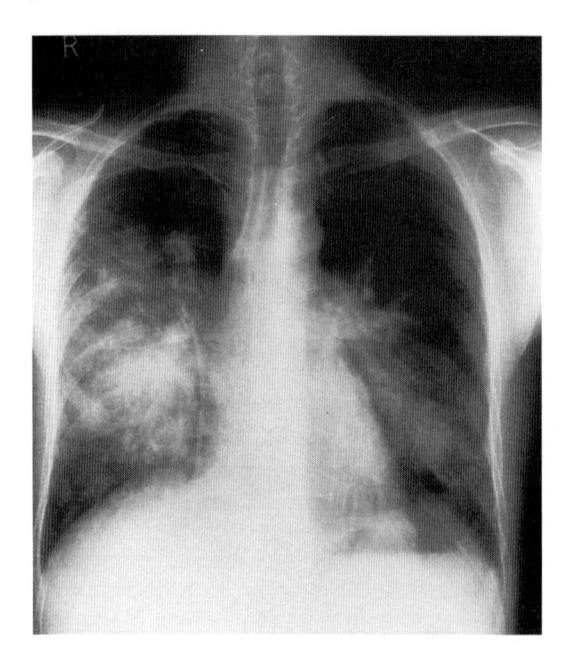

Fig. 4.3. A chest x-ray of a patient with Kaposi's sarcoma, showing extensive intra-alveolar consolidation with hilar lymphadenopathy.

Other Malignancies

B cell lymphomas (Ziegler et al. 1984) and sarcomas (Krown 1988) have an increased incidence in AIDS and can occur in any organ of the body (see Chapter 8). Treatment as appropriate is given with combination chemotherapy.

Lymphocytic Interstitial Pneumonitis and Non-specific Interstitial Pneumonitis

There are increasing reports of pneumonitis in patients who have AIDS (Mayoud and Cadranel 1993).

Lymphoid interstitial pneumonitis (LIP) was not mentioned in the initial major review of pulmonary manifestations of HIV and AIDS in 1984 (Murray et al. 1984) but by the second review in 1987 (Murray et al. 1987) it was described. During that time sporadic case reports of LIP had been described (Solal-Celigny et al. 1985; Grieco and Chinoy-Acharya 1985). This syndrome is not specific to HIV infection or AIDS and has been associated with more than 100 causative agents. LIP is more common in children (30%) and Haitians than others. Long-term effects are poorly documented; in the largest series of 16 patients, 12 remained unchanged throughout follow-up until death. The specific aetiology remains unclear. It seems likely to be viral. Chayt et al. (1986) found high levels of HIV RNA expression in patients with LIP, compared to other HIV-positive patients with pulmonary disease. Several studies have suggested that the recruitment of lymphocytes to the lung is a response to HIV infection (Jeffrey et al. 1991; Autran et al. 1988).

The difference between LIP and non-specific interstitial pneumonitis is a histological rather than a clinical entity.

Non-specific inflammatory pneumonitis is diagnosed by evidence of widespread chronic inflammation (Suffredini et al. 1985): data from transbronchial biopsies is difficult to interpret and open lung biopsy may be needed to differentiate it from LIP. One prospective study of 24 patients (12 with AIDS and 12 with a CD4 count of $<0.2 \times 10^9$/l) in whom there was no abnormal chest x-ray or symptoms, and of whom 23 had TBB, found evidence of non-specific interstitial pneumonitis in 11. Ten of those in whom there was no abnormality were on treatment with zidovudine. The patients had individually normal lung function tests, but the entire group showed a 73 ± 20% predicated DLCO (Ognibene et al. 1988). In a retrospective study looking at this phenomenon, 41 of 110 patients (38%) and 332% of clinical episodes were associated with non-specific inflammatory pneumonitis (Simmons et al. 1987). Thirteen patients had no previous history of lung disease which may potentially induce such pathological changes. In this group no patient developed early pulmonary deterioration after a mean follow-up of 20 weeks, suggesting that they had not missed cases of opportunistic infection. It has been postulated that such changes are related to viral infection; Epstein-Barr and HIV itself are both leading contenders (Agnostini et al. 1993). Azidothymidine (AZT), acyclovir, and anti-CMV agents have been tried as therapeutic agents to no avail. Treatment is symptomatic and palliative, e.g. oxygen.

Research and the Future

The future trends of lung involvement in subjects with HIV infection will change as pharmacological advances are made in producing better tolerated and more effective and specific drug therapies. It is likely that prophylactic drug cocktails will be the way forward.

The application of molecular biological techniques will ease the diagnostic difficulties of infectious complications and answer some of the questions of reinfection/reactivation/cross infection. This is of particular interest in mycobacterial disease and PCP.

More basic scientific research will continue to examine the cellular changes in the lung induced by HIV and other possible infectious agents such as CMV and Epstein-Barr. Several studies have shown changes in the cytokine production of macrophages at various stages of HIV infection and in response to the HIV-1 gp 120 envelope protein as reviewed by Agnostini (1993). There is no doubt that HIV is present in the lung and until we can effectively eradicate it, understanding and perhaps controlling its effects on cell activation and function within the lung are the best ways forward.

References

Advisory committee for the elimination of tuberculosis (1989) Tuberculosis and human immunodeficiency virus infection. MMWR 38: 236–238, 243–250

Agnostini C, Trentin L, Zamballo, Semenzato G (1993) HIV-1 and the lung. Am Rev Respir Dis 147: 1038–49

Allegra CJ, Chabner BA, Tuuazon CU et al. (1987) Trimetrexate for the treatment of *Pneumocystis carinii* pneumonia in patients with acquired immunodeficiency syndrome. NEJM 317: 978–985

Allen JR, Currann JW (1985) Epidemiology of the acquired immunodeficiency syndrome. In: Gallin JI, Fauci AS (eds.) Advances in host defence mechanism, Vol 5. Raven Press, New York, pp 1–17

American Thoracic Society/Centres for Disease Control (1987) Mycobacterioses and the acquired immunodeficiency syndrome. Am Rev Resp Dir 138: 492–496

Autran B, Mayaud B, Guillon JM et al. (1988) Evidence for a cytotoxic T lymphocyte alveolitis in human immunodeficiency-virus infected patients. AIDS 24:179–183

Barta K (1969) Complement fixation test for Pneumocystis. Ann Intern Med 70: 235

Bigby T, Margolskee D, Curtis J et al. (1986) The usefulness of direct sputum in the diagnosis of pneumocystis carinii pneumonia in patients with the acquired immunodeficiency syndrome. Am Rev Resp Dis 133: 515–518

Black JR, Feinberg J, Murphy RL (1994) Clindamycin and primaquine therapy for mild to moderate episodes of pneumocystis carinii pneumonia in patients with AIDS: AIDS clinical trials group 044. Clin Infect Dis 18: 905–913

Bozzette SA, Sattler FR, Chiu J et al. (1990) A controlled trial of early adjunctive treatment with corticosteroids for pneumocystis carinii in the acquired immunodeficiency syndrome. N Engl J Med 323: 1351–1457

Byberg IC, Lund JT, Hording M (1988) Effect of folic and folinic acid on cytopenia occurring during cotrimoxazole treatment of pneumocystis carinii pneumonia. Scand J Infect Dis 20: 685–686.

Cameron W et al. (1992) Rifabutin therapy for the prevention of M avium complex (MAC) bacteraemia in patients with AIDS and CD4 <200. VIII Intl Conf AIDS, Amsterdam, abstract WeB 1052

Centers for Disease Control (1986) Tuberculosis United States, 1985 and the possible impact of human T-lymphotropic virus type III/lymphadenopathy-associated virus infection. MMWR 36: 385–389

Centers for Disease Control (1992) 1993 revised classification system for HIV infection and expanded surveillance case definition for AIDS among adolescents and adults. MMWR 41 (RR-11): 1–19

Chak L et al. (1988) Radiation therapy for acquired immunodeficiency syndrome related Kaposi's sarcoma. J Clin Oncol 6: 863–867

Chaisson RE, Hopewell PC (1989) Mycobacteria and AIDS mortality. Am Rev Respir Dis 139: 1–3

Chaisson RE, Moore RD, Richman DD et al. (1992) Incidence and natural history of Mycobacterium Avium-complex in patients with advanced human immunodeficiency virus disease treated with zidovudine. Am Rev Respir Dis 146: 285–289

Chaisson RE, Schecter GF, Theur CP et al. (1987) Tuberculosis in patients with the acquired immunodeficiency syndrome. Am Rev Resp Dis 136: 570–574

Chayt KS, Harper ME, Marselle LM et al. (1986) Detection of HTLV III RNA in lungs of patients with AIDS and pulmonary involvement 256: 2356–2359

Chew T et al. (1992) A phase II clinical trial of VS103 (liposomal daunorubicin). VIII Intl Conf AIDS, Amsterdam, abstract PoB 3106

Clarke JR, Fleming J, Donegan K et al. (1991) Effect of HIV-1 and cytomegalovirus in bronchoalveolar lavage cells on the transfer factor for lung carbon monoxide in AIDS patients. AIDS 5: 1333–1338

Coker RJ, Nieman R, McBride M et al. (1992) Cotrimoxazole versus dapsone-pyrimethamine for prevention of pneumocystis carinii pneumonia. Lancet 330: 1099

Coleman DL, Hattner RS, Luce JA, Dodek PM, Golden JA, Murray JF (1984) Correlation between gallium lung scans and fibreoptic bronchoscopy in patients with suspected pneumocystis carinii pneumonia and the acquired immune deficiency syndrome. Am Rev Resp Dis 130: 1166–1169

Coleman DL, Dodek PM, Golden JA (1984) Correlation between serial pulmonary function tests and fibreoptic bronchoscopy in patients with pneumocystis carinii pneumonia and the acquired immune deficiency syndrome. Am Rev Resp Dis 129: 491–493.

Collaborative DHPG study group (1986) Treatment of serious cytomegalovirus infection with 9-(1,3-dihydroxy-2-propoxymethyl) guanine in patients with AIDS and other immunodeficiencies. N Engl J Med 314: 801–805

De Lorenzo LJ, Huang CT, Mcguire GP, Stone DJ (1987) Roentgenographic patterns of pneumocystis carinii pneumonia in 104 patients with AIDS. Chest 91: 323–327

Denison DM, Cramer DS, Hanson PJV (1989) Lung function testing and AIDS. Respir Med 83: 133–138

Dormann L et al. (1992) Liposomal-encapsulated cytotoxic agent daunorubicin (LD) versus conventional three drug chemotherapy (cc) in AIDS patients with Kaposi's sarcoma – preliminary results. Third European conference on clinical aspects and treatment of HIV Infection, Paris: abstract 09

Edman JC, Kovacs JA, Masur H, Santi DV, Elwood HJ, Sogun ML (1988) Ribosomal RNA sequences show *Pneumocystis carinii* to be a member of the fungi. Nature 334: 519–522

El-Sadr W, Simberkoff MS (1988) Survival and prognostic factors in severe Pneumocystis carinii pneumonia requiring mechanical ventilation. Am Rev Resp Dis 137: 1264–1267

Engelberg LA, Lerner CW, Tapper ML (1984) Clinical features of pneumocystis pneumonia in patients with the acquired immunodeficiency syndrome. Am Rev Resp Dis 130: 689–694

Fischol MA (1988) Treatment and prophylaxis of Pneumocystis carinii pneumonia. AIDS 2 (Suppl 1): S143-150

Fischl MA, Dickinson GM, La Voie L (1988) Safety and efficacy of sulphamethoxazole and trimethoprim chemoprophylaxis for pneumocystis carinii pneumonia in AIDS. JAMA 259: 1185-1189

Fitzgerald W, Bevalaqua FA, Garay SM, Aranda CP (1987) The role of open lung biopsy in the acquired immunodeficiency syndrome. Chest 135: 422–425

Girard PM, Gaudebout C, Lepetre A et al. (1989) Prevention of pneumocystis carinii pneumonia by pentamadine aerosol in zidovudine-treated AIDS patients. Lancet i: 1348-1352

Girard PM, Landman R, Gaudebout C et al. (1993) Dapsone-pyrimethamine compared with aerosolised pentamadine as primary prophylaxis against pneumocystis carinii pneumonia and toxoplasmosis in HIV infection. N Engl J Med 328: 1514–1520

Golden JA, Sjoerdsma A, Santi DV (1984) Pneumocystis carinii pneumonia treated with α-difluromethylornithine: a prospective study among patients with the acquired immune deficiency syndrome. West J Med 141: 612–623

Goodman JL, Tashki DP (1983) Pneumocystis with normal chest x-ray film and arterial oxygen tension. Early diagnosis in a patient with the acquired immune deficiency syndrome. Ann Intern Med 81: 11–18

Goodman PC, Broaddus VC, Hopewell PC (1984) Chest radiographic patterns in the acquired immune deficiency syndrome. Am Rev Resp Dis 130: 689–694

Gordin FM, Simon GL, Wofsy CB et al. (1984) Adverse reactions to trimethoprim-sulphamethoxazole in patients with the acquired immunodeficiency syndrome. Ann Intern Med 100: 495–499

Gordin FM et al. (1992) Rifabutin monotherapy prevents or delays Mycobacterium avium complex (MAC) bacteraemia in patients with AIDS. VIII Intl Conf AIDS, Amsterdam, abstract PoB 3172

Gottlieb MS, Knight S, Mitsiyasu R, Weisman J, Roth M, Young LS (1984) Prophylaxis of pneumocystis infection in AIDS with pyrimethamine-sulfadoxine. Lancet i: 388–389

Grieco MH, Chinoy-Acharya P (1985) Lymphocytic interstitial pneumonia associated with the acquired immune deficiency syndrome. Am Rev Resp Dis 131: 952–955

Grundy JE, Shenley JD, Griffiths PD (1987) Is cytomegalovirus interstitial pneumonitis in transplant patients an immunopathologic condition. Lancet ii: 996–998

Hanson PJV, Harcourt-Webster JN, Gazzard BG, Collins JV (1987) Fibreoptic bronchoscopy in the diagnosis of bronchopulmonary Kaposi's sarcoma. Thorax 42: 269–271

Hardy WD, Feinberg J, Finkelstein DM et al. (1992) A controlled trial of trimethoprim-sulphamethoxazole or aerosolised pentamadine for secondary prophylaxis of pneumocystis carinii pneumonia in patients with human immunodeficiency virus infection. N Engl J Med 327: 1842-1848

Hartman TE, Primack SL, Muller NL, Staples CA (1994) Diagnosis of thoracic complications in AIDS; accuracy of CT. AJR 162: 547–553

Hattner RS, Solitto RA, Golden JA, Coleman DL, Okerland MD (1984) Sensitivity and specificity of Ga-67 pulmonary scans for the detection of pneumocystis carinii pneumonia in patients with the acquired immunodeficiency syndrome and pulmonary symptoms J Nucl Med 25: 43

Hawkins CC, Gold JWM, Whimbey E et al. (1986) Mycobacterium avium complex infections with the acquired immunodeficiency syndrome. Ann Intern Med 105: 184–188

Helbert M, Robinson D, Buchanan D et al. (1990) Mycobacterial infection in patients infected with the human immunodeficiency virus. Thorax 45: 45–48

Hirsch MS (1992) The treatment of cytomegalovirus in AIDS – more than meets the eye. N Engl J Med 326: 264–266

Hirsch MS, Wormser GP, Schooley RT et al. (1985) Risk of nosocomial infection with human T-cell lymphotropic virus (HLTV-111). N Engl J Med 312: 1–4

Ho DD, Byington RE, Schooley RT, Flynn T, Rota TR, Hirsch MS (1985) Frequency of isolation of HTLV-III from saliva in AIDS. N Engl J Med 313: 1606

Hopewell PC, Luce JM (1985) Pulmonary involvement in the acquired immunodeficiency syndrome Chest 87: 104–112

Horsburgh CR Jr, Selik RM (1989) The epidemiology of disseminated non-tuberculous mycobacterial infection in the acquired immunodeficiency syndrome (AIDS). Am Rev Respir Dis 139: 4–7

Hughes WT, Gray VL, Gutteridge WE, Latter VS, Pudney M (1990) Efficacy of a hydroxynaphthaquone, 566C80, in experimental pneumocystis carinii pneumonia. Antimicrob Agents Chemother 43: 225–228

Hughes W, Leoung G, Kramer F et al. (1993) Comparison of atavaquone (566C80) with trimethoprim-sulphamethoxazole to treat pneumocystis carinii pneumonia in patients with AIDS. N Engl J Med 328: 1521-527

Jacobson MA (1988) Mycobacterial disease: tuberculosis and mycobacterium avium complex. Infect Dis Clin North Am 2: 465-474

Jeffrey AA, Israel-Biet D, Andrieu JM et al. (1991) HIV isolation from pulmonary cell derived from bronchoalveolar lavage. Clin Exp Immunol 85: 488-492

Joint Tuberculous Committee of the British Thoracic Society (1992) Guidelines on the management of tuberculosis and HIV in the United Kingdom. Br Med J 304: 1231-1233

Kesten S, Rebuck AS (1988) Continuous positive airways pressure in Pneumocystis carinii pneumonia. Lancet ii: 1414-1415

Klein N, Duncanson FP, Lenox TH et al. (1992) Trimethoprim-sulphamethoxazole versus pentamadine for pneumocystis carinii pneumonia in AIDS patients: results of a large prospective randomised trial. AIDS 6: 301-305

Kovacs JA, Ng VL, Masur H et al. (1988) Diagnosis of pneumocystis carinii pneumonia: improved detection in sputum with use of monoclonal antibodies. N Engl J Med 318: 589-593

Kramer EL, Sanger JJ, Garay SM (1987) Gallium-67 scans of the chest in patients with acquired immunodeficiency syndrome. J Nucl Med 28: 1107-1114

Krown SE (1988) AIDS-associated Kaposi's sarcoma; pathogenesis, clinical course and treatment. AIDS 242: 426-430

Kvale PA, Rosen MJ, Hopewell PC et al. (1993) A decline in the pulmonary diffusing capacity does not indicate opportunistic lung disease in asymptomatic persons infected with the human immunodeficiency virus. Am Rev Respir Dis 148: 390-395

Leoung GS, Feigal DW Jr, Montgomery AB et al. (1990) Aerosolised pentamadine for prophylaxis against pneumocystis carinii pneumonia - the San Francisco Community prophylaxis trial. N Engl J Med 323: 769-775

Luce JM, Wachter RM, Hopewell PC (1988) Intensive care of patients with the acquired immunodeficiency syndrome: time for a reassessment? Am Rev Resp Dis 137: 1261-1263

Magenat J-L, Nicod LP, Auckenthaler R, Junod AF (1991) Mode of presentation and diagnosis of bacterial pneumonia in human immunodeficiency virus infected patients. Am Rev Respir Dis 144: 917-922

Masur H, Ognibene FP, Yarchoan R et al. (1989) CD4 counts as predictors of the opportunistic pneumonia in human immunodeficiency virus (HIV) infection. Ann Intern Med 111: 223-231

Masur H, Meier P, McCutchen JA et al. (1990) Consensus statement on the use of corticosteroids as adjunctive therapy for pneumocystis pneumonia (PCP) in the acquired immunodeficiency syndrome. N Engl J Med 323: 1500-1514

Mayoud CM, Cadranel J (1993) HIV in the lung: guilty or not guilty? Thorax 48: 1191-1195

Medina I, Mills J, Leoung G et al. (1990) Oral therapy for Pneumocystis carinii pneumonia in the acquired immunodeficiency syndrome. A controlled trial of Trimethoprim-Sulphamoxazole versus trimethoprim-dapsone. New Engl J Med 323: 776-782

Meduri GU, Stover DE, Lee M et al. (1986) Pulmonary Kaposi's sarcoma in the acquired immunodeficiency syndrome. Am J Med 81: 11-18

Meinert CL et al. (1992) Mortality in patients with the acquired immunodeficiency syndrome treated with either foscarnet or gancyclovir for cytomegalovirus retinitis. New Engl J Med 326: 213-220

Meyer JL (1993) Whole lung irradiation for Kaposi's sarcoma. Am J Clin Oncol 16: 372-376

Millar AB, Patou G, Miller RF et al. (1990) Cytomegalovirus in the lungs of patients with AIDS: respiratory passenger or pathogen? Am Rev Respir Dis 145: 1474-1477

Millar AB, Mitchell DM (1990) Non-invasive investigation of pulmonary disease in patients positive for the human immunodeficiency virus. Thorax 45: 57-61

Miller RF, Semple SJG (1991) Continuous positive airway pressure ventilation for respiratory failure associated with Pneumocystis carinii pneumonia. Respir Med 65: 133-138

Miller RF, Godfrey-Fausett P, Semple SJG et al. (1989) Nebulised pentamadine as treatment for Pneumocystis carinii pneumonia in the acquired immune deficiency syndrome. Thorax 44: 565-569

Miller RF, Foley NM, Kessel D, Jeffrey AA (1994) Community acquired lobar pneumonia in patients with HIV infection and AIDS. Thorax 49: 367-368

Milligan SA, Stulbarg MS, Gamsu G, Golden JA (1985) Pneumocystis carinii pneumonia radiographically simulating tuberculosis. Am Rev Resp Dis 132: 1124-1126

Mills J, Leoung G, Medina I et al. (1988) Dapsone treatment of pneumocystis carinii pneumonia in acquired immunodeficiency syndrome. Antimicrob Agents Chemother 32: 1057-1060

Mitchell DM, Fleming J, Pinching AJ et al. (1992) Pulmonary function in human immunodeficiency virus infection. A prospective 18-month study of serial lung function in 474 patients. Am Rev Respir Dis 146: 745–751

Montaner JSG et al. (1991) Aerosol pentamadine for secondary prophylaxis of AIDS-related PCP. A randomised placebo-controlled study. Ann Int Med 114: 948–953

Montgomery AB, Luce JM, Turner J et al. (1987) Aerosolised pentamadine as sole therapy for Pneumocystis carinii pneumonia in patients with acquired immunodeficiency syndrome. Lancet ii: 480–483

Murphy RL et al. (1991) Aerosol pentamadine prophylaxis following PCP in AIDS patients: results of a double blind dose-comparison using an ultrasonic nebuliser. Am J Med 90: 418–426

Murray JF (1989) The white plague: down and out or up and coming? Am Rev Respir Dis 140: 1788–1795

Murray JF, Mills J (1990) Pulmonary infectious complications of human immunodeficiency virus infection. Part I and II. Am Rev Respir Dis 141: 1356–72, 1582–1598

Murray JF, Felton CP, Garay SM et al. (1984) Pulmonary complications of the acquired immune deficiency syndrome: a report of a National Heart, Lung and Blood Workshop. N Engl J Med 310: 1682–1688

Murray JF, Felton CP, Garay S et al. (1987) Pulmonary complications of the acquired immunodeficiency syndrome: an update. Am Rev Resp Dis 135: 504–509

Naidich DP, Garay SM, Lutman BS, McCauley DI (1987) Radiographic manifestations of pulmonary disease in the acquired immunodeficiency syndrome (AIDS). Semin Roentgenol 22: 14–30

Naidich DP, McGuiness G (1991) Pulmonary manifestations of AIDS: CT and radiographic correlations. Radiol Clin N Amer 29: 999–1017

Nieman RB, Fleming J, Coker RJ, Harris JRW, Mitchell DM (1993) Reduced carbon monoxide transfer factor (TLCO) in human immunodeficiency virus type I (HIV-I) infection as a predictor for faster progression to AIDS. Thorax 48: 481–485

O'Doherty MJ, Page CJ, Bradbeer CS et al. (1989) The place of ^{99m}Tc DTPA aerosol transfer in the investigation of lung infections in HIV-positive patients. Respir Med 5: 395–401

O'Doherty MJ, Thomas S, Page C et al. (1990) Pulmonary deposition of nebulised pentamidine isethionate: effect of nebuliser type, dose and volume of fill. Thorax 45: 460–464

O'Doherty MJ, Nunan TO (1993) Nuclear medicine and AIDS. Nucl Med Commun 14: 830–848

Ognibene FP, Steis RG, Macher AM et al. (1985) Kaposi's sarcoma causing pulmonary infiltrates and respiratory failure in the acquired immunodeficiency syndrome. Ann Intern Med 102: 471–475

Ognibene F, Masyr A, Rogers P (1988) Non-specific interstitial pneumonitis without Pneumocystis carinii pneumonia in asymptomatic patients infected with human immunodeficiency virus. Ann Intern Med 109: 874–879

Orenstein M, Weber CA, Cash M, Heurich AE (1986) Value of broncho-alveolar lavage in the diagnosis of pulmonary infection in acquired immune deficiency syndrome. Thorax 41: 345–349

Overland ES, Nolan AJ, Hopewell PC (1980) Alteration of pulmonary function in intravenous drug abusers: prevalence, severity and characterisation of gas exchange abnormalities. Am J Med 68: 231–237

Pifer LL, Hughes WT, Stagno S et al. (1978) Pneumocystis carinii infection: evidence for high prevalence in normal and immunocompromised children. Paediatrics 61: 35–41

Pillay D, Lipman MIC, Lee CA et al. (1993) A clinico-pathological audit of opportunistic viral infections in HIV-infected patients. AIDS 7: 968–974

Pitchenik AE, Ganjei P, Torres A et al. (1986) Sputum examination for the diagnosis of pneumocystis carinii pneumonia in the acquired immunodeficiency syndrome. Am Rev Resp Dis 133: 515–518

Pitkin AD, Grant AD, Foley NM et al. (1993) Changing patterns of respiratory disease in HIV positive patients in a referral centre in the United Kingdom between 1986-7 and 1990-1. Thorax 48: 204–207

Polsky B, Gold JWM, Whimbey E et al. (1986) Bacterial pneumonia in patients with the acquired immunodeficiency syndrome. Ann Intern Med 104: 38–41

Rosso J, Picard C, Mayard C, Revuz J, Meignan M (1986) Comparison of 99 m TC DTPA aerosol and gallium scans in early detection of pneumocystis carinii pneumonia in acquired immune deficiency syndrome. J Nucl Med 27: 951

Ruskin J, LaRiviere M (1991) Low dose cotrimoxazole for prevention of pneumocystis carinii pneumonia in human immunodeficiency virus disease. Lancet 337: 468–471

Sands M, Kron MA, Brown RB (1985) Pentamidine. A review. Rev Infect Dis 7: 625–637

Sattler FR, Frame P, Davis R et al. (1993) Trimetrexate with leucoverin versus trimethoprim-sulphamethoxazole for moderate to severe episodes of pneumocystis carinii pneumonia in patients with AIDS: a prospective, controlled multicentre investigation of the AIDS clinical trials group protocol 029/031. J Infect Dis 170: 165–172

Schneider MME, Hoepelman AIM, Efftink Shattenkerk JKM et al. (1992) A controlled trial of aerosolised pentamadine or trimethoprim-sulphamethoxazole as primary prophylaxis against pneumocystis carinii pneumonia in patients with human immunodeficiency virus infection. N Engl J Med 327: 1826–1841

Selwyn PA, Hartel D, Lewis VA et al. (1989) A prospective study of the risk of tuberculosis among intravenous drug users with human immunodeficiency virus infection. N Engl J Med 320: 545–550

Shaw RJ, Roussak C, Forster SM, Harris JW, Pinching AJ, Mitchell DM (1988) Lung function abnormalities in patients infected with the human immunodeficiency virus with and without overt pneumonitis. Thorax 43: 436–440

Simmons JT, Suffredini AF, Lack EE et al. (1987) nonspecific interstitial pneumonitis in patients with SIDS: radiologic features. AJR 149: 265–268

Small PM et al. (1991) Treatment of tuberculosis in patients with advanced human immunodeficiency virus infection. New Engl J Med 324: 289–294

Smith DE, McLuckie A, Wyatt J, Gazzard B (1988) Severe exercise hypoxaemia with normal or near normal x-rays: a feature of pneumocystis carinii infection. Lancet ii: 1049–1051

Smith D, Davies S, Nelson M et al. (1990) Pneumocystis carinii pneumonia treated with eflornithine in AIDS patients resistant to conventional therapy. AIDS 4: 1019–1021

Smith RL, Ripps CS, Lewis ML (1988) Elevated lactate dehydrogenase values in patients with pneumocystis carinii pneumonia. Chest 93: 987–992

Solal-Celigny P, Coudere LJ, Herman D et al. (1985) Lymphoid interstitial pneumonitis in the acquired immunodeficiency syndrome–related complex. Am Rev Resp Dis 131: 956–960

Squire SB, Lipman MCI, Bagdades EK et al. (1992) Severe cytomegalovirus pneumonitis in HIV infected patients with higher than average CD4 counts. Thorax 47: 301–304

Staikowsky F, Lafon B, Guidet B, Denis M, Mayaud C, Offenstadt G (1993) Mechanical ventilation for pneumocystis carinii pneumonia in patients with the acquired immunodeficiency syndrome: is the prognosis really improved? Chest 104: 756–762

Stern RG, Gamsu G, Golden JA (1984) Intrathoracic adenopathy: differential features of AIDS and diffuse lymphadenopathy syndrome. AJR 142: 689–692

Stover DE, White DA, Romano PA et al. (1985) Spectrum of pulmonary disease associated with the acquired immunodeficiency syndrome. Am J Med 78: 429–437

Stover DE, Greeno RA, Gagliardi AJ (1989) The use of a simple exercise test for the diagnosis of pneumocystis carinii pneumonia in patients with AIDS. Am Rev Resp Dis 139: 1343–1346

Stover DE, White DA, Roomano PA, Gellene RA (1984) Diagnosis of pulmonary disease in acquired immune deficiency syndrome (AIDS). Role of bronchoscopy and broncho-alveolar lavage. Am Rev Resp Dis 131: 659–662

Suffredini AF, Ognibene FP, Lack EE et al. (1987) Nonspecific interstitial pneumonitis. A common cause of pulmonary disease in the acquired immunodeficiency syndrome. Ann Intern Med 107: 7–13

Suster B, Ackerman M, Orenstein M, Wax MR (1986) Pulmonary manifestation of AIDS: review of 106 episodes. Radiology 161: 87–93

Tanabe K, Fuchimoto M, Egawa K et al. (1988) Use of pneumocystis carinii genomic DNA clones for hybridisation analysis of infected human lungs. J Infect Dis 157: 593–596

Thuer CP, Chaisson RE, Sheckter GF, Hopewell PC (1988) Human immunodeficiency virus infection in tuberculosis patients in San Francisco. Am Rev Respir Dis 137: 121 (abstract)

Toma E, Fournier S, Poisson M et al. (1989) Clindamycin with primaquine for Pneumocystis carinii pneumonia. Lancet i: 1046–1048

Wakefield AE, Guiver L, Miller RF, Hopkin JM (1991) DNA amplification on induced sputum samples for the diagnosis of pneumocystis carinii pneumonia. Lancet 337: 1378–1379

Wakefield AE, Peters SE, Baberji S et al. (1992) Pneumocystis carinii shows DNA homology with the ustomycetous red yeast fungi. Mol Microbiol 6: 1903–1911

Wallace JM, Hannah JB (1988) Pulmonary disease at autopsy in patients with the acquired immunodeficiency syndrome. West Med J 149: 167–171

Wallace JM, Rao AV, Glassroth et al. (1993) Respiratory illness in persons with human immunodeficiency virus infection. Am Rev Respir Dis 148: 1523–1529

Walzer PD (1988) Diagnosis of pneumocystis carinii pneumonia. J Infect Dis 157: 629–632

Walzer PD, Cuslion MT, Juranek D et al. (1987) Serology and *Pneumocystis carinii*. Chest 91: 935

Warren JB, Shaw RJ, Weber JN, Holt DA, Keel EE, Pinching AJ (1985) Role of fibreoptic bronchoscopy in management of pneumonia in acquired immune deficiency syndrome. Br Med J 291: 1012–1013

Watson JM, Fern KJ, Porter JDH, Whitmore SE (1991) Notifications of tuberculosis in England and Wales, 1982-1989. Communicable Diseases Report 1: R13-16

Watson JM, Meredith SK, Whitmore-Overton E, Bannister B, Darbyshire JH (1993) Tuberculosis and HIV: estimates of the overlap in England and Wales. Thorax 48: 199-203

Webster A et al. (1989) CMV infection and progression towards AIDS in patients with HIV infection. Lancet i: 63-66

Wharton M, Coleman DL, Wofsy C et al. (1986) Prospective randomised trial of trimethoprim-sulphamethoxole versus pentamidine for pneumocystis carinii pneumonia in the acquired immune deficiency syndrome. Ann Intern Med 105: 37-44

Youle M, Chanas A, Gazzard B (1990) Treatment with foscarnet of presumed CMV pneumonitis in patients with AIDS; a double-blind controlled study. J Infect 20: 41-50

Young LS (1987) Antigen detection in Pneumocystis carinii infection. Serodiagnosis Immunotherapy 1: 163-167

Zaman MK, Wooten OJ, Supra Manya B et al. (1988) Rapid non-invasive diagnosis of Pneumocystis carinii from induced liquefied sputum. Ann Intern Med 109: 7-10

Zaman MK, White DA (1988) Serum lactate dehydrogenase levels and pneumocystis carinii pneumonia. Diagnostic and prognostic significance. Am Rev Resp Dis 137: 796-800

Ziegler JL, Beckstead JA, Volberding PA et al. (1984) Non-Hodgkin's lymphoma in 90 homosexual men. Relation to generalized lymphadenopathy and the acquired immune deficiency syndrome. N Engl J Med 311: 565-570

5 Gastroenterological Problems of HIV Infection and AIDS

Ian McGowan and Duncan Churchill

Introduction

Gastrointestinal disease occurs in the majority of patients with the acquired immunodeficiency syndrome (AIDS). Opportunistic gut infection and neoplasia occur throughout the gut. The differential diagnosis of HIV-related gastrointestinal symptoms is large and includes tumours and a variety of opportunistic infections. Multiple pathology is common. Investigation of gastrointestinal symptoms is important as many pathogens will respond to specific therapy, although relapse is common and long-term treatment may be necessary. Where specific treatment for gastrointestinal disease is not available or has been unsuccessful it is always possible to palliate patients' symptoms and improve their quality of life. This chapter aims to describe some of the more common gastrointestinal problems that physicians are likely to encounter and to provide guidelines for investigation and management.

Presentation of Gastroenterological Problems

Oral Lesions

Oral disease is common in patients with HIV infection and AIDS. It is important to recognise the presence of oral disease for three reasons. Firstly, it may be the cause of treatable symptoms. Secondly, the nature of lesions seen in the mouth may suggest the nature of disease elsewhere in the gut (e.g., oral herpes and candida may be associated with similar lesions in the oesophagus). Thirdly, some oral lesions such as oral hairy leukoplakia and oral candidiasis are important prognostic markers.

The commonest oral disease seen is candidiasis. In the pseudomembranous form, white plaques are seen on the mucosa of the mouth (Fig. 5.1). The appearance is characteristic, and diagnosis is usually straightforward. An atrophic form of oral candidiasis is also encountered, with smooth red patches on the palate, tongue, or buccal mucosa. This is often missed without careful examination. Oral candidiasis is an important marker of disease progression: in a cohort of

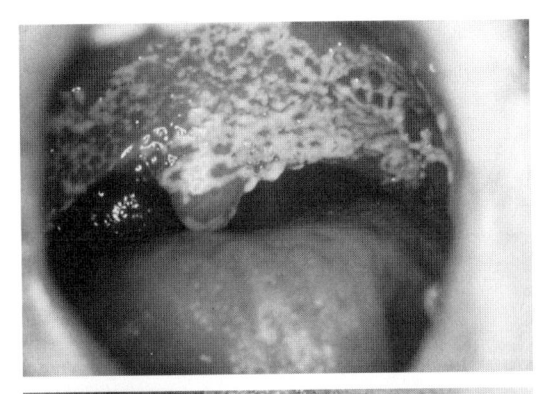

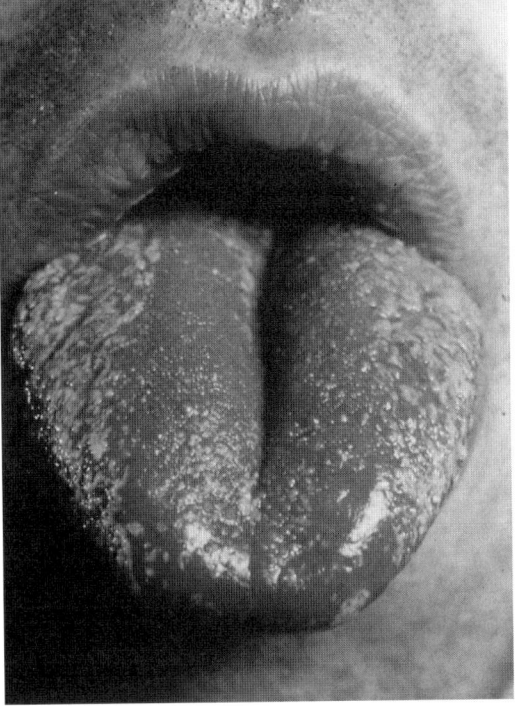

Fig. 5.1. Oral candidiasis.

seropositive homosexual men in London, 50% progressed to AIDS within a year of the onset of oral candidiasis (Kelly et al. 1990). In an American series 59% of HIV-positive patients with pseudomembranous candidiasis developed AIDS within 3 months of diagnosis (Klein et al. 1984). Candidiasis commonly causes oral discomfort, and although it may initially respond to topical therapy, the majority of patients will require systemic therapy (Table 5.4).

Oral hairy leukoplakia is another characteristic lesion seen in patients with HIV. It is recognised as ribbed white areas on the lateral part of the tongue, or less commonly on the buccal mucosa or dorsum of the tongue (Fig. 5.2). It is due to infection with Epstein–Barr virus (EBV) (Greenspan et al. 1985). In homosex-

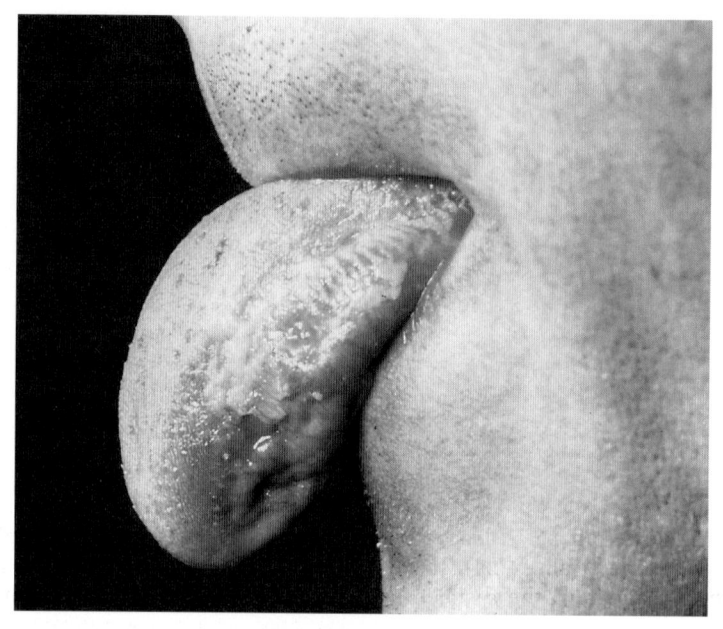

Fig. 5.2. Oral hairy leukoplakia.

ual men oral hairy leukoplakia is associated with a risk of approximately 40% of progression to AIDS within one year (Kelly et al. 1990). It is usually asymptomatic, but if particularly painful can be treated with acyclovir (Resnick et al. 1988).

Kaposi's sarcoma (KS) can occur anywhere in the mouth, and is often associated with cutaneous KS. In particular palatal KS is strongly associated with visceral disease. Radiotherapy is effective treatment for symptomatic or unsightly local lesions, but may produce severe mucositis (Watkins et al. 1989).

The differential diagnosis of oral ulceration in HIV disease is wide. Examination of the mucosa can give clues to the cause of the ulceration, but additional investigations are needed to confirm the diagnosis. Infection with Herpes simplex virus (HSV) presents with crops of small, painful, vesicular ulcers on the fauces or palate, and may be associated with circumoral ulcers. The diagnosis can be confirmed by viral culture. Cytomegalovirus (CMV) infection is less common in the mouth, and causes isolated ulcers. Viral culture is unhelpful, as this virus is frequently shed from the mucosal surfaces of asymptomatic patients with HIV infection (Quinnan et al. 1984). Biopsy may reveal characteristic histopathological features of CMV infection. Oro-pharyngeal ulceration not associated with HSV or CMV is usually classified as aphthous ulceration; however, controversy exists as to whether this form of ulceration should more correctly be called HIV-associated ulceration. If there is no response to treatment for HSV or aphthous ulceration, biopsy should be considered to exclude CMV and lymphoma, which are rarer causes of mucosal ulceration.

Oral warts, due to infection with human papilloma virus (HPV), are seen on occasion on the buccal mucosa of patients with HIV. Xerostomia, the sensation

Oesophageal Symptoms

At least 10% of all patients with HIV infection will experience oesophageal symptoms at some stage of their illness (Fauci et al. 1984) (Table 5.1). Symptoms include pain on swallowing both solids and liquids, or a sensation of food sticking in the oesophagus. Some patients also describe epigastric or retrosternal pain unrelated to swallowing. (The causes of oesophageal symptoms are listed in Table 5.1). The combination of oral candidiasis and oesophageal symptoms is highly predictive of oesophageal candidiasis (Tavitian et al. 1986; Connolly et al. 1989a), and this underlies the practice of giving empirical treatment with antifungal drugs, without further investigation.

Oesophageal candidiasis causes odynophagia, or pain on swallowing, although it may be clinically silent (Clotet et al. 1986). It is almost always associated with oral candidiasis, but may also be seen in association with other oesophageal pathology (Laine et al. 1992a). It has a characteristic endoscopic appearance, with white plaques in the distal oesophagus (Fig. 5.3) or a white membrane extending circumferentially around the oesophageal mucosa. Biopsies are not usually needed but may be helpful if there is doubt about the diagnosis. Treatment is with systemic antifungal agents.

In patients with oesophageal symptoms but without oral candidiasis, those who fail to respond to antifungal treatment, and those without an AIDS diagnosis, endoscopy supplemented by biopsy is the investigation of choice. Barium swallows have an inferior sensitivity, especially for oesophageal candidiasis, and lack specificity in the diagnosis of oesophageal ulceration (Connolly et al. 1989b).

Cytomegalovirus (CMV) is a less common cause of oesophageal pathology (Jacobson et al. 1988; Wilcox et al. 1990). Characteristically it produces large shallow ulcers in the distal oesophagus, although other presentations include lesions in the mid and upper oesophagus, multiple small ulcers throughout the oesophagus and diffuse oesophagitis. Evidence of CMV infection at other sites is seen in a minority of patients. The diagnosis must be confirmed by endoscopic biopsy. Large intranuclear inclusions are seen on haematoxylin and eosin (H&E)

Table 5.1. Causes of oesophageal symptoms in patients with AIDS

Candida
Cytomegalovirus
Herpes simplex virus
Epstein–Barr virus
Aphthous ulceration
Mycobacterium avium intracellulare
Cryptosporidium
Kaposi's sarcoma
Non-Hodgkin's lymphoma
Peptic oesophagitis
Primary HIV seroconversion illness

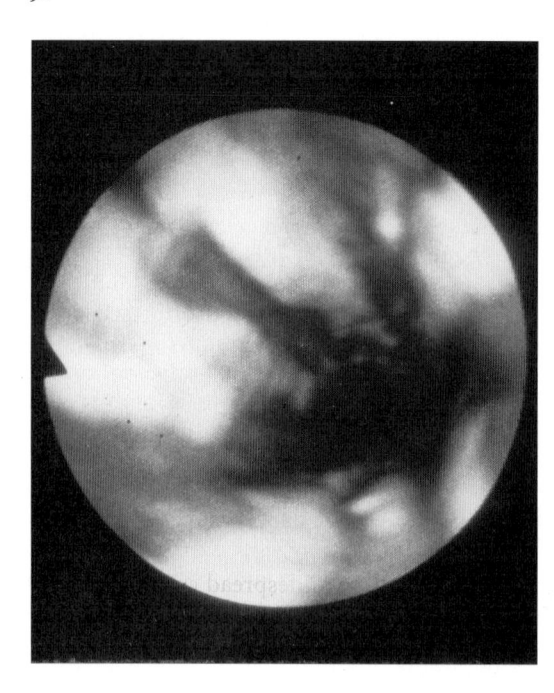

Fig. 5.3. Endoscopic view of oesophageal candidiasis.

staining of biopsy specimens, predominantly in endothelial cells in the submucosa (Weber et al. 1987). Immunohistochemical staining can be helpful if H&E staining of a suspicious ulcer is negative (Francis et al. 1989; Theise et al. 1991). CMV oesophagitis usually develops late in the course of HIV infection; most patients have had an AIDS diagnosis by the time they develop CMV oesophagitis. The prognosis is consequently poor, with a median survival of 4–6 months from the time of diagnosis (Wilcox et al. 1990).

Herpes simplex oesophagitis is usually accompanied by oral herpes, and produces multiple superficial, fluid-filled vesicles or shallow ulcers. Biopsies show characteristic multinucleated cells.

A syndrome of acute symptomatic oesophageal ulceration complicating HIV seroconversion has been described (Rabenek et al. 1990). Oesophageal symptoms are accompanied by malaise, fever, myalgia, and often a macular rash. Endoscopy shows single or multiple small oesophageal ulcers with characteristic histological changes seen on light microscopy. Under electron microscopy, HIV-like particles can be seen in the mucosa. The ulceration heals spontaneously without treatment. On occasion, oesophageal candidiasis may complicate seroconversion, but this also heals without treatment.

EBV has been recognised as a cause of oesophageal ulceration in patients with HIV infection (Kitchen et al. 1990). There are macroscopic similarities with aphthous ulcers, but biopsies show specific histological features which resemble those seen in oral hairy leukoplakia, with EBV detected in tissue from these ulcers by *in-situ* hybridisation (Kitchen et al. 1990). The ulcers may be endoscopically distinguishable from CMV- and HSV-associated ulcers, and are said to be deep, linear, and usually in the mid oesophagus. Similar lesions can be found in the pharynx in some patients, although interestingly no association with oral hairy leukoplakia has been reported.

Other, less common, causes of oesophageal symptoms in HIV infection include oesophageal cryptosporidiosis (Kazlow et al. 1986), and *Mycobacterium avium-intracellulare* (Grayand Rabenek 1989). Non-Hodgkin's lymphoma may affect the oesophagus. Kaposi's sarcoma of the oesophagus does not usually cause symptoms, unless there is associated mucosal ulceration.

Abdominal Pain

The differential diagnosis of abdominal pain in patients with HIV infection is similar to that in patients without HIV infection, but specific diagnoses including extensive visceral KS, CMV ulceration affecting the oesophagus, stomach or duodenum, mesenteric adenopathy, and AIDS sclerosing cholangitis (ASC) should also be considered.

Gastrointestinal Bleeding

This is an uncommon problem, perhaps due to the widespread empirical use of H_2 receptor antagonists. Non-Hodgkin's lymphoma, KS and CMV disease may all cause gastrointestinal haemorrhage. Patients with thrombocytopenia are at increased risk of bleeding (Parente et al. 1991).

Jaundice

Frank jaundice is rarely seen in association with HIV disease. Homosexual men and injecting drug users are still the most common groups infected with HIV in Europe, and viral hepatitis and the late sequelae of chronic viral hepatitis are the most common causes of jaundice. Occasionally jaundice is seen in patients with AIDS sclerosing cholangitis (Cello 1989) or secondary to drugs (Table 5.5). Patients may be asymptomatic, or present with fever, abdominal pain or hepatomegaly.

Weight Loss/Anorexia

Weight loss is a major problem in AIDS and directly influences survival (Kotler et al. 1989a). The causes of weight loss are multifactorial and include anorexia, malabsorption, and chronic diarrhoea. In addition disturbance of cytokine production associated with opportunistic infections such as tuberculosis may contribute to further weight loss. "Enteropathic" AIDS is a more extreme form seen in Africa, where it is known as "slim disease" (Serwadda et al. 1985). Patients may complain specifically of weight loss, or more commonly clinicians notice a gradual decline in body mass in patients attending clinic.

Diarrhoea

Diarrhoea is a significant problem in 50%–90% of HIV patients. The differential diagnosis is very wide (Table 5.2). Patients may only complain of diarrhoea, or

Table 5.2. Pathogens in HIV associated diarrhoea

Bacteria
  Salmonella sp
  Shigella sp
  Campylobacter jejuni
  Mycobacterium avium-intracellulare

Viruses
  Cytomegalovirus
  Adenovirus
  Human immunodeficiency virus

Protozoa
  Cryptosporidium
  Giardia lamblia
  Isospora belli
  Microsporidium
  Cyanobacterium-like bodies

may have other symptoms such as fever, weight loss, or abdominal pain. A careful history may not elucidate the cause of the diarrhoea, but it may provide clues as to the site of infection and will enable the clinician to assess the severity of the problem. Cramps, bloating and nausea suggest small intestinal or gastric pathology. Haematochezia points towards colonic disease, whilst tenesmus is associated with proctitis or a rectal lesion.

Perianal Problems

Anorectal disease is particularly common in sexually active homosexual men, and so may be found in association with HIV disease. Some of the causes are listed in Table 5.3, and all male homosexual patients presenting with anorectal symptoms such as irritation, itching, pain, or rectal discharge should be screened for sexually transmitted infections. Clinical examination with proctoscopy is important, but specific diagnosis depends on microbiological confirmation.

Kaposi's Sarcoma/Lymphoma

Kaposi's sarcoma (KS) is the commonest tumour associated with HIV infection, and is commonly seen in the gastrointestinal tract. In a series from San Francisco, KS was found at post mortem in the gut of 70% of patients dying of AIDS (Friedman et al. 1985). KS is commoner in homosexual men and patients from developing countries than in patients from other risk groups, and it has been suggested that another sexually transmitted agent may be involved in the pathogenesis of KS (Beral et al. 1990, 1991). In the majority of patients, gastrointestinal KS is asymptomatic; however, it may be the cause of bleeding, obstruction, perforation, and protein-losing enteropathy (Perrone et al. 1981). The presence of gastrointestinal KS should be considered if there is cutaneous or palatal disease. Diagnosis is by endoscopy; the lesions are characteristic, but it is prudent to take biopsies for histological confirmation.

Table 5.3. Causes of ano rectal symptoms in HIV disease

Bacteria
   Chlamydia trachomatis
   Neisseria gonorrhoeae
   Treponema pallidum

Viruses
   Herpes simplex
   Cytomegalovirus
   Human papilloma virus

Neoplasia
   Lymphoma
   Kaposi's sarcoma
   Anal carcinoma

Lymphoma is much less common than KS. With the advent of effective prophylaxis against common opportunistic infections such as *Pneumocystis*, patients are surviving longer, and the incidence of lymphoma is increasing. HIV-associated lymphomas are usually high grade non-Hodgkin's type of B-cell origin (Knowles et al. 1988; Pluda et al. 1990). Extranodal involvement is typical and the gut is the commonest site involved.

Investigation of Gastroenterological Problems

Stool Culture and Microscopy

The differential diagnosis of HIV-associated diarrhoea includes many unusual organisms (Table 5.2), and in addition more common organisms such as *Salmonella* species may present atypically with septicaemia or disseminated infection (Nelson et al. 1992)

    Diarrhoea lasting in excess of 2 weeks warrants investigation. Stool samples should be collected and sent for routine culture, parasitological examination, and culture for *Mycobacteria*. It is important that the laboratory is notified of the patient's HIV seropositivity since examination for organisms such as *Cryptosporidium* may not otherwise be carried out. Identifying the oocysts of *Cryptosporidium* remains difficult. The organism is small (4.5 μm), and may be shed intermittently. Ma and colleagues have described a three-stage examination to improve the diagnostic yield (Ma and Soave 1983), but most laboratories use a modified Ziehl–Neelsen technique as a screening test. Concentration techniques such as Sheather's sugar flotation method (Sheather 1953) may be helpful in follow-up of patients excreting small numbers of oocysts. Monoclonal antibodies directed against oocyst wall antigens are now available and may in the future become a routine test to identify *Cryptosporidium* in faecal smears.

    Pathogen-negative diarrhoea (PND) is a difficult clinical problem in patients with HIV disease. PND is diagnosed on the basis of 6 negative stool examinations together with a normal rectal biopsy (Connolly et al. 1989c). Upper gastrointestinal endoscopy with microscopic examination of duodenal aspirate and mucosa is sometimes helpful in patients with PND. Histopathological examination of duodenal tissue may show evidence of colonisation with organisms such as *Cryptosporidium* (Fig. 5.4). Greenson et al. (1991) showed that when conventional laboratory practice was augmented by examination of duodenal mucosal biopsies with light and electron microscopy, it was possible to identify pathogens in 11/22 patients with PND. The organisms most commonly identified by electron microscopy were *Microsporidia*, thought to be *Enterocytozoon bienusi*. Stool samples and duodenal smears stained with Giemsa are being evaluated for use in identifying *Microsporidium* (Van Gool et al. 1990; Weber et al. 1992).

Antibiotic-associated diarrhoea, including pseudomembranous colitis due to *Clostridium difficile* is occasionally seen in patients with HIV infection. It is important to look for *C. difficile* toxin in the stools of patients whose diarrhoea is otherwise unexplained.

Radiology/Ultrasound

Plain abdominal radiographs have a limited role in the investigation of HIV-related abdominal symptoms. They can demonstrate the presence of renal calculi (if radiopaque), calcification associated with chronic pancreatitis, or gas under the diaphragm associated with a perforated viscus. In patients with diarrhoea and abdominal pain, a plain radiograph may show toxic dilatation of the bowel, or conversely may establish that the diarrhoea is in fact due to faecal impaction with overflow.

Double contrast barium studies lack sensitivity and specificity and are rarely performed in AIDS patients. A study comparing endoscopy with double

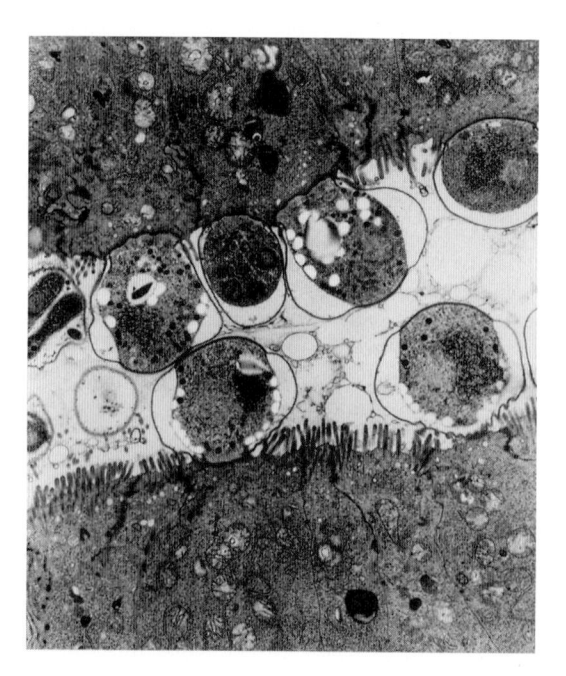

Fig. 5.4. Electron micrograph of *Cryptosporidium* oocysts attached to small bowel surface epithelium cells from a patient with chronic diarrhoea.

contrast barium examination in the investigation of upper gastrointestinal symptoms in AIDS patients showed that endoscopy combined with appropriate microbiological and histological sampling provided the correct diagnosis in 95.5% of cases, compared with 31% from barium studies (Connolly et al. 1989a).

Ultrasound is most useful in imaging the biliary tree, examining intraabdominal lymph nodes, looking for ascites, and directing percutaneous biopsies.

Endoscopy

Fibre-optic endoscopy is of considerable value in investigating HIV-positive patients with gastroenterological complaints. It is especially useful in patients with oesophageal symptoms, most of whom will have a diagnosis made after a single investigation. Endoscopy with biopsy of the duodenum and duodenal aspiration has a role in the investigation of diarrhoea. Other indications for upper gastrointestinal endoscopy include the assessment of gastrointestinal KS, and the investigation of abdominal pain. Peptic ulcers should always be biopsied, as CMV may cause ulceration throughout the gastrointestinal tract.

Sclerosing cholangitis has been found to occur in patients with HIV. The aetiology remains uncertain, but there is a strong association with *Cryptosporidium* and CMV (Cello 1989). Patients present with right upper quadrant pain, elevated alkaline phosphatase, and occasionally fever. There is a characteristic beading and variable stenosis of the biliary tree, which becomes more marked as the disease progresses (Fig. 5.5). These changes may be seen with ultrasound examination, but ERCP is probably more sensitive. There is some evidence that the pain associated with AIDS sclerosing cholangitis (ASC) may be improved by performing an endoscopic sphincterotomy (Dowsett et al. 1988; Schneiderman et al. 1987), and it is probably this group of patients who should be investigated with ERCP.

In the investigation of patients with diarrhoea, repeated stool examinations and rigid sigmoidoscopy with rectal biopsy are the most helpful procedures (Connolly et al. 1989c). The roles of flexible sigmoidoscopy and colonoscopy are less well defined but are the only way to diagnose proximal CMV colitis/ileitis.

It is important to take multiple biopsies from any lesion seen at endoscopy. When taking biopsies from oesophageal ulcers, it is usually easiest to biopsy the edge of the ulcer rather than the base. Deep biopsies are needed if Kaposi's sarcoma or CMV are suspected, as there is a high false-negative rate. This is due to the submucosal situation of KS lesions and the cells infected with CMV (Friedman et al. 1985; Connolly et al. 1989b; Theise et al. 1991). CMV cultures from ulcer biopsies are unhelpful as CMV viraemia is seen in up to 50% of patients with AIDS (Quinnan et al. 1984). Some patients with immunohistochemically proven CMV ulceration may have negative cultures (Wilcox et al. 1990). The diagnosis depends on histological demonstration of CMV inclusion bodies.

Brush cytology of lesions seen at endoscopy may help to increase the yield. Saline washes of the cytology brush have been shown to be a sensitive method of diagnosing oesophageal *Candida* (Connolly et al. 1989a) but this is not usually needed.

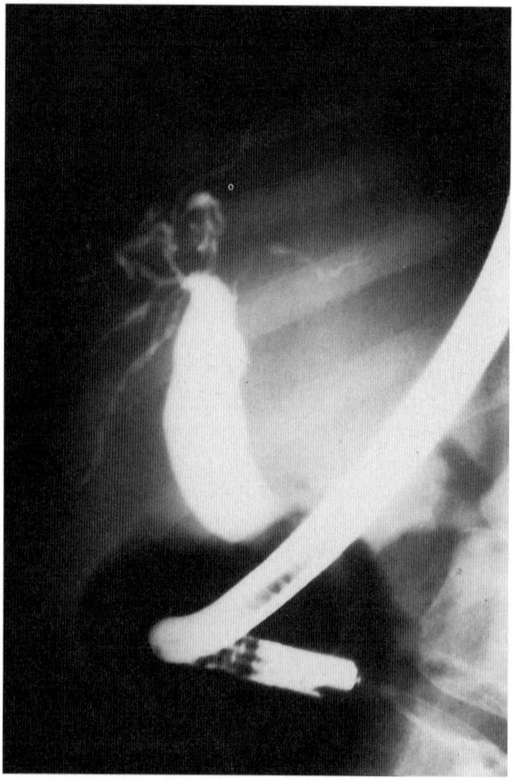

Fig. 5.5. ERCP study showing widespread stricturing of intrahepatic biliary tree in a patient with AIDS sclerosing cholangitis.

All patients undergoing endoscopy should be treated as being potentially HIV positive, and appropriate care taken to avoid the risk to staff (British Society of Gastroenterology Working Party Report 1989). Manual cleaning of endoscopes is the most important step in ensuring sterilisation of the instruments after procedures. Following thorough manual cleaning, the majority of pathogens (including HIV) are inactivated by a 4-minute soak in 2% glutaraldehyde. Procedures on patients who are immunosuppressed, including those with HIV infection, should be carried out after a 1-hour soak of the instrument in 2% glutaraldehyde, in order to ensure inactivation of more persistent organisms including *Mycobacteria* and *Cryptosporidium*. Dedicated instruments are not needed.

Nuclear Medicine

^{99m}Tc-Iminodiacetic acid scans of the liver and biliary tree may be of use in the diagnosis of ASC, especially in early cases where ultrasound and/or CT scans of the abdomen have failed to give a precise diagnosis or to demonstrate dilatation of the biliary tree (Fig. 5.6). This method has a high sensitivity in the detection of abnormality in the biliary tree (Miller et al. 1990), and is useful in deciding which patients should be referred for ERCP.

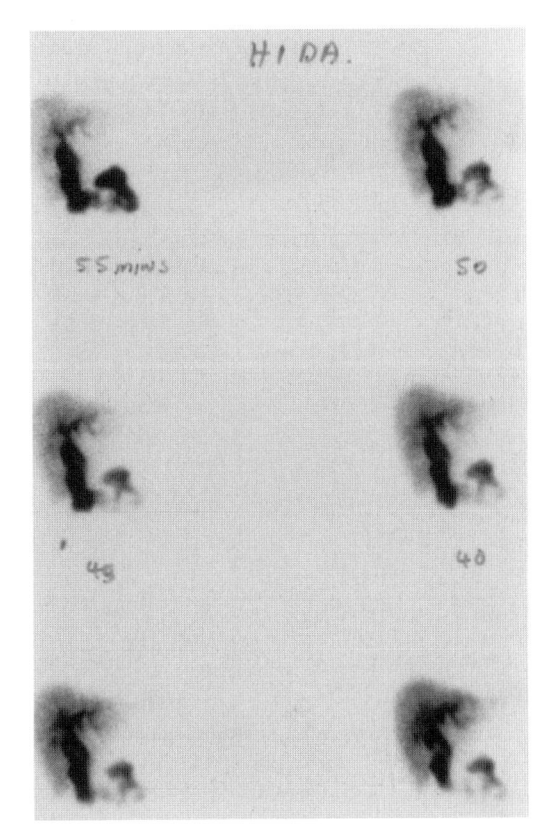

Fig. 5.6. Serial ^{99m}Tc-iminodiacetic acid scans of the liver, showing marked delay in excretion of tracer from the intrahepatic biliary tract and common bile duct in a patient with AIDS sclerosing cholangitis.

Management of Specific Problems

Oral Disease

Maintenance of oral hygiene is an important part of caring for patients who are HIV-positive. Gingivitis is common and of variable severity. Patients with gingivitis are best managed jointly with oral physicians and dentists. Therapy includes improved dental hygiene, antiseptic mouthwashes and the use of antibiotics such as metronidazole.

Oral candidiasis may respond to local therapy with antifungals such as amphotericin lozenges, or nystatin in the form of suspension or pastilles. Patients often relapse and need systemic therapy. Ketoconazole, fluconazole, and itraconazole can all be used (Table 5.4). Ketoconazole is cheaper than fluconazole but may be less effective (Laine et al. 1992b). Resistance to systemic antifungals is a common problem. Symptoms may initially be controlled by increasing the dose of antifungal therapy, but often parenteral amphotericin is the only useful form of therapy (Table 5.4).

Culture-proven HSV ulceration should be treated with acyclovir (Table 5.4). Five-day courses can be given, but most patients with AIDS require long-term suppressive therapy.

Table 5.4. Drugs used in the management of HIV-related gastrointestinal disease

Problem	Drug	Dose	Side effects	Comments
Infections				
Fungal				
Candida	Nystatin pastilles	prn		Topical preparations are of limited value in severe oral disease
	Amphotericin lozenges	prn		
	Ketoconazole	200–400 mg/day	Nausea, hepatitis, thrombocytopenia	Use with caution in patients with abnormal liver function
	Fluconazole	50–100 mg/day	Nausea	
	Itraconazole	200 mg/day	Nausea	
	Amphotericin	250 microgram/kg daily iv	Nausea, diarrhoea, headache, fever, anaemia, renal failure, hepatitis, convulsions	Used in patients with candidal infections not responding to oral systemic therapy. Needs to be given with careful renal, hepatic and haematological monitoring
Viral				
HSV	Acyclovir			
	Short course	200 mg 5 × daily	Rashes, abnormal liver function	Short courses often followed by symptomatic relapse and maintenance needed
	Maintenance	200 mg qds		
	Parenteral	5–10 mg/kg tds	Crystalluria if patient is dehydrated	Resistance to acyclovir emerging
CMV	Ganciclovir			
	Induction	10 mg/kg/day iv	Fever, rash, neutropenia, anaemia thrombocytopenia	Zidovudine needs to be stopped during induction
	Maintenance	5 mg/kg/day iv		Maintenance therapy usually requires a central line such as a Hickman line. Many patients are on domiciliary therapy
	Foscarnet	20–60 mg/kg tds 3 weeks iv	Nausea, vomiting, rash, convulsions, hypocalcaemia	Dose needs to be titrated against renal function
Protozoal				
Cryptosporidium	Paromomycin	1 g bd for 1 month Maintenance therapy 0.5–1 g bd	Abdominal cramps, flatulence; may worsen diarrhoea	
Microsporidium	Albendazole	400 mg bd	Changes in liver enzymes, nausea, vomiting, headache, pancytopenia	
Isospora belli	Cotrimoxazole	960 mg qds	Rashes	Maintenance needed to prevent relapse

Table 5.4. *Continued*

Problem	Drug	Dose	Side effects	Comments
Giardia lamblia	Metronidazole	2 g for 3 days, 400 mg bd 5 days	Nausea, vomiting, ataxia, disulfiram-like reaction with alcohol	Warn patients about alcohol interaction
	Tinidazole	2 g single dose Repeat after 1 week	Nausea, vomiting, ataxia, disulfiram-like reaction with alcohol	Better tolerated than metronidazole
Aphthous ulcers	Topical			
	Difflam mouthwash spray	prn		All topical preparations must be applied carefully to maximise effect. Oral hygiene very important. Other causes of oral ulceration must be excluded
	Hydrocortisone pellets	tds		
	Triamcinolone in orabase	tds		
Systemic therapy	Thalidomide	50–100 mg/day	Rashes	Generalised erythematous rashes may limit drugs use. Peripheral neuropathy
	Prednisolone	60 mg/day reducing dose	Euphoria, insomnia, increased immunosuppression, Cushing's syndrome	Concern has been expressed about the use of potent steroids in the context of HIV related immunosuppression. Few data are available and so steroids when used should be reduced as soon as clinical response allows
Nausea	Prochlorperazine	20 mg stat then 5–10 mg tds	Extrapyramidal symptoms, hypotension insomnia, depression	Antiemetic medication is best started im/iv/pr in patients with severe symptoms
	Metoclopramide	10 mg tds	Extrapyramidal symptoms	
	Ondansetron	8 mg tds	Constipation, flushing	Valuable in chemotherapy induced nausea
	Nabilone	1–2 mg bd	Drowsiness, hypotension euphoria, hallucinations	Combinations of drugs can be tried in intractable nausea, as long as they come from different pharmacological groups as suggested above
Diarrhoea	Loperamide	4 mg stat, then 2 mg after each motion, max dose 16 mg/day	Abdominal cramps, urticarial rashes	
	Codeine phosphate	10–16 mg qds		
	Lomotil	4 tabs stat, then 2 tabs qds	Anticholinergic symptoms	
	Morphine (MST)	10–60 mg bd	Nausea, vomiting, drowsiness	Used when no response to 1st line agents listed above

Mild cases of aphthous ulceration may be helped by gargles with chlorhexidine gluconate, or application of topical steroids such as triamcinolone in orabase. Oral thalidomide has been used to treat patients with giant aphthae, but one report has suggested that in HIV patients, thalidomide is associated with a high incidence of allergic rashes (Williams et al. 1991). High dose systemic steroids may achieve the same result more safely, but should be reduced as soon as possible.

Intraoral warts are best treated with cryotherapy but may be recurrent. In HIV associated xerostomia artificial saliva substitutes can be used, and citrus sweets provide a simple alternative.

Oesophageal Disease

Management of oesophageal candidiasis is with systemic antifungal drugs (Table 5.4). As discussed above, treatment is often empirical and in uncomplicated oesophageal candidiasis symptoms usually respond in under a week. Failure to respond to treatment is an indication for endoscopy to exclude a second pathology. In general, higher doses of antifungal therapy are required in oesophageal rather than oral candidiasis. Controversy exists as to the optimal duration of therapy, both for induction and maintenance. Induction therapy should be continued until there is resolution of oesophageal symptoms. The patients can then be kept under observation until symptoms recur, at which time long-term therapy should be started. Alternatively patients can be put on long-term therapy at first presentation. The advantage of the first policy is that patients will require less drug, which is both cheaper and may also reduce the incidence of drug toxicity.

CMV ulceration of the gastrointestinal tract is uncommon. Treatment of CMV oesophagitis is outlined in Table 5.4. Ganciclovir or foscarnet may be used (Dietrich et al. 1988; Nelson et al. 1991). Both must be given intravenously, and often necessitate the insertion of a central line, although many patients are able to administer their medication at home. There have been no comparative trials of foscarnet and ganciclovir in CMV oesophagitis; both drugs have been demonstrated to be effective in healing oesophageal disease, and the major difference between the two drugs is in their spectrum of toxicity (Table 5.4). Treatment is usually given as a 2–3-week induction course or until symptomatic and endoscopic resolution have occurred. 77% of patients responded completely to 3 weeks' treatment with foscarnet in one study, and the response to ganciclovir is similar (Blanshard 1992; Peters et al. 1991). A placebo-controlled trial of ganciclovir in AIDS patients with CMV colitis demonstrated improvement in 20/32 patients on the active drug. However a similar result was obtained in 11/30 patients on placebo (Dieterich et al. 1990). The role of maintenance therapy in CMV oesophagitis is also open to question. In one study, 13/17 patients who responded to an induction course of foscarnet for CMV oesophagitis without subsequent maintenance therapy did not experience relapse (Nelson et al. 1991). Zidovudine potentiates the myelotoxic effects of ganciclovir, and should not be prescribed during ganciclovir induction therapy. Healing of large ulcers may be complicated by stricture formation (Goodgame et al. 1991; Churchill et al. 1992).

Herpetic oesophagitis is treated with acyclovir (Table 5.4). Maintenance treatment is advised.

Often ulceration is seen in the oesophagus without a clear histological diagnosis. Repeat endoscopy is worthwhile, as CMV inclusions are sometimes seen in subsequent biopsies (Connolly et al. 1989b). Despite repeat endoscopy, some patients will fail to have a specific diagnosis, and aphthous ulcers may thus be diagnosed by exclusion. These are treated in a similar manner to oral aphthous ulcers. Dexamethasone combined with sucralfate has also been successfully used to treat oesophageal aphthous ulceration in patients with HIV (Sokol-Anderson et al. 1991).

Abdominal Pain

Management of abdominal pain depends on the results of clinical examination augmented by ancillary tests such as ultrasound and endoscopy. Epigastric pain may respond to an empirical course of an H_2 antagonist, but symptoms which persist beyond 2 weeks of therapy require further investigation. Right upper quadrant pain together with raised alkaline phosphatase, or a dilated biliary tree suggests ASC.

Gastrointestinal Bleeding

The management of gut haemorrhage is no different to that of non-HIV patients. Bleeding KS is best managed conservatively. The role of chemotherapy or other modalities of therapy in advanced visceral KS remains unclear.

Abnormal Liver Function and Jaundice

Biochemical evidence of hepatitis in AIDS patients is very common. The aetiology may be multifactorial including acute or chronic carriage of hepatotropic viruses: hepatitis A virus (HAV), hepatitis B virus (HBV), hepatitis C virus (HCV/Non-A, Non-B), and hepatitis D virus (HDV/delta). Opportunistic infections such as *Mycobacterium avium intracellulare*, infiltration with tumour, or hepatotoxic drugs (Table 5.5), may also present with abnormal liver function tests.

Hepatitis A, which is spread by oro-faecal transmission, occurs with increased frequency in homosexual men. Oro-anal contact (rimming) has been shown to be a risk factor. The infection may rarely be associated with prolonged cholestasis, but a chronic carrier state does not occur. HIV does not appear to alter the natural history of hepatitis A. A vaccine is now available for the prevention of hepatitis A, but data about its use in patients with HIV are lacking.

HIV infection may alter the natural history of HBV in a number of ways. A cytotoxic T-cell response to HBV core proteins expressed on the surface of hepatocytes is thought to be important in the hepatic parenchymal inflammatory response to HBV replication, and in the eradication of infection. Pre-existing HIV infection with quantitative and/or qualitative CD4 cell defects may favour the establishment of chronic infection (Underhill et al. 1986). Following a course of HBV vaccine there is a lower anti-HBs response rate in the presence of HIV (Carne et al. 1987). HBV replication may be potentiated in the presence of HIV infection. The rate of spontaneous loss of HBe antigen with time may be reduced (Krogsgaard et al. 1987), and reactivation of viral replication may occur. HIV

Table 5.5. Hepatotoxic drugs used in HIV disease

Antifungals
  Ketoconazole
  Fluconazole
  Amphotericin

Antituberculous
  Isoniazid
  Rifampicin

Antivirals
  Acyclovir
  Ganciclovir

Antibiotics
  Cephalosporins
  Cotrimoxazole
  Ciprofloxacin
  Pentamidine

Antiprotozoal
  Pyrimethamine

infection in the chronic HBV carrier may decrease hepatic inflammatory activity as measured by the levels of transaminases and histology (MacDonald et al. 1987; Krogsgaard et al. 1987). Finally, HIV may diminish the response to therapy in chronic HBV infection.

Following the development of serological tests for HCV, it has become possible to study the epidemiology of this virus (Kuo et al. 1989). Initial tests lacked specificity, but the development of second generation ELISA and confirmatory RIBA tests has improved the diagnosis of HCV infection. It appears that although HCV is often associated with parenteral modes of transmission, usually following blood transfusion or in intravenous drug users, it is also sexually transmitted with an increased prevalence in homosexual men. A recent study from London looking at 1064 serum samples obtained from a sexually transmitted disease clinic, showed that 6.9% of homosexual men, compared with 1.0% of heterosexuals, had evidence of infection (Tedder et al. 1991). Carriage of antibodies to HCV was strongly associated with HIV and HBV seropositivity. It is possible that HIV can modify the natural history of HCV infection and further data is awaited.

HDV is an incomplete RNA virus that requires HB surface antigen for replication. HDV infection most commonly occurs in injecting drug users, or in patients subjected to repeated parenteral exposure such as haemophiliacs. The virus appears to be uncommon in homosexual men. Like HBV, HDV can present as a self-limiting viral infection, or may develop into a chronic carrier state. In this case there is a 70% chance of the patient developing cirrhosis. Currently there are no data on the possible interaction between HIV and HDV.

Investigation will be directed by the nature of the biochemical abnormalities, and the patient's other problems and treatment. It is important to exclude biliary obstruction with abdominal ultrasound. The role of percutaneous liver biopsy remains uncertain, with many conditions being diagnosed by other means including blood culture or bone marrow examination. A number of studies have shown the diagnostic rate of liver biopsy to vary between 24% and 80% (Cappell et al. 1990), and subsequent treatment may be of uncertain benefit. Liver biopsy may be more useful in certain subgroups of patients with HIV infection. A study from Harlem (New York) reviewed 48 biopsies from a group of patients, of whom 82% had a history of injecting drug use. Within this selected population, 33.3% of the biopsies had evidence of *Mycobacterium tuberculosis* infection and this information led to the initiation of anti-tuberculous chemotherapy (Comer et al. 1989).

Pancreatobiliary Disease

A syndrome which resembles primary sclerosing cholangitis is recognised as a cause of abnormal liver function in AIDS patients (Schneiderman et al. 1987; Viteri and Greene 1987; Dowsett et al. 1988; Cello et al. 1989). The typical presentation is with right upper quadrant pain, accompanied by a raised alkaline phosphatase. Approximately 50% of patients with AIDS sclerosing cholangitis (ASC) have fever, although only 15% are jaundiced. Ultrasound scans of the abdomen are abnormal in the majority, and show biliary tract dilatation. ^{99m}Tc-labelled iminodiacetic acid (IDA) scans of the hepatobiliary system typically demonstrate delayed excretion of tracer, or strictures, but endoscopic retrograde cholangio-pancreatography (ERCP) is the definitive investigation. A number of different patterns of abnormality in the biliary tract are recognised. Papillary stenosis, and intrahepatic disease with beading and stricturing of the bile ducts, are each seen in around 15% of patients. A combination of these two abnormalities is seen in half the patients, whilst the remainder have extrahepatic strictures. The disease is commonly associated with cryptosporidiosis, microsporidiosis and CMV infection (Forbes et al. 1993; Pol et al. 1993). Endoscopic sphincterotomy may give pain relief in a proportion of patients with papillary stenosis. Liver function tests do not usually improve, and the prognosis is poor, with most patients dying within 6 months of diagnosis. The majority of patients can be managed conservatively with opiates (Forbes et al. 1993).

A syndrome of acalculous cholecystitis is also encountered in patients with HIV infection, either with or without co-existing sclerosing cholangitis (Kavin et al. 1986). The presentation is with right upper quadrant pain and tenderness, typically accompanied by fever and weight loss. Liver enzymes are often markedly elevated. Abdominal ultrasound may show thickening of the gallbladder wall and biliary dilatation. IDA scans and oral cholecystograms often show non-filling of the gallbladder. Cholecystectomy is effective in relieving symptoms in this condition. There is often evidence of CMV infection of the biliary tree, and CMV inclusions may be seen in the wall of the resected gallbladder.

Hyperamylasaemia and pancreatic duct abnormalities are frequently seen but are not usually associated with symptoms. Acute pancreatitis occurs in AIDS, most commonly as a result of treatment with dideoxyinosine (DDI) or intravenous pentamidine. CMV, *Toxoplasma gondii*, KS and lymphoma have all been implicated in acute pancreatitis in patients with AIDS (Brivet et al. 1987). Diabetes mellitus has been reported in two HIV-positive intravenous drug users without the usual immunological markers of type 1 diabetes, and a viral aetiology has been proposed (Vendrell et al. 1987).

Weight Loss/Anorexia

Weight loss is a common symptom associated with HIV infection and individuals who lose more than 10% of their baseline weight within 6 months are said to have AIDS wasting syndrome (Centers for Disease Control 1987). In general, patients in developed countries tend to lose weight on an intermittant basis possibly as a result of active secondary infection (Grunfeld et al. 1992). In contrast AIDS patients from developing countries have progressive weight loss "slim disease" (Serwadda et al. 1985) resulting from untreated secondary infection. Weight loss is an important problem as prognosis is related to the degree of weight loss (Kotler et al. 1989).

The causes of weight loss are complex and several different factors may coexist in individual patients.

Anorexia may occur secondary to drug therapy, opportunistic infection, taste disturbance or oral discomfort resulting in inadequate food intake.

Malabsorption of fat, lactose, vitamin B_{12} and bile acids has been demonstrated (Miller et al. 1988; Kapembwa et al. 1989, 1990) and may occur throughout all stages of HIV infection. The mechanisms of malabsorption remain unclear but villous atrophy of varying severity has been described by many authors (Kotler et al. 1984; Cummins et al. 1990) (Fig. 5.7). This has been variably associated with crypt hyperplasia, or increase in crypt mitotic figures (Kotler et al. 1984; Cummins et al. 1990). Chronic inflammatory cells in the *lamina propria* are increased, together with intraepithelial lymphocytes (Greenson et al. 1991). When mucosal cellular infiltrates are examined immunocytochemically, it is found that the CD4/CD8 ratio is reversed in a similar manner to peripheral blood lymphocytes. This is caused by a selective depletion in CD4 helper lymphocytes, and an increase in CD8 cytotoxic lymphocytes; an increase in activated macrophages in the *lamina propria* is also seen (Jarry et al. 1990). Mucosal plasma cell production of immunoglobulin A has been shown to be reduced when examined using polyclonal rabbit anti-human immunoglobulin antibody (Kotler et al. 1987), and Ullrich (1989) has demonstrated the reduction or absence of β glucosidase in the duodenal brush border in biopsies from HIV patients. Using electron microscopy a number of ultrastructural abnormalities have been identified, including damage to jejunal autonomic nerves in the *lamina propria* (Griffin et al. 1988). All of these changes may result from the presence of HIV in the mucosa, or HIV-infected lymphocytes migrating through the *lamina propria* and epithelium releasing cytokines which in turn affect epithelial cell kinetics.

Diarrhoea is discussed below and may result in profound weight loss especially in patients with cryptosporidiosis.

Active secondary infection may precipitate weight loss by inducing anorexia but metabolic disturbance has also been described. Basal energy expenditure is increased by up to 60% in AIDS patients with *Mycobacterium avium-intracellulare* infection (Kotler et al. 1989a). Treatment of active infection may lead to improved nutritional status (Kotler et al. 1989b). Increased α-interferon production and disturbed lipid metabolism with hypertriglyceridaemia has been reported in AIDS patients (Grunfeld et al. 1992) but there is no direct relationship with wasting.

Management of weight loss necessitates a multidisciplinary approach involving clinicians and dieticians. Clinical examination and appropriate investigations

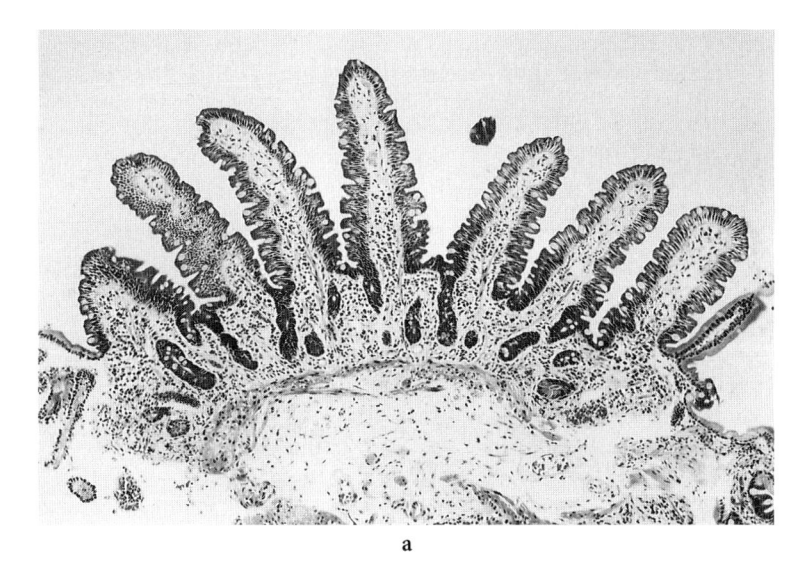

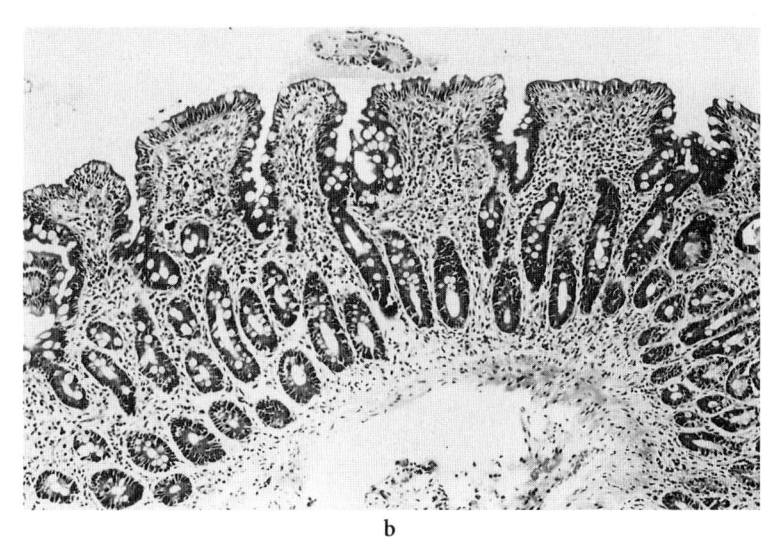

Fig. 5.7a,b. Small bowel biopsy from healthy control patient (a) and from an AIDS patient with diarrhoea and malabsorption showing increased chronic inflammatory cells in the lamina propria and crypt hyperplasia with villous atrophy (b).

will enable any secondary infection to be treated. In addition it may be possible to elucidate the likely factors leading to weight loss. A detailed dietary history will provide information necessary to plan a nutritional programme suitable for individual patients. Simple measures such as encouraging smaller, more frequent meals may be helpful. A wide variety of nutritional supplements are also available. Megestrol acetate (Megace) has been shown to be a useful appetite stimulant when given at a dose of 800 mg/day (Van Roenn et al. 1988; Flynn et al. 1992). In patients unable to tolerate oral feeding enteral and parenteral feeding are alternative forms of nutrition but their efficacy and clinical indications are still evolving (Kotler et al. 1991; Singer et al. 1991). Enteral nutrition offers a safer and cheaper alternative to total parenteral nutrition (TPN). TPN is perhaps most useful in patients with severe diarrhoea, nausea and vomiting in whom fluid balance and control of symptoms has been difficult. In this case the perceived benefits may be due to fluid replacement rather than nutritional support. There is a need for controlled trials before further advice can be given.

Diarrhoea

Patients with symptoms lasting more than 2 weeks should be investigated. Some of the more common causes are discussed below.

Bacterial Enteric Infections

Bacterial enteric infections account for less than 5% of opportunistic infections in AIDS patients. One study from San Francisco showed a twentyfold increase in *Salmonella* infections (Celum et al. 1987). Non-typhoidal salmonellas such as *S. typhimurium* and *S. enteritidis* are particularly common. *Shigella* and *Campylobacter* infections are also more common. Patients present with severe diarrhoeal symptoms, and 45% of the patients in the San Francisco study had bacteraemia (Celum et al. 1987). It is important to exclude toxic megacolon with plain abdominal radiography (Fig. 5.8). Patients with toxic megacolon should be treated with aggressive medical therapy including intravenous fluid

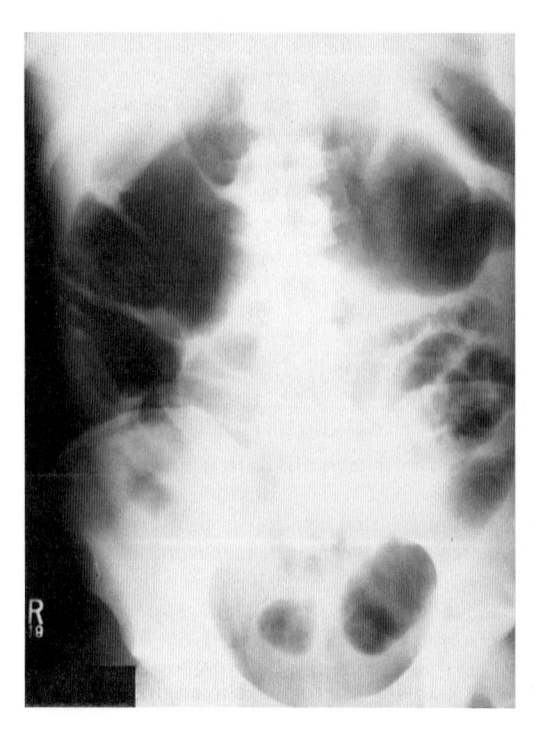

Fig. 5.8. Plain abdominal radiograph, showing toxic dilatation of proximal and transverse colon associated with CMV colitis.

and antibiotics; surgery appears to carry a poor prognosis (Beaugerie et al. 1991). Organisms are usually sensitive to conventional therapy, but drugs may need to be given parenterally. Relapse of invasive salmonellosis following cessation of treatment is common and is an indication for secondary prophylaxis.

Post mortem studies of patients with *Mycobacterium avium-intracellulare* or other atypical mycobacterial infections show the gut is involved in 60% of cases. A characteristic endoscopic duodenal mucosal appearance has been described (Gray and Rabenek 1989). These organisms are commonly found in the environment and a single isolation from stool samples is probably not significant. In patients with diarrhoea and repeated positive samples, disseminated mycobacterial disease should be considered, especially if *Mycobacteria* are found at a second site, and if other findings such as fever and anaemia are present. Treatment regimens are still evolving, but the aim of treatment is symptomatic relief rather than cure of infection. A regimen of intravenous amikacin accompanied by oral ciprofloxacin, ethambutol and rifampicin has been effective in our unit (Scoular et al. 1991).

Intestinal spirochaetes occur in 36% of homosexual men (McMillan and Lee 1981), and have been traditionally regarded as non-pathogenic. However one case report suggested that in AIDS patients the organism, like so many other "non-pathogens", may cause symptoms (Nathwani et al. 1990). However, treatment of intestinal spirochaetosis makes little difference to diarrhoeal symptoms (Connolly et al. 1989c).

Protozoa

One of the manifestations of the "Gay Bowel" syndrome was the high prevalence of intestinal parasites. The pathogenicity of these organisms has been questioned, especially in the context of HIV infection. *Entamoeba histolytica* has been subspeciated on the basis of the electrophoretic mobility of its iso-enzymes into 22 zymodemes. The zymodemes found in homosexual men appear to be non-pathogenic even in HIV-positive individuals (Allason-Jones et al. 1988). *Entamoeba coli, Entamoeba hartmanni, Endolinax nana* and *Iodamoeba buetschlii* do not produce disease in humans. *Blastocystis hominis* is usually not associated with disease.

Cryptosporidium, a small 4.5 μm organism, is one of the most common pathogens isolated from HIV-infected patients with diarrhoea. The parasite may be transmitted via a number of different routes. Initially the disease was thought to be a zoonosis, but water contamination, sexual and nosocomial transmission have all been reported (Current et al. 1983; D'Antonio et al. 1985; Soave et al. 1984; Ravn et al. 1991). Cryptosporidiosis occurs in both immunocompetent and immunosuppressed populations, although the disease is often more severe in the latter group. The degree of immunosuppression influences patient prognosis and HIV-infected patients with reasonable immune function may recover spontaneously from their cryptosporidial infection (Blanshard et al. 1992; McGowan et al. 1993). Clinically, patients present with watery diarrhoea which may vary in volume from 1 to 17 l per day, together with abdominal pain and fever. *Cryptosporidium* has also been associated with sclerosing cholangitis (Dowsett et al. 1988). Diagnosis is discussed elsewhere. Treatment is supportive as no agent has shown convincing efficacy. *Cryptosporidium* is difficult to eradicate from the water supply as it is resistant to most agents used in conventional concentrations, and its small size allows it to pass through most filtration systems. The organism is heat-sensitive and immunosuppressed patients should be advised to boil water for drinking purposes.

Giardia lamblia is a common cause of diarrhoea. Patients present with watery diarrhoea, abdominal pain and flatulence. Trophozoites may be identified in faeces, but occasionally the organism is identified in duodenal aspirate, or on routine histopathology of duodenal biopsies. Treatment is with metronidazole or tinidazole, but relapse may occur.

Isospora belli is an opportunistic protozoan that produces diarrhoea in AIDS patients. Isosporiasis is uncommon in developed countries, but has been reported in 15% of AIDS patients in Haiti (Pape et al. 1989). The organism can be treated with trimethoprim-sulphamethoxazole, but relapse is common. Pyrimethamine may be used as secondary prophylaxis.

Microsporidia are perhaps the most recent organisms to be associated with HIV-related diarrhoea (Muscat 1990; Eeftink Schattenkirk et al. 1991). There are over 700 species although only six have been associated with disease in immunocompromised humans. Hepatitis, peritonitis, keratopathy, conjunctivitis, nasal obstruction, and sclerosing cholangitis have all been reported in association with *Microsporidia*. *Enterocytozoon bieneusi* is the most common species associated with diarrhoea. Diagnosis is difficult as the spores are only 1.5 μm in diameter and are best seen using electron microscopy. Stool samples and duodenal smears stained with Giemsa are being evaluated for use in identifying *Microsporidia* (Van Gool et al. 1990; Weber et al. 1992). Treatment is difficult. Chloroquine, tetracycline, and spiramycin have all shown some efficacy in suppressing *Encephalitozoon cuniculi* spore production *in vitro* (Waller 1979). Albendazole has shown promise in AIDS patients with microsporidiosis (Blanshard et al. 1991).

Coccidian parasites variously described as blue-green algae or cyanobacterium-like bodies have been described as an important cause of prolonged diarrhoea in travellers returning from the tropics (Pollok et al. 1992). These organisms may also affect patients with HIV infection and produce a prolonged illness characterised by watery diarrhoea and weight loss. Treatment with cotrimoxazole may be effective.

Fungal Enteric Infections

The isolation of yeasts from stool samples is a common laboratory finding of uncertain significance. Gupta and Ehrinpreis (1990) have described 10 cases of diarrhoea in a heterogeneous population of critically ill patients with non-HIV disease, which was characterised by the presence of *Candida albicans* in stool culture and a rapid therapeutic response to anti-fungal therapy. There are no similar reports in patients with AIDS.

Viral Enteric Infections

By 50 years of age 50% of the population will have been exposed to the CMV and developed immunity. In homosexual men almost 90% have evidence of previous infection. As with other herpes viruses CMV remains latent within the host. The immunosuppression associated with HIV infection allows the virus to reactivate and cause symptoms. In AIDS patients CMV has been associated with choroidoretinitis, pneumonitis, encephalitis, oesophagitis, sclerosing cholangitis, hepatitis and adrenalitis. CMV colitis occurs in less than 5% of patients with AIDS (Jacobson et al. 1988). A recent case report demonstrated CMV proctitis associated with an HIV seroconversion illness (Gupta 1993). Symptoms of CMV colitis include bloody diarrhoea, abdominal pain and fever. Colonic perforation has also been reported (De Riso et al. 1989). Sigmoidoscopy may show diffuse erythema and mucosal ulceration. Occasionally the mucosal lesions which may be segmental are only found at colonoscopy. Diagnosis is histopathological and is made on the basis of characteristic CMV inclusion bodies, or detection of CMV antigen with monoclonal antibodies (Culpepper-Morgan et al. 1987). Treatment is with ganciclovir or foscarnet (Table 5.4). Response to induction therapy is relatively poor and early relapse common despite maintenance treatment (Dieterich et al. 1988; Peters et al. 1991; Blanshard 1992).

Adenovirus has been identified in 7.4% of HIV-infected homosexual men with diarrhoea, by using a combination of virus culture and transmission electron microscopy (Janoff et al. 1991). Only one of the patients had a potential copathogen to explain the diarrhoea. No specific treatment is available.

KS and Lymphoma

Visceral Kaposi's sarcoma and lymphoma can both involve the gastrointestinal tract and present with diarrhoea. In clinical practice this is not a major problem. In rare cases patients may abuse laxatives. Pseudomembranous colitis in HIV-infected patients is treated in the same way as in seronegative patients with oral vancomycin or metronidazole.

Symptomatic Treatment

The effective management of HIV-related diarrhoea depends on appropriate investigation to identify pathogens. Although in many cases this is possible, many organisms are of uncertain pathogenicity, and others respond poorly to specific treatment. Symptomatic treatment is therefore an important component of management in all cases. Fluid can be given orally in the form of glucose and electrolyte solutions. In patients with severe diarrhoea and vomiting, intravenous fluids may be needed. In all cases it is important to be aware of patients' home circumstances. The appropriate use of commodes and incontinence pads can do much to improve patients' quality of life.

It is possible to control the vast majority of diarrhoea by using anti-diarrhoeal agents in a step-wise manner as suggested below. There is no fixed regimen, and one can combine 1st line agents before moving on to more potent opiates.

Antidiarrhoeal Agents

1st Line Therapy.   Loperamide, diphenoxylate, codeine phosphate.

2nd Line therapy.   Morphine (slow release preparation).

3rd Line Therapy.   Intractable diarrhoea may respond to subcutaneous administration of diamorphine. Somatostatin and interleukin 2 have been used on an experimental basis without clear evidence of efficacy.

Perianal Problems

HSV is a difficult problem in the context of HIV-associated immunosuppression. Attacks tend to become more frequent, the symptoms are more severe, and the lesions more widespread. Response to short courses of acyclovir are often unsatisfactory, and most patients require maintenance therapy (Table 5.4). In spite of adequate suppressive therapy, some individuals develop resistant ulceration which fails to respond to intravenous acyclovir (Erlich et al. 1989). This has been found to be partially due to the emergence of thymidine kinase-deficient strains of HSV. Foscarnet is not phosphorylated by viral thymidine kinase, and may be helpful in this situation.

HPV infection is common in homosexual men. Perianal warts tend to be more resistant to therapy in immunosuppressed patients with HIV, but more worrying is the association between HPV infection, anal intra-epithelial neoplasia (AIN), and HIV. It has been suggested that the incidence of anorectal cancer in homosexual men is 25–50 times that of heterosexual controls (Daling et al. 1982). In a more recent study anorectal dysplasia in homosexual men was associated with a history of anal warts, frequent receptive anal intercourse, antibody to HIV and a low CD4/CD8 lymphocyte ratio (Frazer et al. 1986). Perianal warts can be treated with local application of podophyllin, or cryotherapy. Resistant lesions may be removed surgically, but recurrence is common. Anal intra-epithelial neoplasia may be diagnosed on biopsy, but it is uncertain what percentage will develop local carcinoma. Careful proctoscopic examination and follow-up is important, but no specific treatment is recommended.

Kaposi's Sarcoma/Lymphoma

Treatment of gastrointestinal KS is indicated if there are major symptoms (Spittle 1989). Local lesions in the mouth may respond to radiotherapy, but chemotherapy is the main modality of treatment. A variety of chemotherapy regimes have been used. Complex combination chemotherapy has the disadvantage of causing increased immunosuppression and increased risk of opportunistic infections. Simple regimes using vincristine and bleomycin alone or in combination produce a response in up to 75% of patients with a low risk of bone marrow suppression (Gill et al. 1990). Alpha interferon may be used to induce remission of KS in patients with CD4 counts of 200 or more, but high doses are needed, and side effects such as fatigue, fever and alopecia are common. This form of treatment is not beneficial in more immunosuppressed patients. The outlook with lymphoma is generally poor, but depends on the histological characteristics of the tumour, with large non-cleaved cell tumours having the best prognosis. Treatment with modified combination chemotherapy regimes may produce a clinical response, at the expense of increased immunosuppression.

Future Developments

With the advent of laboratory techniques such as immunohistochemistry, *in-situ* hybridisation and polymerase chain reaction, it has become possible to study HIV enteropathy in much more detail. Villous atrophy has been described using standard histopathological methods, and immunohistochemical staining has identified a number of features such as selective depletion of T4 lymphocytes within the lamina propria. Current research may clarify how HIV interacts with the various cellular components of the gut mucosa, and whether local release of cytokines mediates enterocyte damage.

Improved health care and the use of antiretroviral therapy has meant that patients with AIDS are surviving for longer periods of time. One consequence of this has been the emergence of drug resistance. Oro-pharyngeal candidiasis, peri-anal herpes simplex infection and CMV ulceration have shown resistance to treatment with conventional agents.

Gastrointestinal CMV disease is a late manifestation of AIDS and has a poor prognosis. Consequently it has been difficult to assess the impact of anti-CMV therapy. Ganciclovir has been used (Dieterich et al. 1988), and now there is evidence that foscarnet may be efficacious (Hawkins et al. 1991). A novel form of therapy with TI-23 (a human monoclonal anti-CMV antibody) may offer hope for the future (Petersen et al. 1991).

KS is known to occur in homosexual men without any evidence of HIV infection (Safai et al. 1991). This and other epidemiological evidence suggests that an enteric sexually transmitted agent, possibly viral, may be responsible (Beral et al. 1992; Soriano et al. 1991). Treatment of visceral KS remains difficult. Combination chemotherapy and interferon have both been tried, but studies tend to be small with poorly defined end points. DAB_{486} IL-2 is a recombinant fusion protein composed of human IL-2 and cytotoxic fragments of *diphtheria* toxin. It is thought to act by binding to IL-2 receptors on KS cells. A preliminary study in 2 patients with chemotherapy-resistant KS demonstrated a 30% reduction in cutaneous lesions (LeMaistre et al. 1991).

Following the development of serological tests for HCV antibodies, several centres are carrying out sero-epidemiological studies. Chirianni investigated 206 Italian HIV seropositive patients. 47% of intravenous drug users (74/155), 62% of post transfusion patients (5/8), 20% of homosexual men (4/20) and 8.7% of heterosexuals (2/23) were HCV seropositive (Chirianni et al. 1991). In the near future we are likely to see a rapid growth in information about the natural history of HCV and its interactions with HIV and HBV.

References

Allason-Jones E, Mindel A, Sargeaunt P et al. (1988) Outcome of untreated infection with *Entamoeba histolytica* in homosexual men with and without HIV antibody. Br Med J 297: 654–657

Bartelsman JF, Sars PR, Tygat GN (1989) Gastrointestinal complications in patients with acquired immunodeficiency. Scand J Gastroenterol 24: 112–117

Beaugerie L, Goujard F, Gharakhanian et al. (1991) Etiology and Management of Toxic Megacolon in AIDS Patients. VII International Conference on AIDS, Florence (abstract M.B. 2204)

Beral V, Peterman TA, Berkelman RL, Jaffe HN (1990) Kaposi's sarcoma among persons with AIDS: a sexually transmitted infection? Lancet 335: 123–128

Beral V, Bull D, Jaffe H et al. (1991) Is the risk of Kaposi's sarcoma in AIDS patients in Britain increased if sexual partners came from the United States or Africa. Br Med J 302: 624–625

Beral V, Bull D, Darby S, et al. (1992) Risk of Kaposi's sarcoma and sexual practices associated with faecal contact in homosexual or bisexual men with AIDS. Lancet 339: 632–635

Blanshard C (1992) Treatment of HIV-related cytomegalovirus disease of the gastrointestinal tract with foscarnet. J Acq Imm Defic Syn 5 (Suppl 1): S25–S28

Blanshard C, Peacock C, Ellis D, Gazzard B (1991) Treatment of intestinal microsporidiosis with Albendazole. VII International Conference on AIDS, Florence (abstract W.B. 2265)

Blanshard C, Jackson AM, Shanson DC, Francis N, Gazzard BG (1992) Cryptosporidiosis in HIV-seropositive patients. Q J Med 85: 813–823

Bourinbaiar AS, Phillips DM (1991) Transmission of human immunodeficiency virus from monocytes to epithelia. J Acq Imm Defic Syn 4: 56–63

British Society of Gastroenterology (1989) Cleaning and disinfection of equipment for gastro-intestinal flexible endoscopy: recommendations of a working party of the British Society of Gastroenterology. Gut 29: 1134–1151

Brivet F, Coffin B, Bedossa P et al. (1987) Pancreatic lesions in AIDS. Lancet ii: 570

Cappell MS, Schwartz MS, Biempica L (1990) Clinical utility of liver biopsy in patients with serum antibodies to the human immunodeficiency virus. Am J Med 88: 123–130

Carne CA, Weller IVD, Waite J et al. (1987) Impaired responsiveness of homosexual men with HIV antibodies to plasma derived hepatitis B vaccine. Br Med J 294: 866–868

Cello JP (1989) Acquired immunodeficiency syndrome cholangiopathy: spectrum of disease. Am J Med 86: 539–546

Celum CL, Chaisson RE, Rutherford GW, Barnhart JL, Echenberg DF (1987) Incidence of salmonellosis in patients with AIDS. J Infect Dis 156; 6:998–1001

Centers for Disease Control (1987) Revision of the CDC surveillance case definition for acquired immunodeficiency syndrome. MMWR 36 (Suppl 2S): 3S–15S

Chirianni A, Abrescia N, Tullio Cataldo et al. (1991) Anti-HCV prevalence in HIV infected patients. VII International Conference on AIDS, Florence (abstract W.B. 87)

Churchill DR, Kenton-Smith J, Malin A (1992) Oesophageal stricture complicating cytomegalovirus ulceration in a patient with AIDS. J Infect 25: 108–109

Clotet B, Grifol M, Parro O et al. (1986). Asymptomatic esophageal candidiasis in the acquired-immunodeficiency-syndrome-related-complex. Ann Intern Med 105: 145

Comer GM, Mukherjee S, Scholes JV, Holness LG, Clain DJ (1989) Liver biopsies in the acquired immunodeficiency syndrome: influence of endemic disease and drug abuse. Am J Gastroenterol 84; 12: 1525–1531

Connolly GM, Forbes A, Gleeson JA (1989a) Short communication: investigation of upper gastrointestinal symptoms in patients with AIDS. AIDS 3: 453–456

Connolly GM, Hawkins D, Harcourt-Webster JN, et al. (1989b) Oesophageal symptoms, their causes, treatment, and prognosis in patients with the acquired immunodeficiency syndrome. Gut 30: 1033–1039

Connolly GM, Shanson D, Hawkins DA, Harcourt-Webster JN, Gazzard BG (1989c) Non-cryptosporidial diarrhoea in human immunodeficiency virus (HIV) infected patients. Gut 30: 195–200

Culpepper-Morgan JA, Kotler DP, Scholes DP, Tierney AR (1987) Evaluation of diagnostic criteria for mucosal cytomegalic inclusion disease in the acquired immunodeficiency syndrome. Am J Gastroenterol 82; 12: 1264–1270

Cummins AG, La Brooy JT, Stanley DP, Rowland R, Shearman DJC (1990) Quantitative histological study of enteropathy associated with HIV infection. Gut 31: 317–321

Current WL, Reese NC, Ernst JV et al. (1983) Human cryptosporidiosis in immunocompetent and immunodeficient persons. N Engl J Med 308: 289–296

Daling JR, Weiss NS, Klopfenstein LL et al. (1982) Correlates of homosexual behaviour and the incidence of anal cancer. JAMA 247: 1988–1990

D'Antonio RG, Winn RE, Taylor JP et al. (1988) A waterborne outbreak of cryptosporidiosis in normal hosts. Ann Int Med 103: 886–888

De Riso AJ, Kemeny MM, Torres RA, Oliver JM (1989) Multiple jejunal perforations secondary to cytomegalovirus in a patient with acquired immunodeficiency syndrome. Dig Dis Sci 34: 623–629

Dieterich DT, Chachoua, LaFleur F, Worrell C (1988) Ganciclovir treatment of gastrointestinal infections caused by cytomegalovirus in patients with AIDS. Rev Inf Dis 10 (Suppl 3): 532–537

Dieterich D, Kotler D, Busch D et al. (1990) Randomized, placebo-controlled study of ganciclovir treatment of cytomegalovirus (CMV) colitis in AIDS patients (PTS). VI International Conference on AIDS, San Francisco (abstract F.B.94)

Dowsett JF, Miller R, Davidson R et al. (1988) Sclerosing cholangitis in acquired immunodeficiency syndrome. Scand J Gastroenterol 23: 1267–1274

Eeftink Schattenkirk JKM, van Gool T, van Ketel RJ et al. (1991) Clinical significance of small intestinal microsporidiosis in HIV-1-infected individuals. Lancet 337: 895–898

Erlich KS, Mills J, Chatis P et al. (1989) Acyclovir resistant herpes simplex virus infections in patients with the acquired immunodeficiency syndrome. N Engl J Med 320: 293–296

Fauci AS, Macher AM, Longo DC et al. (1984) Acquired immunodeficiency syndrome: epidemiologic, clinical, immunologic and theraputic considerations. Ann Intern Med 100: 92–106

Flynn N, Enders S, Oster M, Cone L, Hooten T (1992) Megestrol acetate 800mg/day vs placebo for treatment of weight loss and anorexia in AIDS patients. VIIIth International Conference on AIDS, Amsterdam, (abstract PoB 3687)

Forbes A, Blanshard C, Gazzard B (1993) Natural history of AIDS related sclerosing cholangitis: a study of 20 cases. Gut 34: 116–121

Francis ND, Boylston AW, Roberts AHG, Parkin JM, Pinching AJ (1989) Cytomegalovirus infection in gastrointestinal tracts of patients infected with HIV-1 or AIDS. J Clin Pathol 42: 1055–1064

Frazer IH, Crapper RM, Medley G et al. (1986) Association between anorectal dysplasia, human papilloma virus and human immunodeficiency virus in homosexual men. Lancet i: 657–660

Friedman SL, Wright TL, Altman DF (1985) Gastrointestinal Kaposi's sarcoma in patients with acquired immunodeficiency syndrome. Endoscopic and autopsy findings. Gastroenterology 89: 102–108

Gill P, Rarick M, Bernstein-Singer M et al. (1990) Treatment of advanced Kaposi's sarcoma using a combination of bleomycin and vincristine. Am J Clin Oncol 13: 315–319

Goodgame RW, Ross PG, Kim HS, Hook AG, Sutton FM (1991) Esophageal stricture after cytomegalovirus ulcer treated with ganciclovir. J Clin Gastroenterol 13: 678–681

Gray JR and Rabenek L (1989) Atypical mycobacterial infection of the gastrointestinal tract in AIDS patients. Am J Gastroenterol 84: 1521–1524

Greenson JK, Belitsos PC, Yardley JH, Bartlett JG (1991) AIDS enteropathy: occult enteric infections and duodenal mucosal alterations in chronic diarrhoea. Ann Intern Med 114: 366–372

Greenspan JS, Greenspan D, Lennette ET et al. (1985) Replication of Epstein-Barr virus within the epithelial cells of oral "hairy" leukoplakia, an AIDS-associated lesion. N Engl J Med 313: 1564–1571

Griffin GE, Miller A, Batman P et al. (1988) Damage to jejunal intrinsic autonomic nerves in HIV infection. AIDS 2: 379–382

Grunfeld C, Pang M, Shimizu L, Shigenaga JK, Jensen P, Feingold KR (1992) Resting energy expenditure, caloric intake, and short term weight change in human immunodeficiency virus infection and the acquired immunodeficiency syndrome. Am J Clin Nutr 55: 455–460

Grunfeld C, Pang M, Doerrier W, Shigenaga JK, Jensen P, Feingold KR (1992) Lipids, lipoproteins, triglyceride clearance and cytokines in human immunodeficiency virus infection and the acquired immunodeficiency syndrome. J Clin Endocrinol Metab 74: 1045–1052

Gupta KK (1993) Acute immunosuppression with seroconversion. N Engl J Med 328: 288–289

Gupta TP and Ehrinpreis MN (1990) *Candida* associated diarrhoea in hospitalised patients. Gastroenterology 98: 780–785

Hawkins D, Nelson M, Connolly G, Francis N, Gazzard B (1991) Foscarnet in the treatment of cytomegalovirus infection of the oesophagus and colon. VII International Conference on AIDS, Florence (abstract W.B. 2262)

Hillman RJ, Gopal Rao G, Harris JRW, Taylor-Robinson D (1990) Ciprofloxacin as a cause of *Clostridium difficile*-associated diarrhoea in an HIV antibody positive patient. J Infect 21: 205–207

Jacobson MA, O'Donnell JJ, Porteous D, Brodie HR, Feigal D, Mills J (1988) Retinal and gastrointestinal disease due to cytomegalovirus in patients with the acquired immune deficiency syndrome: prevalence, natural history and response to ganciclovir therapy. Q J Med 67: 473–486

Janoff EN, Orenstein JM, Manischewitz JF, Smith PD (1991) Adenovirus colitis in the acquired immunodeficiency syndrome. Gastroenterology 100: 976–979

Jarry A, Cortez A, Renee A, Muzeau F, Brousse N (1990) Infected cells and immune cells in the gastrointestinal tract of AIDS patients. An immunohistochemical study of 127 cases. Histopathology 16: 133–140

Kapembwa MS, Batman PA, Fleming SC et al (1989) HIV enteropathy. Lancet ii: 1521–1522

Kapembwa MS, Bridges C, Joseph AE, Fleming SC, Batman P, Griffin GE (1990) Ileal and jejunal absorptive function in patients with AIDS and enterococcidial infection. J Infect 21: 43-53

Kavin H, Jonas RB, Chowdhury L, Kabin S (1986) Acalculous cholecystitis and cytomegalovirus infections in the acquired immunodeficiency syndrome. Ann Intern Med 104: 53-54

Kazlow PG, Shah K, Benkov KJ, Dische R, Leleiko NS (1986) Oesophageal cryptosporidiosis in a child with the acquired immunodeficiency syndrome. Gastroenterology 91: 1301-1303

Kelly GE, Stanley BS, Weller IVD (1990) The natural history of human immunodeficiency virus infection: a five year study in a London cohort of homosexual men. Genitourin Medicine 66: 238-243

Kitchen VS, Helbert M Francis ND et al (1990) Epstein-Barr virus associated oesophageal ulcers in AIDS. Gut 31: 1223-1225

Klein RS, Harris CA, Small CB et al (1984) Oral candidiasis in high risk patients as the initial manifestation of the acquired immunodeficiency syndrome. N Engl J Med 311: 354-358

Knowles DM, Chomilak GA, Subar M et al. (1988) Lymphoid neoplasia associated with the acquired immune deficiency syndrome (AIDS). Ann Intern Med 108: 744-753

Kotler DP (1989) Intestinal and hepatic manifestations of AIDS. Adv Intern Med 34: 43-71

Kotler DP, Gaetz JP, Lange M, Klein EB, Holt PR (1984) Enteropathy associated with the acquired immunodeficiency syndrome. Ann Intern Med 101: 421-428

Kotler DP, Scholes JV, Tierney AR (1987) Intestinal plasma cell alterations in acquired immunodeficiency syndrome. Dig Dis Sci 32: 129-138

Kotler DP, Tierney AR, Wang J, Pierson RN (1989a) Magnitude of body-cell-mass depletion and the timing of death from wasting in AIDS. Am J Clin Nutr 50: 444-447

Kotler DP, Tierney AR, Altilio D et al. (1989b) Body mass repletion during ganciclovir treatment of cytomegalovirus infections in patients with acquired immunodeficiency syndrome. Arch Intern Med 149: 901-905

Kotler DP, Tierney AR, Ferraro R, Cuff P, Wang J, Pierson RN (1991) Enteral alimentation and repletion of body cell mass in malnourished patients with acquired immunodeficiency syndrome. Am J Clin Nutr 53: 149-154

Krogsgaard K, Lindhart BO, Nielsen JO et al (1987) The influence of HTLV-III infection on the natural history of hepatitis B virus infection in male homosexual HBsAg carriers. Hepatology 1: 37-41

Kuo G, Choo QL, Alter HJ (1989) An assay for circulating antibodies to a major etiologic virus of human non-A, non-B hepatitis. Science 244: 362-364

Laine L, Bonacini M, Sattler F, Young T, Sherrod A (1992a) Cytomegalovirus and *Candida* esophagitis in patients with AIDS. J Acq Imm Defic Syn 5: 605-609

Laine L, Dretler R, Conteas C et al. (1992b) Fluconazole compared with ketoconazole for the treatment of *Candida* esophagitis in AIDS. Ann Intern Med 117: 655-660

LeMaistre CF, Craig F, Smith J et al. (1991) Phase I/II evaluation of an IL-2 receptor targeted fusion toxin, $DAB_{486}IL-2$, for treatment of AIDS-associated Kaposi's sarcoma. VII International Conference on AIDS, Florence (abstract TU.B.85)

Levy JA, Margaretten W, Nelson J (1989) Detection of HIV in enterochromaffin cells in the rectal mucosa of an AIDS patient. Am J Gastroenterol 84; 7: 787-789

Ma P, Soave R (1983) Three-step stool examination for cryptosporidiosis in 10 homosexual men with protracted watery diarrhoea. J Infect Dis 147: 824-828

McDonald JA, Harris S, Waters JA, Thomas HC (1987) Effect of human immunodeficiency virus (HIV) infection on chronic hepatitis B viral antigen display. J Hepatol 4: 337-342

McGowan I, Hawkins AS, Weller IVD (1993) The natural history of cryptosporidial diarrhoea in HIV-infected patients. AIDS 7: 349-354

McMillan A, Lee FD (1981) Sigmoidoscopic and microscopic appearance of the rectal mucosa in homosexual men. Gut 22: 1035-1041

Miller ARO, Griffin GE, Batman P et al. (1988) Jejunal mucosal architecture and fat absorption in male homosexuals infected with human immunodeficiency virus. Q J Med 69: 1009-1119

Miller RF (1990) Nuclear medicine and AIDS. Eur J Nucl Med 16: 103-118

Muscat I (1990) Editorial: Human microsporidiosis. J Infect Dis 21: 125-129

Nathwani D, McWhinney PHM, Green ST, Boyd JD (1990) Intestinal spirochaetosis in a man with the acquired immune deficiency syndrome (AIDS). J Infect 21; 3: 318-319

Nelson J, Reynolds-Kohler C, Margaretten W, Wiley CA, Reese CE, Levy JA (1988) Human immunodeficiency virus detected in bowel epithelium from patients with gastrointestinal symptoms. Lancet i: 259-262

Nelson MR, Connolly GM, Hawkins DA, Gazzard BG (1991) Foscarnet in the treatment of cytomegalovirus infection of the esophagus and colon in patients with the acquired immunodeficiency syndrome. Am J Gastroenterol 86: 876–881

Nelson M, Shanson D, Hawkins D, Gazzard B (1992) *Salmonella, Campylobacter* and *Shigella* in HIV-seropositive patients. AIDS 6: 1495–1498

Pape JW, Verdier R, Johnson WD (1989) Treatment and prophylaxis of *Isospora belli* infection in patients with the acquired immunodeficiency syndrome. N Eng J Med 320: 1044–1047

Parente F, Cernushi M, Rizzardini G, Lazzarin A, Valsecchi L, Bianchi-Porro G (1991) Opportunistic infections of the oesophagus not responding to oral systemic antifungals in patients with AIDS: their frequency and treatment. Am J Gastroenterol 86: 1729–1734

Perrone V, Pergola M, Abate G et al. (1981) Protein-losing enteropathy in a patient with generalised Kaposi's sarcoma. Cancer 47: 588–591

Peters BS, Beck EJ, Anderson et al. (1991) Cytomegalovirus infection in AIDS. Patterns of disease, response to therapy and trends in survival. J Infect 23: 129–137

Petersen E, Gray J, Grayson J et al. (1991) Therapy with human monoclonal antibody (Mab) to cytomegalovirus (TI-23). VII International Conference on AIDS, Florence (abstract W.B. 2291)

Pluda JM, Yarchoan R, Jaffee ES et al. (1990) Development of non-Hodgkin lymphoma in a cohort of patients with severe HIV infection on long term anti-retroviral therapy. Ann Intern Med 113: 276–282

Pol S, Romana CA, Richard S et al. (1993) Microsporidia infection in patients with the human immunodeficiency virus and unexplained cholangitis. N Engl J Med 328: 95–99

Pollok RCG, Bendall RP, Moody A, Chiodini PL, Churchill DR (1992) Traveller's diarrhoea associated with cyanobacterium-like bodies. Lancet 340: 556–557

Quinnan GV, Masur H, Rook AH et al. (1984) Herpes virus infections in the acquired immune deficiency syndrome. JAMA 252: 72–77

Rabeneck L, Popovic M, Gartner S et al. (1990) Acute HIV infection presenting with painful swallowing and esophageal ulcers. JAMA 263; 7: 2318–2322

Ravn P, Lundgren JD, Kjaeldgaard P et al. (1991) Nosocomial outbreak of cryptosporidiosis in AIDS patients. Br Med J 302: 277–280

Resnick L, Herbst JS, Ablastin DV et al. (1988) Regression of oral hairy leukoplakia after orally administered acyclovir therapy. JAMA 259: 384–388

Safai B, Peralta H, Menzies K et al. (1991) Kaposi's sarcoma amongst HIV-seronegative high risk population. VII International Conference on AIDS, Florence (abstract TU.B. 83)

Schneiderman DJ, Cello JP, Laing FC (1987) Papillary stenosis and sclerosing cholangitis in the acquired immunodeficiency syndrome. Ann Intern Med 106: 546–549

Scoular A, French P, Miller RF (1991) *Mycobacterium avium-intracellulare* infection in the acquired immunodeficiency syndrome. Br J Hosp Med 46: 295–300

Serwadda D, Mugerwa RD, Sewankambo KN et al. (1985) Slim disease: a new disease in Uganda and its association with HTLV-III infection. Lancet 2: 849–852

Sheather AL (1953) The detection of intestinal protozoa and mange parasites by a flotation technique. J Comp Pathol 36: 268–275

Singer P, Rothkopf MM, Kvetan V, Kirvela O, Gaare J, Askanazi J (1991) Risks and benefits of home parenteral nutrition in the acquired immunodeficiency syndrome. J Parenter Enteral Nutr 15: 75–79

Soave R, Danner RL, Honig CL et al. (1984) Cryptosporidiosis in homosexual men. Ann Intern Med 100: 504–511

Sokol-Anderson ML, Prelutsky DJ, Westblom TU. (1991) Giant esophageal aphthous ulcers in AIDS patients: treatment with low-dose corticosteroids. AIDS 5: 1537–1538

Soriano V, Hewlett I, Friedman-Kien AE, Tor J, Huang X, Epstein L (1991) Definitive exclusion of HIV infection in a Kaposi's sarcoma bisexual man. Suggestions on a pathogenic model of KS. VII International Conference on AIDS, Florence (abstract TU.B. 82)

Spittle MF (1989) Diagnosis and treatment of Kaposi's sarcoma. J Antimicrob Chemother 23 Suppl A: 127–135

Tavitian A, Raufman JP, Rosenthal LE (1986) Oral candidiasis as a marker for oesophageal candidiasis in the acquired immunodeficiency syndrome. Ann Intern Med 104: 54–55

Tedder RS, Gilson RJC, Briggs M et al. (1991) Hepatitis C virus: evidence for sexual transmission. Br Med J 302: 1299–1302

Theise ND, Rotterdam H, Dieterich D (1991) Cytomegalovirus esophagitis in AIDS: diagnosis by endoscopic biopsy. Am J Gastroenterol 86: 1123–1126

Ullrich R, Zeitz M, Heise W, L'age M, Hoffken G, Riecken EO (1989) Small intestinal structure and function in patients infected with human immunodeficiency virus (HIV): Evidence for HIV induced enteropathy. Ann Intern Med 111: 15–21

Underhill GS, Jeffries DJ, Forster GE, Harris JR (1986) Correlation between fulminant form of viral hepatitis and retrovirus infection associated with AIDS. Br Med J 292: 1080–1081

Van Gool T, Hollister WS, Eeftinck Schattenkerk J et al. (1990) Diagnosis of *Enterocytozoon bienusi* microsporidiosis in AIDS patients by recovery of spores from faeces. Lancet 336: 697–698

Van Roenn JH, Murphy RL, Weber KM, Williams LM, Weitzman SA (1988) Megestrol acetate for treatment of cachexia associated with human immunodeficiency virus (HIV) infection. Ann Intern Med 109: 840–841

Vendrell J, Nubiola A, Goday A et al. (1987) HIV and the pancreas. Lancet ii: 1212

Viteri AL and Greene JF (1987) Bile duct abnormalities in the acquired immune deficiency syndrome. Gastroenterology 92: 2014–2018

Waller T (1979) Sensitivity of *Encephalitozoon cuniculi* to various temperatures, disinfectants and drugs. Lab Anim 13: 227–230

Watkins EB, Findlay P, Gelmann E, Lane HC, Zabell A (1989) Enhanced mucosal reactions in AIDS patients receiving oropharyngeal irradiation. Int J Radiation Oncol. Biol. Phys 13: 1403–1408

Weber JN, Thom S, Barrison I et al. (1987) Cytomegalovirus colitis and oesophageal ulceration in the context of AIDS: clinical manifestations and preliminary report of treatment with Foscarnet (phosphonoformate). Gut 28: 482–487

Weber R, Bryan RT, Owen RL, Wilcox CM, Gorelkin L, Visvesvara GS (1992) Improved light-microscopical detection of *microsporidia* spores in stool and duodenal aspirates. N Engl J Med 326: 161–166

Wilcox CM, Diehl, Cello JP, Margaretten W, Jacobson MA (1990) Cytomegalovirus esophagitis in patients with AIDS. A clinical, endoscopic, and pathologic correlation. Ann Intern Med 113: 589–593

Williams I, Weller IVD, Malin A, Anderson J, Waters RSM (1991) Thalidomide hypersensitivity in AIDS. Lancet 337: 436–437

6 Neurological Complications of HIV Infection and AIDS

Hadi Manji, Ruth McAllister, Sean Connolly and Alan Thompson

Introduction

In 1981, as the first cases of the acquired immunodeficiency syndrome (AIDS) were being reported, it soon became apparent that the nervous system was frequently affected. Initially, it seemed as if most of these neurological complications were a consequence of the immunosuppressive effects of the human immunodeficiency virus (HIV) resulting in opportunistic infections (OI) and tumours. However, as the epidemic unfolded, it was obvious that these presentations could account for only up to 30% of the neurological problems seen. In particular, a progressive decline in cognitive function associated with motor deficits was frequently observed, especially in the later stages of the disease. These observations were supported by the experience in paediatric AIDS where children, who are less susceptible to opportunistic infections, were noted to suffer a progressive deterioration in intellectual abilities with the loss of developmental milestones. There is now a substantial body of evidence to suggest that HIV itself may cause damage to the central and peripheral nervous systems.

Neurological problems occur in up to 40% of patients with AIDS and may be the AIDS-defining illness in 10% of such patients (Levy et al. 1988) (Table 6.1). These include opportunistic infections such as toxoplasmosis, cryptococcal meningitis and progressive multifocal leukoencephalopathy (PML). Primary central nervous system lymphoma (PCNSL) is the commonest tumour found in the central nervous system of HIV-infected patients.

Table 6.1. CNS complications of HIV infection

Focal*	Diffuse*
Toxoplasmosis	Cryptococcal meningitis
Lymphoma (PCNSL and NHL)	HIV encephalopathy
PML	CMV encephalitis
Other abscesses, e.g. tuberculoma	
Cerebrovascular disease: infarction, vasculitis	
Herpes simplex encephalitis	

*Considerable overlap exists.

The relative risk of developing a specific complication depends upon a number of factors including the degree of immunosuppression, HIV risk group, race and geographic location. Cytomegalovirus retinitis, for example, is rare with a CD4 count above 0.1×10^9/l. Similarly, cryptococcal meningitis is more prevalent in intravenous drug users (IVDU) and Afro-Americans in the USA than in other risk groups. In Africa, cryptococcal meningitis is the third most common AIDS-defining opportunistic infection after oesophageal candidiasis and extrapulmonary tuberculosis (Taelman et al. 1991). Toxoplasmosis is more common in France than in the UK because of the higher background seroprevalence rate.

In AIDS, as a result of defects in both cellular and humoral immunity, a new spectrum of diseases is being encountered in neurological as in other organ systems. The clinical presentation of these illnesses is often different to that seen in the everyday practice of medicine. For example, in cryptococcal meningitis, only 30% of patients will have the clinical signs of meningism (Chuck and Sande 1989). This, together with the possibility of multiple pathologies occurring simultaneously, requires that a high index of suspicion for neurological disease needs to be maintained by physicians looking after patients with AIDS. However, it should also be stressed that other diagnostic possibilities unrelated to HIV must always be considered.

In the sections that follow the differential diagnoses of some frequently encountered neurological presentations will be considered. Subsequent sections deal with investigations, pathophysiology and management of the common neurological complications. A final section describes the complications due to HIV itself.

Common Neurological Presentations

Headache (Table 6.2)

This common symptom requires careful consideration within the context of HIV infection. It may herald serious, but eminently treatable, complications such as toxoplasmosis and cryptococcal meningitis.

As in everyday neurological practice, a strict adherence to the classic symptoms suggestive of intracranial space-occupying lesions, such as recent onset of

Table 6.2. Differential diagnosis of headache

Meningitis
   Cryptococcal
   Lymphomatous
   HIV-related
   Other infections e.g. tuberculous, listeria

Intracranial mass lesions
   Toxoplasmosis
   Primary CNS lymphoma or metastatic systemic
   Lymphoma
   Other abscesses e.g. tuberculomas

Other causes
   Sinusitis, tension, migraine, drug-induced (e.g. zidovudine) NSAIDs

early-morning headaches which are made worse by coughing or stooping, will result in some of these treatable complications being missed. In HIV infection, these difficulties are compounded by a blunted inflammatory response. Furthermore, especially in the later stages of HIV disease, when cerebral atrophy may be present, it may take longer for signs and symptoms suggestive of raised intracranial pressure such as papilloedema to develop (Luxton and Harrison 1979).

Headache secondary to infection or lymphoma may not be severe, particularly in the early stages, and may respond to analgesics. Sinusitis seems to be commoner in HIV-infected individuals and may cause headaches associated with facial pain and tenderness. Migraine and tension headaches have the same features as in non-infected patients but each may be triggered or exacerbated by intracranial infections or neoplasms.

Tension or stress-related muscle contraction headaches are described as a superficial band-like sensation round the head with a specific tender spot over temporalis or at the insertion of the trapezius muscle. Often the patient may recognise an association with stress. Treatment with analgesics in the long term has little benefit. Simply recognising the headaches for what they are and practising relaxation exercises may be helpful.

Sometimes it can be very difficult to distinguish between organic and non-organic headaches in patients with HIV infection. In any case, the patient should be fully investigated if there is doubt. The following features should alert a physician that urgent investigations are necessary: a recent onset of headaches; a change in character of headaches; focal symptoms or signs and fever with systemic illness. Cranial computed tomography (CT) or magnetic resonance imaging (MRI) should be performed first, and should this prove unhelpful, examination of the cerebrospinal fluid is necessary to look particularly for evidence of cryptococcal meningitis and lymphoma.

In the out-patient clinic, a serum cryptococcal antigen test is a useful screening measure for cryptococcal meningitis. It is positive in over 95% of cases of meningitis (Dismukes 1988), and the result can be obtained in a few hours. A negative result should not, however, lead to a false sense of security.

Headaches are a symptom to be taken seriously. On the other hand, it should be realised that serious intracranial pathology such as toxoplasmosis can exist in patients without headache.

Difficulty in Walking (Table 6.3)

When confronted with a patient who complains of difficulty in walking, it is important initially to assess whether this is due to the general disability which is common in advanced AIDS or due to an underlying neurological disorder. The two may co-exist. The examination must take into account the physical condition of the patient. If the patient is unwell, then frequent rests should be allowed during the examination. The importance of exerting maximum power even for one second should be emphasized - normal power against resistance for that short duration excludes any significant weakness. Debilitated patients may have difficulty in heel-toe walking, but this is usually of no significance. Often, it is only with repeated examinations that any deterioration becomes apparent and the importance of this needs to be stressed.

Table 6.3. Differential diagnosis of difficulty in walking

Central nervous system
  Brain (cerebrum, cerebellum, brainstem)
    toxoplasmosis, lymphoma, PML
    Other abscesses e.g. cryptococcoma, tuberculoma
    Infarcts e.g. vasculitis

  Spinal cord
    Vacuolar myelopathy
    Myelitis (HVZ, HS)
    Toxoplasmosis, lymphoma
    HTLV1 (coinfection)

Peripheral nervous system
  Nerve roots
    Cauda equina syndrome
    CMV polyradiculopathy, lymphoma, syphilis, HIV

  Single nerve lesions
    Mononeuritis multiplex
    Pressure palsies e.g. lateral popliteal nerve palsy

  Neuropathies
    Distal symmetrical neuropathy
    Demyelinating neuropathy
    Drugs e.g. vincristine, isoniazid, ddI, ddC

  Muscle disease (myopathy)
    autoimmune
    HIV-related
    zidovudine induced
    Steroids

After the history and examination, it should be possible to locate the site(s) of pathology in the majority of cases. For example, the presence of some of the following features should raise the possibility of spinal cord involvement: weakness of proximal and distal muscles in the lower limbs but without upper limb involvement (an important other cause being a parasaggital intracranial lesion); involvement of the upper and lower limbs but with no abnormal signs above the neck (with a normal jaw jerk); the presence of a sensory level or sensory disturbance on the chest, abdomen or perineum; sphincter problems and back pain. Lhermitte's phenomenon (neck flexion producing an electrical shock sensation down the back and sometimes into the legs) suggests cervical cord pathology. The usual cause of a myelopathy in a patient with AIDS is the vacuolar myelopathy. Although, to date, myelography and spinal MRI have failed to reveal abnormalities in this condition, imaging of the spinal cord and analysis of cerebrospinal fluid (CSF) is mandatory to exclude disease due to malignancy and infection. Vitamin B12 deficiency and coinfection with HTLV-I should also be considered in the differential diagnosis.

A progressive hemiparesis should raise the possibility of an intracranial lesion. Unsteadiness may relate to involvement of the cerebellum, the brain stem or the dorsal columns. CT or MRI is usually indicated in these cases.

In addition to myalgia, symptoms which should alert one to the possibility of a myopathy include: difficulty in rising from the sitting, lying or squat positions;

difficulty ascending (but not descending) stairs; weakness of the neck muscles and dysphagia. Alternatively, patients may simply complain of loss of muscle bulk around the buttocks and thighs.

Primary muscle involvement in HIV disease is being encountered with increasing frequency. Aetiological factors which have been implicated include HIV itself (directly or indirectly via immune mediated mechanisms), zidovudine or an as yet unidentified infectious agent. The investigation of such patients should include serial creatine phosphokinase measurements, electromyographic (EMG) studies and muscle biopsies. The clinical indications for a muscle biopsy include the presence of definite signs of a proximal myopathy, particularly if there are myopathic features on EMG studies.

Peripheral neuropathies, which may be investigated by nerve conduction studies (NCS), can present with walking difficulties due to severe discomfort in the soles of the feet. This may be compounded by an associated weakness, particularly in patients with the inflammatory demyelinating neuropathies. Apart from HIV and cytomegalovirus (CMV), which have been implicated in the pathophysiology of these neuropathies, drugs are an important cause of neuropathy. An example is vincristine, a chemotherapeutic agent used in the treatment of Kaposi's sarcoma. Some of the newer anti-retroviral drugs are also known to cause a dose-dependent peripheral neuropathy. These include both 2',3'-dideoxyinosine (ddI) and 2',3'-dideoxycytidine (ddC).

Visual Problems

Visual problems in patients with HIV may result from primary retinal vascular disease, opportunistic infections, neoplasms or the neuro-ophthalmic complications of intracranial disease.

The most common ocular manifestations of HIV disease are the non-specific "cotton-wool spots" resulting from a retinal vasculopathy and focal necrosis. These are asymptomatic and usually resolve in 4 to 6 weeks. Rarely, retinal haemorrhages may be associated with cotton-wool spots.

In patients with AIDS, CMV retinitis is the most common cause of loss of vision. The prevalence is estimated at 15%–46% (Bloom and Palestine 1988). Patients may complain of floaters, loss of peripheral vision, visual field defects or reduced acuity. Pain, redness or photophobia are not associated features. Often patients may be asymptomatic since the retinitis may start in the periphery and constant vigilance for this complication is necessary, particularly in patients with low CD4 counts. On fundoscopy, perivascular yellow exudates and haemorrhages may be visible – the so-called "crumpled cheese and ketchup" appearance.

Visual field defects due to a hemisphere disturbances are usually caused by space-occupying lesions but may occasionally be vascular in origin. Visual inattention due to parietal lobe lesions may also present with symptoms such as recurring accidents on one side.

Diplopia may be due to a cranial nerve palsy or be part of a more extensive brain stem disorder. The causes of cranial nerve palsies that need to be considered include cryptococcal, tuberculous, lymphomatous, neurosyphilitic and HIV meningitis. Such patients should be fully assessed with cranial CT or MRI. If this is not diagnostic, examination of the CSF is necessary. Causes of ocular palsies not due to HIV disease, such as diabetes mellitus, intracranial aneurysms, myasthenia gravis and thyrotoxicosis should always be considered.

Seizures

Neurological advice is often sought in the management of seizure disorders in HIV seropositive patients. The incidence of this symptom in HIV infection has been estimated to be 12% in one hospital-based series (Wong et al. 1990). Epileptic seizures have been reported as a presenting symptom in up to 40% of patients with toxoplasmosis, 15% of PCNSL patients, 8% of cryptococcal meningitis patients and 7% of patients with HIV encephalopathy. Less commonly, seizures may complicate the clinical picture in PML. In about half the patients who present with seizures one of the above identifiable causes for the seizures is found. The remainder, in whom all investigations are normal, are presumed to be due to a HIV parenchymal disease (Wong et al. 1990).

A patient who presents with a seizure, either partial or generalised, needs to be investigated urgently with a CT or MRI scan and if this is unhelpful, an examination of the CSF is necessary. A normal interictal EEG does not rule out an epileptic-type seizure. This is usually a clinical diagnosis based on an eyewitness account of the episode(s). The metabolic causes of seizures, for example, hypoxia, hypocalcaemia and hypoglycaemia also need to be excluded. Alcohol excess and drug-related causes should not be forgotten.

Retrospective studies have suggested that the incidence of recurrent seizures and of status epilepticus in this group of patients is higher than expected. Hence, treatment after a single seizure has been recommended. The incidence of hypersensitivity reactions with phenytoin has been high, at between 14%–26% (Holtzman et al. 1989; Wong et al. 1990). There are no data available comparing the various anticonvulsants in patients with HIV disease and therefore specific recommendations cannot yet be made as to the drug of first choice.

Altered Mental Status

This term embraces changes in consciousness, cognition and personality ranging from mild forgetfulness to an acute toxic confusion. These are the common neurological symptoms in HIV infection and AIDS but they are entirely non-specific. They may accompany any central nervous system or systemic complication and be mimicked or exacerbated by anxiety and depression. Complaints of poor memory and concentration naturally give rise to dread that they signify the onset of dementia. Lovers, friends, relatives and workmates can provide valuable insights into changes in the patient's personality and behaviour over time. Whenever altered mental status is suspected, the patient's permission should be sought to interview as many of these observers as appropriate, bearing in mind that there is no need to mention HIV in such enquiries. Bedside testing of higher cerebral function is, by contrast, very insensitive and even the most experienced clinician can miss significant deficits especially when orientation is well preserved. If there is doubt it is best to be guided by the patient and relatives and arrange a formal neuropsychiatric assessment.

Associated features which call for urgent admission and full investigation, usually with cranial CT or MRI and lumbar puncture, are drowsiness, disorientation in time or place, constitutional symptoms, such as malaise, weight loss or fever, and seizures, since they denote an increased risk of intracranial infection or tumour. Occasionally, an EEG may be helpful in demonstrating non-convulsive status epilepticus or an encephalitic process to account for a patient's confusion or drowsiness. If these features are absent and neurological examination is normal, the best approach is neuropsychological and mood assessment. The object is to see whether the patient's mental function is demonstrably poorer than his educational level would predict, and if so whether his mood state is likely to account for it. The results also provide a baseline for comparison with follow-up assessments to establish clearly whether there is a declining trend in performance. Patients with confirmed cognitive deficit or significant deterioration over time need investigation for CNS opportunistic infection or tumour. HIV encephalopathy cannot be diagnosed clinically and there are no characteristic CT/MRI, CSF or EEG features.

AIDS patients run a high risk of toxic confusional states to which subclinical encephalopathy may render them more susceptible. Whether or not there is underlying encephalopathy, an acute deterioration in mental function is likely to have at least one, perhaps several, reversible underlying causes (Table 6.4). Neuropsychological testing is inappropriate unless these factors have been sought and corrected.

Psychiatric symptoms such as mood disorder, personality change, hallucinations and delusions may be the presenting features of a toxic confusional state in patients with AIDS-related complex (ARC) or AIDS. Intracranial infections sometimes produce psychiatric rather than neurological symptoms. Mania, for example, may be due to cryptococcal meningitis or cerebral toxoplasmosis. No psychiatric diagnosis should be made in an immunosuppressed patient without searching for an underlying physical cause.

Table 6.4. Causes of diffuse cerebral dysfunction in HIV infection

Infections
   CNS
      Toxoplasmosis, cryptococcal meningitis, PML, CMV, Herpes encephalitis, neurosyphilis tuberculosis, HIV encephalopathy
   Systemic
      Septicaemia, pneumonia, urinary tract infection

Neoplasms
   Lymphoma – primary or metastatic; rarely Kaposi's sarcoma

Metabolic
   ↓ pO_2 (pneumonia)
   ↓ Hb (zidovudine, marrow infiltration)
   ↑ Urea (dehydration, ganciclovir, diarrhoea)
   ↓ Na (IADH secretion – pneumonia meningitis, drugs)
   ↓ glucose (pentamidine)

Psychological
   Depression, psychosis

Recreational drugs
   Alcohol, cannabis, opiates

Medication
   Steroids (euphoria, depression, psychosis); opiates (confusion); vincristine (depression)

Sensory Symptoms

Sensory symptoms are often vague, and sensory examination is as notoriously unreliable as in everyday neurological practice. The commonest mistake is to attribute symptoms to anxiety or hysteria when the signs are inconsistent, patchy, or not in a clear-cut anatomical distribution. Myelopathy and neuropathy may produce slight sensory impairment which few patients can report consistently, especially as few examiners can give a consistent stimulus repeatedly. The history is the best guide. If the patient complains of altered (not necessarily diminished) sensation which is persistent, unfamiliar and not clearly related to pressure (e.g. pins and needles in the feet only when the legs are crossed), it should be investigated. If there is a discrepancy, the patient's account of the distribution of his symptoms is likely to be more reliable than the sensory signs.

Sensory symptoms in AIDS commonly arise from peripheral neuropathies, the most common being a distal sensory neuropathy. Other neuropathies encountered include a demyelinating inflammatory neuropathy, a mononeuritis multiplex, a radiculopathy due to CMV or pressure palsies. These may be investigated with nerve conduction studies and EMG. Meralgia paraesthetica, characterised by paraesthesiae, pain and numbness on the outer aspect of the thigh, is not uncommon. It is associated with marked fluctuations in body weight and is due to compression of the lateral cutaneous nerve of the thigh.

The detection of a sensory level, which implies spinal cord pathology, is unusual in HIV-related myelopathy, so urgent investigation with myelography or spinal MRI for a compressive cord lesion is indicated. Hemianaesthesia or hemisensory inattention is occasionally seen in patients with intra-cerebral lesions due to toxoplasmosis, lymphoma or PML.

Investigation of Neurological Problems

In HIV-infected patients with neurological problems, routine investigations often lack specificity. For example, there are no radiological features on CT scan to differentiate mass lesions due to toxoplasmosis from those due to primary CNS lymphoma. Brain biopsy is the only method for obtaining a definitive diagnosis. Cerebrospinal fluid abnormalities are found in up to 60% of asymptomatic HIV-infected individuals. These changes include mildly elevated protein levels, a slight excess of mononuclear cells and the presence of oligoclonal bands. HIV may be cultured from the CSF in up to one third of well, asymptomatic HIV individuals (McArthur et al. 1988). Therefore, these CSF abnormalities must be taken into account when interpreting the results of a diagnostic lumbar puncture. They cannot be used to diagnose meningitis or HIV encephalopathy.

Blood Serology

Over 95% of cases of toxoplasmosis in HIV infection are due to reactivation of latent toxoplasma cysts as a result of immunosuppression. Hence, specific IgM indicating de novo infection is rarely detected. Most patients with toxoplasmosis will be seropositive for IgG antibody, suggesting previous exposure, but often the four-fold rise in an acute infection which is diagnostic in an immunocompetent individual does not occur. It has therefore been suggested that all patients diagnosed as being HIV seropositive should have baseline toxoplasma serology performed to identify those patients at greatest risk of developing this complication. The risk of developing cerebral toxoplasmosis in an HIV-infected individual who is IgG seropositive for *Toxoplasma gondii* is estimated at between 12% and 30% (Grant et al. 1990). A negative IgG test does not exclude a diagnosis of toxoplasmosis but makes it less likely (McArthur 1987; Porter and Sande 1992). The background seroprevalence of IgG antibodies to toxoplasma varies from country to country reflecting dietary habits and exposure to cats: 20% of British and 90% of French adults being toxoplasma seropositive.

In cryptococcal meningitis, the serum cryptococcal titre is usually positive. Serum and CSF titres should be measured concurrently as in rare fulminating cases, the CSF may be negative and the serum positive (Dismukes 1988). After a course of treatment for cryptococcal meningitis, the serum titre may remain persistently elevated and is therefore not a useful marker of efficacy of therapy or relapse. This may be due to a defect in antigen clearance or to a continued release of antigen from dead yeast cells.

Progressive multifocal leukoencephalopathy (PML) is caused by reactivation of a human DNA virus (designated JC virus, after the first patient from whom the virus was isolated). This is distinct from the Jacob–Creutzfeld agent. Seroepidemiological studies show that 70% to 80% of adults are JC-virus antibody-positive and therefore serological studies are unhelpful in making the diagnosis.

It appears that within the context of HIV infection, *Treponema pallidum* infection is more aggressive and may present with more atypical signs than in immunocompetent individuals. Patients with HIV infection who present with neurological disease should routinely have blood and CSF serological testing for this spirochaete. Negative results should be regarded cautiously as there have been reported cases of active neurosyphilis with negative serological tests.

Cerebrospinal Fluid Examination

In patients with HIV infection or even patients in whom HIV infection is suspected, a cranial CT scan or MRI should be performed prior to lumbar puncture because of the possibility of silent intracranial mass lesions or cerebral oedema.

In cryptococcal meningitis, cytochemical investigations on the CSF are unhelpful. They may be normal in up to 50% of cases. Greater emphasis is therefore placed on the specific tests for *Cryptococcus neoformans*, in addition to routine culture. India ink staining is positive in 70%–80% of cases. CSF cryptococcal antigen titres are positive in over 90%. Occasionally the initial CSF studies may be negative and repeat lumbar punctures are necessary to confirm the diagnosis. Following a course of treatment for cryptococcal meningitis a repeat examination of the CSF should be carried out. The CSF culture should be sterile. For suspected relapses a repeat lumbar puncture is indicated for restaining with

India ink staining, reculturing and measurement of the antigen titre which can be compared to previous levels.

Unlike systemic non-Hodgkin's lymphoma with meningeal spread, where CSF examination is positive for lymphoma cells in up to 70% of cases, in primary CNS lymphoma the yield is much lower, at around 25% (So et al. 1988a). In situations where lumbar puncture can be safely performed, repeated examinations of the CSF may be warranted as a relatively non-invasive method for establishing the diagnosis when compared to the potential risks of brain biopsy.

To date, serological and cytochemical tests on the CSF in cases of PML and toxoplasmosis are unhelpful although the technique of polymerase chain reaction (PCR) may have a role to play in the future.

As with blood, CSF should be routinely sent for syphilis serology. Cytochemical markers however, are valueless in making a diagnosis of active neurosyphilis in HIV seropositive individuals since HIV itself can result in similar changes. This is in contrast to patients not infected with HIV. The presence of a reactive VDRL test in the CSF would be diagnostic, and although a reactive TPHA or FTA antibody test increases the likelihood of active neurosyphilis, these tests may result in overdiagnosis, as they may remain positive from a previous adequately-treated episode.

In HIV-infected individuals, the threshold for performing lumbar punctures is necessarily low. In non-HIV-related clinical practice, the incidence of post-lumbar puncture headache is about 30%. The headache results from leakage of spinal fluid at the puncture site faster than it is formed. In the upright position the reduction in volume allows downward shift of the brain which stretches the basal meninges which contain pain fibres/receptors, resulting in headache. Characteristically, this is a severe headache associated with nausea and vomiting which is made worse by sitting or standing and is alleviated by lying flat. It may start within 24 h or come on a few days after the procedure. To date, the only factors which seem to influence the incidence of these headaches is the gauge of needle used, smaller-bore needles decreasing the incidence of headache. Management of this complication, should it occur, consists of reassurance that this is a benign self-limiting condition, with bed rest, simple analgesia and an adequate fluid intake.

Neuroradiological Studies

Imaging studies of the CNS are essential in the evaluation of patients with HIV disease who are neurologically symptomatic. However, it should be emphasised that both CT and MRI scanning lack specificity.

Toxoplasmosis is the commonest cause of multiple mass lesions within the central nervous system of patients with HIV infection (Holliman 1988). Cranial CT scans with contrast enhancement characteristically show lesions with a predilection for the basal ganglia or straddling the corticomedullary junction in the frontoparietal and occipital lobes. The lesions usually show ring enhancement, mass effect and surrounding oedema (De la Paz and Enzman 1988; Figs 6.1, 6.2). However, these features may be mimicked by lymphoma (Fig. 6.3), metastatic Kaposi's sarcoma (KS) and other abscesses such as cryptococcoma, aspergilloma and candida (Holliman 1988).

Neurological Complications of HIV Infection and AIDS

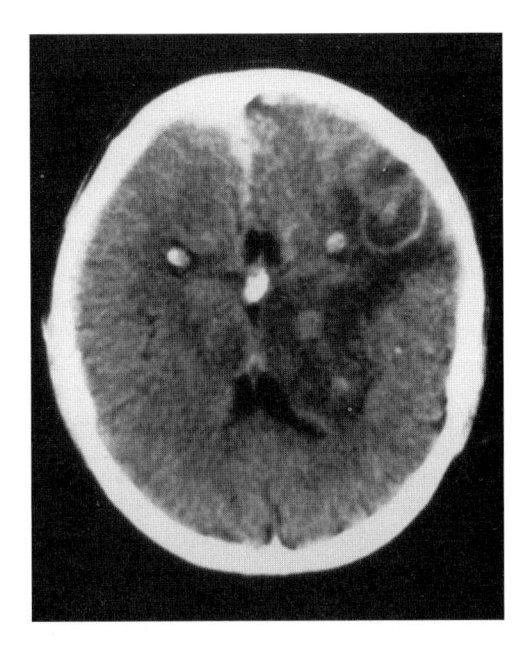

Fig. 6.1. CT scan showing ring enhancing lesion with oedema and mass effect. Diagnosis: toxoplasmosis.

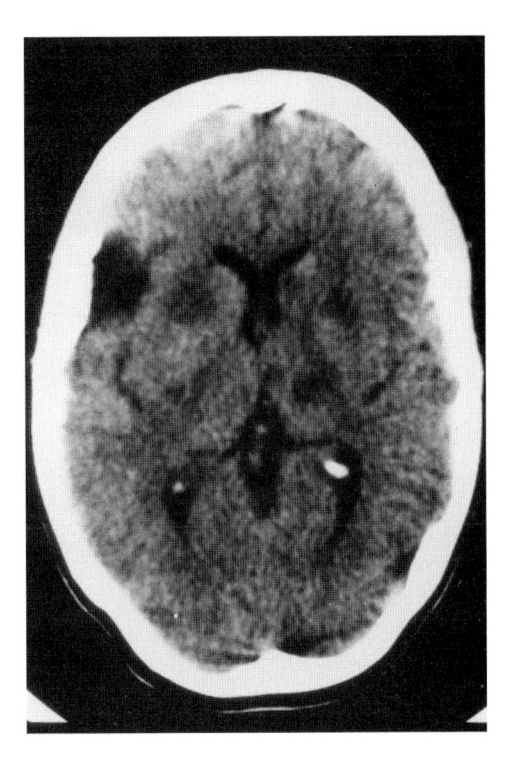

Fig. 6.2. CT scan showing multiple low density non-enhancing lesions. Diagnosis: toxoplasmosis.

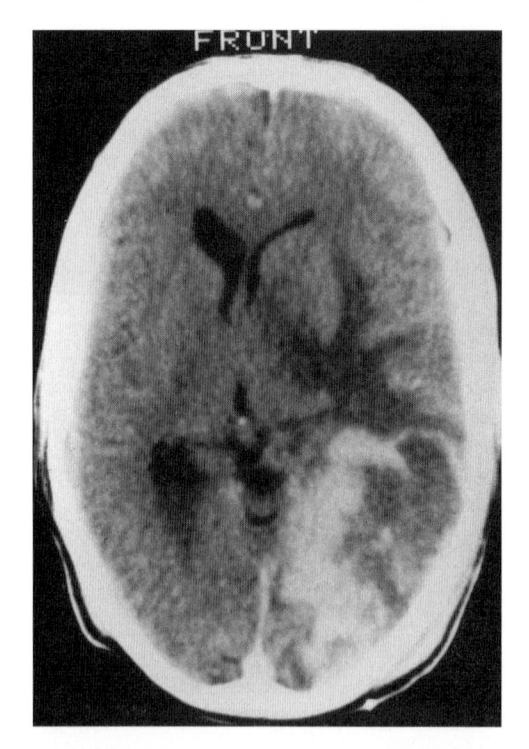

Fig. 6.3. CT scan showing occipito-parietal lesion with mass effect and surrounding oedema. Diagnosis: primary CNS lymphoma.

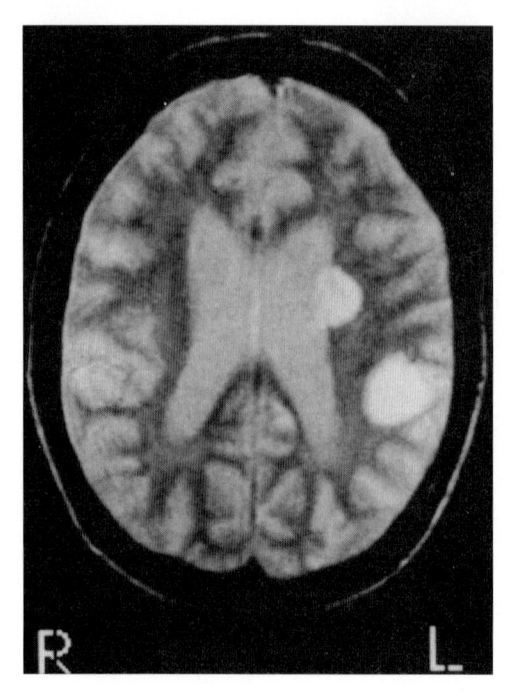

Fig. 6.4. MRI scan showing lesions in the corona radiata and parietal lobe. Diagnosis: toxoplasmosis.

MRI scanning, which has proven to be relatively more sensitive, may influence management by the demonstration of multiple lesions after only a single lesion has been visualised on CT scan (Fig. 6.4). Multiple lesions make a diagnosis of toxoplasmosis more likely, whereas a single lesion on MRI is most probably lymphoma. In one series, 71% of solitary lesions on MRI proved to be lymphoma at biopsy or at autopsy. Furthermore, MRI may reveal lesions which are more accessible to biopsy, should it become necessary (Levy et al. 1990a).

Cranial CT scans in patients with PML typically show non-enhancing, hypodense, white matter lesions without mass effect (Fig. 6.5). These are located periventricularly, in the cerebellum and in the parieto-occipital regions (Fig. 6.6). Recent MRI studies have shown evidence of additional grey matter involvement in up to 50% of cases (Mark and Atlas 1989). Often, only single rather than multifocal lesions are apparent. This serves as an illustration that, with increasing experience with HIV disease, previously held tenets, such as PML being restricted to white matter or only being multifocal, no longer apply.

Cerebral infarcts are recognisable by their site and, if the cortex is involved, by their wedged shape. In the acute phase, gyral enhancement may be seen. Haemorrhage into mass lesions may rarely be seen in toxoplasmosis or metastatic Kaposi's sarcoma.

In patients presenting with symptoms and signs suggestive of spinal cord or cauda equina disease, imaging with myelography or spinal MRI is indicated. This may reveal lymphomatous deposits, extradural abscesses or nerve root nodules as in CMV polyradiculopathy. To date, no neuroradiological correlates of the HIV-associated vacuolar myelopathy have been reported.

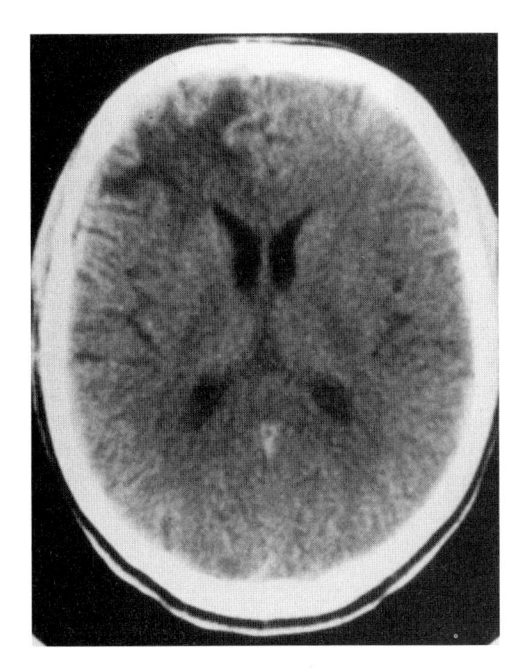

Fig. 6.5. CT scan showing diffuse frontal low intensity white matter lesion. Diagnosis: progressive multifocal leucoencephalopathy.

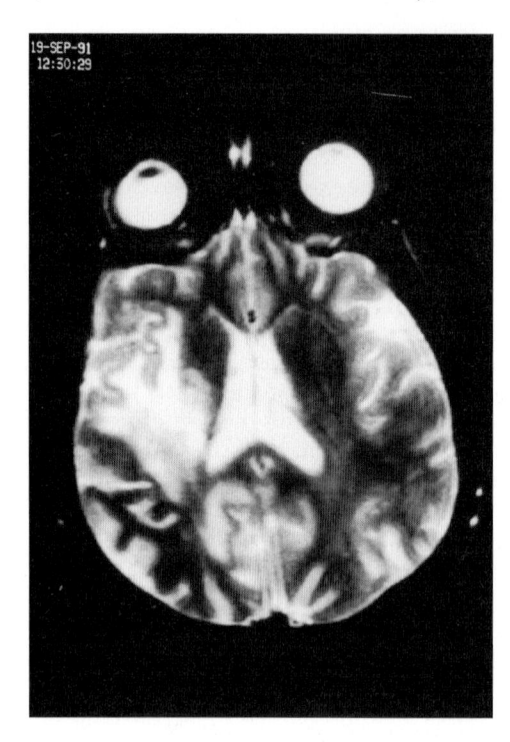

Fig. 6.6. MRI scan showing diffuse white matter abnormality in the temporal and occipital areas. Diagnosis: progressive multifocal leucoencephalopathy.

Tissue Biopsy

Brain Biopsy

In the early phase of the AIDS epidemic, brain biopsy of all intracerebral mass lesions was advocated, as CT scan appearances were non-specific and serological tests unhelpful. It is now established practice to treat patients with focal lesions with anti-toxoplasma therapy. A response, clinically and radiologically, within 14–21 days is regarded as diagnostic. A lack of response or a continued deterioration is an indication for biopsy. Negative toxoplasma serology and intolerance to the available anti-toxoplasma therapy may be other factors that need to be taken into consideration for early biopsy. A recently published series in this group of patients has shown CT or MR guided stereotactic biopsy to be safe in experienced hands with a high diagnostic yield (Levy et al. 1990b).

A definitive diagnosis of PML can only be made histopathologically: the characteristic features include focal demyelination with axonal sparing, bizarre enlarged astrocytes and abnormal oligodendrocytes with inclusions which stain for JC viral antigens (Richardson 1988).

Muscle Biopsy

Muscle biopsy is indicated in patients presenting with clinical or neurophysiological evidence of a myopathy. Prior to the introduction of zidovudine, muscle disease seemed to occur only rarely in HIV-infected patients. After the introduction of the anti-retroviral agent, increasing reports implicated its role in a myopathy. Although it has not yet been possible to identify a specific clinical myopathic syndrome attributable to the drug, Dalakas and colleagues were able to distinguish the muscle biopsies from myopathic patients who had been on zidovudine by the presence of ragged red fibres. On electron microscopy (EM) studies, these showed the presence of abnormal mitochondria with paracrystalline inclusions. Inflammatory cells were present in similar numbers in the zidovudine-exposed and non-exposed groups (Dalakas et al. 1990).

From the practical point of view, inflammatory cells on muscle biopsy should lead to the consideration of prescribing steroids, and the presence of ragged red fibres, withdrawal of zidovudine.

Further studies are clearly required to unravel this problem in order that appropriate practical management decisions can be made.

Neurophysiological Investigations

Electrophysiological studies can have an important role in the evaluation of the complications of HIV infection, helping in the diagnosis of many conditions and in the evaluation of response to treatment.

Motor and sensory nerve conduction studies (NCS) are of value in the accurate assessment of the neuromuscular complications. The presence of a peripheral neuropathy can be confirmed and the probable pathophysiology determined in most cases. It is particularly important to detect evidence of significant demyelination, which will influence the management since steroids and plasmapheresis have been shown to be effective therapies. The outcome can be objectively monitored by repeated testing. These studies also provide information about the sites of focal pathology. For example, active denervation in lower limb muscles supplied by individual roots can be indicative of the CMV polyradiculopathy syndrome. Also, multifocal neuropathies in mononeuritis multiplex can be diagnosed by careful NCS and EMG.

Electromyographic (EMG) examination of muscles is useful in the diagnosis of myopathic disorders. It is possible to indicate if a significant degree of active muscle fibre degeneration is occurring which could be due to an inflammatory process e.g. polymyositis. This would have therapeutic implications for the patient, and as inflammation can only be confirmed histopathologically, a muscle biopsy should then be performed in all such cases. EMG in conjunction with nerve conduction studies can also help distinguish neurogenic muscle weakness form a myopathic process.

The investigation of new-onset seizures in patients with HIV infection should include a routine electroencephalogram (EEG) which may reveal epileptogenic discharges, and indicate whether these are focal or generalised. An EEG should also be considered in patients who develop a significant change in mental status, especially if non-convulsive status epilepticus is to be excluded. To date, the routine EEG has been found to be unhelpful in the diagnosis of HIV encephalopathy, mild excessive generalised slowing being documented in a minority of demented patients.

Somatosensory evoked potentials (SEPs) can be useful in investigation of spinal cord pathology, where they complement neuroradiological tests such as MRI scanning. Investigations such as the P300 auditory evoked potential, which has been claimed to be a neurophysiological measure of cognitive function, have no clinical utility at present and are only applicable for research purposes.

Pathophysiology and Management

Toxoplasmosis

Toxoplasma gondii is an obligate intra-cellular parasite which is ubiquitous in the human population. The cat is the definitive host. Transmission is mainly by the faecal-oral route by eating under-cooked meat infected with cysts. In man, the primary infection is usually asymptomatic or it may present as a glandular fever-like illness. The organism encysts in all tissues and reactivation in the brain of an immunocompromised host results in the most common opportunistic infection of the central nervous system in HIV infection (Holliman 1988). The incidence of toxoplasmosis varies between 5% and 30%, depending on the background seroprevalence in a particular country.

Clinically, the features of toxoplasmosis result from multifocal brain abscesses with or without a diffuse meningoencephalitis (Navia et al. 1986c; Pons et al. 1988) (Table 6.5). On rare occasions, patients may present with a meningoencephalitis without focal symptoms or signs (Gray et al. 1989). The symptoms may evolve over 1 or 2 weeks or acutely with a confusional state or a focal deficit mimicking a cerebrovascular accident. It should be emphasised that primary CNS lymphoma may present in a similar fashion and there are no specific clinical features which distinguish the two conditions. Rarely, toxoplasma abscesses may involve the spinal cord presenting as a transverse myelitis (Mehren et al. 1988) or a cauda equina syndrome (Kayser 1990).

In patients with a compatible history and a scan showing multiple lesions a combination of sulphadiazine and pyrimethamine together with folinic acid supplements should be instituted immediately as anti-toxoplasma therapy (Table 6.6) The combination therapy acts by blocking folate metabolism in the free trophozoites but not within the latent cysts. However, the incidence of side effects with this regimen is high, up to 40% of patients manifesting signs of serious toxicity (Haverkos 1987; Leport et al. 1988). Prospective trials have shown a combination of clindamycin and pyrimethamine to be as effective as the sulphadiazine/pyrimethamine regimen. Although the haematological side-effect profile is less with the former combination, the incidence of gastrointestinal toxicity is higher (Dannemann et al. 1992). A response clinically and radiologically, within 14 to 21 days, is regarded as diagnostic although clinical improvement is often seen earlier (Fig. 6.7).

Patients who present with a single lesion on CT scan should be treated similarly, but if MRI is available and this confirms that the lesion is truly solitary then

Table 6.5. Clinical presentation of toxoplasmosis in AIDS (Pons et al. 1988)

	%
Focal symptoms (hemiparesis, aphasia, ataxia, movement disorder)	70
Headache	45
Lethargy/confusion	40
Seizures	38
Fever	35
Neck stiffness	5

Table 6.6. Drug treatment of opportunistic infections in AIDS

Infection	Drug	dose	Duration	Side effects	Notes
Toxoplasmosis					
Acute	Pyrimethamine[1]	Day 1: 75 mg; then 25–50 mg/day po [1]	4–6 weeks	Myelosuppression, nausea and vomiting	[1]Loading dose 100–200 mg followed by 50–75 mg also used.
	+				
	Sulphadiazine[2,3]	6–8 g/day po	4–6 weeks	Nausea, vomiting, anorexia, rashes, blood dyscrasias	[2]Adverse reaction rate 40% Clindamicin 1200 mg/day an alternative to sulphadiazine. S/E diarrhoea and occasionally pseudomembranous colitis, rashes
	+				
	Folinic acid	10–20 mg/day po	4–6 weeks		[3]Sulphadiazine desensitisation
Maintenance	Pyrimethamine	25–50 mg/day po	Indefinitely		
	+				
	Sulphadiazine	2–4 g/day po	Indefinitely		
	+				
	Folinic acid	5–10 mg/day po	Indefinitely		
Cryptococcal meningitis					
Acute	Amphotericin B[1]	0.5–0.8 mg/kg/day IV	6 weeks Total dose of 1.0–2.0 g	Nausea, vomiting, nephrotoxic, hypokalaemia, hypomagnesia, arrhythmias, convulsions, hepatotoxic	[1]Alternatively high risk – amphotericin B; Low risk – fluconazole. See text
	±				
	5[1] Flucytosine[2]	100 mg/kg/day		Myelosuppression, rashes	[2]Check serum levels
Maintenance	Amphotericin B or	100 mg/week IV			
	Fluconazole	200 mg/day po		Nausea, vomiting, abnormal LFTs	

Table 6.6. Continued

Infection	Drug	Dose	Duration	Side effects	Notes
CMV retinitis and polyradiculopathy					
Acute	Ganciclovir[1]	5 mg/kg/BD IV	2–3 weeks + stabilisation of retinitis	Myelosuppression, abnormal LFTs	[1]Combination with zidovudine not recommended because of severe myelosuppression
	or				
	Foscarnet[2,3,4]	60–70 mg/kg TDS IV	As above	Nephrotoxic, penile ulceration, anaemia, thrombocytopenia	[2]Combination with zidovudine possible because of less myelosuppression
Maintenance	Ganciclovir	5 mg/kg OD IV	Indefinitely		[3]Predose hydration suggested
	or				
	Foscarnet	60–120 mg/kg OD IV	Indefinitely		[4]No data for polyradiculopathy

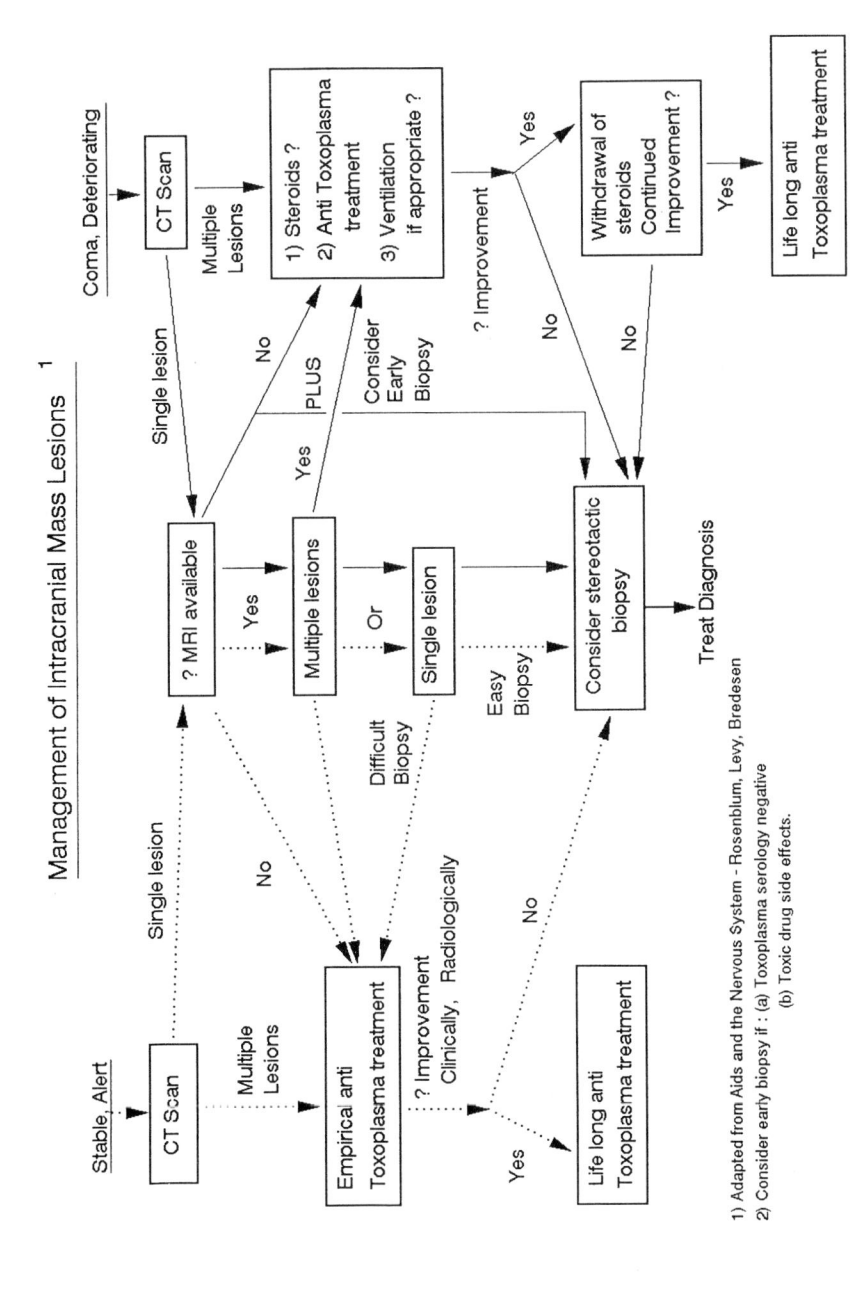

Fig. 6.7. Management of intracranial mass lesions. Scheme adapted from Rosenblum et al. (1988).

1) Adapted from Aids and the Nervous System - Rosenblum, Levy, Bredesen
2) Consider early biopsy if : (a) Toxoplasma serology negative
   (b) Toxic drug side effects.

biopsy should be considered since almost two-thirds of such lesions are due to lymphoma (Circillo and Rosenblaum 1991).

A response to anti-toxoplasma therapy can be expected in up to 90% of patients, even those who present in coma. If indicated, and considered appropriate, ventilation as a supportive measure may be necessary. High dose steroids, because of their mass reducing effect, are indicated in cases where there is significant raised intracranial pressure with symptoms such as a diminished level of consciousness. However, as steroids may jeopardise immune function further and pose practical difficulties in the interpretation of the empirical trial of anti-toxoplasma therapy, they should be withdrawn as soon as is clinically reasonable. A deterioration at that stage should lead to consideration of biopsy to exclude the possibility of lymphoma or an abscess such as a tuberculoma.

The majority of patients survive the acute episode and make a good recovery. Since the chemotherapeutic agents used are only effective against the rapidly proliferating stage but not against the encysted form, life long prophylaxis is necessary. Without this, relapse occurs in 50% of patients (Luft and Hafner 1990; Klein 1989). Trials are in progress to determine whether primary prophylaxis would be effective in HIV patients with positive toxoplasma serology.

Cryptococcal Meningitis

Cryptococcus neoformans is an encapsulated fungus commonly found in the soil and is the most common fungal infection of the CNS in HIV infection. In man, infection occurs via aerial inhalation with the respiratory infection usually being asymptomatic. Blood-borne spread to any organ can occur but the organism has a predilection for the CNS where it causes a meningitis. The occurrence of cryptococcomas is rare. In HIV-infected individuals the incidence of cryptococcal meningitis is between 5 and 10% (Chuck and Sande 1989). In up to 40% of these cases this complication will be the AIDS-defining illness.

The clinical presentation may be acute or more commonly indolent with symptoms such as headache being present for weeks or months before diagnosis. The mean interval between the onset of symptoms and diagnosis was 31 days in one study (Zuger et al. 1986) (Table 6.7). Only one-third of patients show the classical signs of meningism (Chuck and Sande 1989). Some patients present with non-specific signs and symptoms not implicating the nervous system and hence the diagnosis must be considered in any HIV seropositive individual presenting with unexplained fever, malaise or headache (Chuck and Sande 1989; Zuger et al. 1986).

Table 6.7. Clinical presentation of cryptococcal meningitis (Chuck and Sande 1989; Zuger et al. 1986)

	%
Malaise	76
Headache	73
Temperature above 38.4°	56
Meningism	27
Altered mental status	17
Focal signs	15
Seizures	4

Treatment of cryptococcal meningitis is with amphotericin B usually aiming for a target dose of 1–2 g over 4–6 weeks (Table 6.6). In spite of this the mortality rate in the acute stages remains high, at around 20% (Chuck and Sande 1989; Zuger et al. 1986). Amphotericin B has a number of drawbacks, needing to be infused into a central vein via a Hickman line as it readily causes a phlebitis. Serious side effects include renal impairment, hypokalaemia and hypomagnesaemia. These may be minimised by keeping the patient well hydrated and prescribing mineral supplements. If renal toxicity becomes a problem, the regimen can be changed to alternate-day therapy provided that the target dose has been reached and the patient is improving.

The response to treatment is assessed by clinical improvement and a repeat CSF examination at about 6 weeks, when the CSF should be sterile on culture. In common with other infections in AIDS, relapses can be expected in up to 65% of patients on cessation of treatment. Relapse is associated with a higher mortality. However, it is becoming increasingly apparent that this high relapse rate may reflect a high incidence of clinically silent infection even after a course of therapy has rendered the CSF sterile. The prostate, in particular, seems an important reservoir of infection. Thus, it may be prudent to ensure that as well as rendering the CSF and blood sterile, a urine sample after prostatic massage should also be culture-negative before maintenance therapy is started (Bozzette et al. 1991). Maintenance treatment regimens used with some success include amphotericin B 100 mg/ week.

5-Flucytosine in combination with amphotericin B is standard treatment in non-AIDS patients with cryptococcal meningitis. However, in AIDS, its role has not been clearly defined. Some studies suggest it has no benefit in terms of increased survival or a reduced relapse rate. Furthermore, it is often poorly tolerated, causing vomiting, renal and hepatic impairment, leucopenia and thrombocytopenia (Chuck and Sande 1989).

Fluconazole, a new oral fungistatic triazole compound, is a long-awaited alternative to amphotericin. It has good CNS penetration, low toxicity and a long half-life. The most recent trials comparing amphotericin B at a dose of 0.3–0.5 mg/kg/day versus fluconazole 200 mg daily showed no statistically significant differences in outcome. However, the rate of early deaths was higher in the fluconazole group and this may have been related to the more rapid clearing of cryptococcus from the CSF found in the amphotericin group (Saag et al. 1992). It has been possible to identify high- and low-risk groups of HIV-infected patients with cryptococcal meningitis. Factors associated with the high-risk group included a reduced consciousness level, a CSF cryptococcal antigen titre of greater than 1:1024 and CSF white blood count of less than 20 cells/mm^3 (Saag et al. 1992). Current opinion favours the use of amphotericin with or without 5-FC for the high risk group for at least 2 weeks or until the patient is clinically stable. The low-risk group can be treated with fluconazole (Stansall and Sande 1992). As with other infective complications of AIDS, maintenance treatment is mandatory. In contrast to acute therapy, fluconazole 200 mg a day seems to be as effective as amphotericin B 100 mg/week (Galgiani 1990).

Progressive Multifocal Leukoencephalopathy (PML)

This previously rare condition occurs in immunosuppressed indivuduals. The central nervous system demyelination is caused by the reactivation of a DNA virus – the JC virus. The incidence of PML in HIV infection is around 2%–4% (Richardson 1988).

PML usually presents insidiously with focal neurological symptoms and signs including limb weakness, gait abnormalities, incoordination, visual loss and cognitive dysfunction (Berger et al. 1987). Although primarily affecting the white matter, there are reports of cases with extensive grey matter involvement.

Attempts at treatment of PML with prednisolone and HLA-matched lymphocytes have proved largely unsuccessful. In a review of 28 patients by Berger et al, survival ranged from 0.3 to 18 months (Berger et al. 1987). Death was usually due to one of the other complications of immunosuppression. Two patients improved without specific treatment and were alive at 20 and 23 months. Hence, without properly-controlled trials, the true implications of anecdotal reports of improvement with, for example, radiotherapy (De Bouchier 1990), zidovudine (Conway et al. 1990) and cytosine arabinoside, both systemic (Portegies et al. 1991) and intrathecal (Britton et al. 1992), are difficult to assess. A multicentre prospective trial evaluating cytosine arabinoside is in progress.

Cytomegalovirus (CMV) Infection

Over 90% of HIV-infected individuals have serological evidence of CMV infection. As AIDS patients live longer, this infection is becoming increasingly common. In the nervous system it is responsible for a retinitis, a polyradiculopathy syndrome, a multifocal peripheral neuropathy and an encephalitis.

In AIDS patients, CMV retinitis is the commonest cause of blindness. Patients may often be asymptomatic in the early stages and it is essential to screen patients for this complication in the clinic. A patient who presents with a CMV complication at another site, such as colitis or polyradiculopathy, requires careful ophthalmological assessment as the presence of retinitis may lengthen the duration of induction therapy required.

CMV retinitis begins with cotton-wool spots close to the vascular arcades and is at first indistinguishable from benign HIV retinopathy. However, the cotton-wool spots enlarge and coalesce into a yellow-white infiltrate followed by irregularities in calibre of the nearby vessels. Flame-shaped haemorrhages appear close to the abnormal vascular segments and eventually a full thickness haemorrhagic retinitis develops. Without treatment, progression to blindness is inevitable. 9-(1,3,-dihydroxy-2-propoxymethy (DHPG, gancyclovir) and trisodium phosphonoformate hexahydrate (foscarnet) (Laskin et al. 1987; Fanning et al. 1990) have been shown to be effective in halting progression of the disease. More recently, in vitro and in vivo studies suggest there may be some synergistic effect in combination therapy of these two drugs. Life-long maintenance therapy is necessary although relapses may occur in spite of this (Table 6.6).

CMV polyradiculopathy in patients with AIDS is a well-recognised syndrome with over 25 cases now reported in the literature. It is estimated to occur in up to 2% of AIDS patients presenting with neurological problems (De Gans and Portegies 1989). It is characterised by a subacute cauda equina-like syndrome with back pain, a progressive lower motor neurone weakness in the legs and sphincter disturbance. Myelography or MRI, essential to rule out a compressive mass lesion such as lymphoma, may be normal or show nodules on the nerve roots. Characteristically, the cerebrospinal fluid shows a neutrophil leucocytosis, which is unusual in a viral infection. It is postulated that an initial monocyte response results in a secondary neutrophil chemotaxis due to the release of cytokines (de Gans et al. 1990). The differential diagnosis is syphilitic polyradiculopathy and lymphomatous infiltration of the nerve roots. Without treatment, there is usually a progression of the neurological deficit with death in 2–3 months. In 1989, the first reports of treatment with DHPG (ganciclovir) were published and subsequent reports in two small series suggested that earlier recognition of the syndrome, when the neurological deficit is milder, and treatment with DHPG result in a better outcome (Graveleau et al. 1990; de Gans et al. 1990). However, the optimum dose and duration of induction therapy has not been determined. At present, induction doses of 10 mg/kg/day are recommended for 2–3 weeks although it may be appropriate to continue this at least until no further neurological improvement occurs (Manji et al. 1992). Maintenance regimens seem fairly standard at 5mg/kg/day for 5 out of 7 days a week. There have been no trials of foscarnet therapy in the treatment of this CMV complication.

Said et al. (1991) have reported a rapidly progressive multifocal peripheral neuropathy in patients with profound immunosuppression and evidence of active CMV disease, such as retinitis, pneumonitis or colitis. Nerve biopsy specimens revealed multifocal necrotic lesions with a mainly polymorphonuclear cell infiltrate. Some patients responded to anti-CMV therapy (Said et al. 1991)

Although evidence of CMV may be found in the brains of up to one-third of patients dying of AIDS, the clinical correlates of a CMV encephalitis remain unclear. Anecdotal reports suggest this to be a disorder characterised by fever, a deterioration in conscious level (which may be rapid) and seizures. There are as yet no specific diagnostic tests. However, this may be a diagnosis worth considering and treating with DHPG or foscarnet when faced with a patient for whose rapidly deteriorating condition no cause can be found.

Syphilis

Routine syphilis serological tests include the venereal disease research laboratory tests (VDRL). This is a non-specific lipoidal antigen test which is positive in 75% of cases of primary syphilis. The titre gradually declines in the secondary stages and is negative in 30% of untreated latent and late cases. After treatment, the VDRL tends to become negative. The treponema pallidum haemagglutination test (TPHA) is the usual specific antitreponemal test used for screening purposes. In cases of problem sera, the fluorescent treponemal antigen antibody test (FTA–ABS) is the most sensitive and most specific test available. It is the first test to become positive in early untreated syphilis.

Invasion of the central nervous system occurs early in the course of syphilis infection. *T. pallidum* has been isolated from the CSF of up to 25% of neurologically asymptomatic patients with early syphilis (Chesney and Kemp 1924). Thirteen percent of untreated primary syphilis patients and 25%–40% of patients with secondary syphilis without neurological symptoms have CSF abnormalities (Lukehart et al. 1988; Hahn and Clerk 1946; Merritt 1940). However, in the majority of patients this is asymptomatic. Rarely, patients may present with an acute syphilitic meningitis in the secondary stage.

After an interval of 2 years, complications due to meningovascular syphilis may occur. The essential feature is an endarteritis of the vessels of the brain, cord and meninges. Parenchymatous neurosyphilis, which includes general paralysis of the insane and tabes dorsalis, usually develops 10–15 years after the primary infection (Catterall 1975). Even in the pre-AIDS era, the diagnosis and treatment of syphilis proved, at times, to be difficult. However, with standard therapy with either a single intramuscular dose of 2.4 million units (1800 mg) benzathine penicillin G commonly prescribed in the USA, or 10 days of 600,000 units (600 mg) procaine penicillin intramuscularly, progression to neurosyphilis is rare, in spite of subtherapeutic levels of penicillin within the CSF (Collart et al. 1980; Goh et al. 1984). It seems as if an intact immune system plays an integral role in the response to therapy.

The clinical manifestations of neurosyphilis are protean and enter within the differential diagnosis of most of the neurological complications seen in HIV infection. These include acute and chronic meningitis, cranial nerve palsies, focal intracerebral lesions, seizures, retinitis, the cauda equina syndrome and cognitive dysfunction. One retrospective study estimated the incidence of neurosyphilis in AIDS patients to be 1.5% (Katz and Berger 1989).

Within the context of HIV infection, the difficulties in diagnosis and treatment of syphilis are compounded by four factors. Firstly, as a result of the depressed cellular immunity it appears as if infection with *T. pallidum* may be more aggressive and may present with more atypical signs than in the immunocompetent individual (Muscher et al. 1990; Lanska et al. 1988). However, most HIV-infected patients present with typical dermatological features of primary and secondary syphilis with positive serological tests. In the USA, there have been anecdotal reports of rapid progression to neurosyphilis (Muscher et al. 1990) and of relapses with meningovascular syphilis in spite of standard treatment for secondary syphilis with 2.4×10^6 units benzathine penicillin (Berry et al. 1987). The chronic aseptic meningitis associated with HIV infection may, in theory, increase the risk of developing neurosyphilis. Secondly, altered B cell function may result in suppression of serological markers which may remain negative or be delayed in the presence of active neurosyphilis (Hicks et al. 1987). Recently, Haas showed that treponemal antibody tests may revert to negative with progressive HIV disease – loss of reactivity to FTA–ABS in 7% of asymptomatic seropositives and in 38% of those with symptomatic HIV disease (Haas et al. 1990). However, a majority of HIV-infected cases with neurosyphilis will have a positive CSF VDRL (Matlow and Rachlis 1990). On the other hand, HIV-related polyclonal B cell activation could result in an increased rate of false-positive serological tests and also make the monitoring of serial titres as a marker of treatment efficacy obsolete (Drabick and Tramont 1990). Thirdly, it is not possible to use the CSF cytochemical parameters as markers for active neurosyphilis in HIV-infected patients since 40%–60% of these individuals may have changes as a result of the HIV infection. Finally, HIV infection may itself produce a wide spectrum of neurological manifestations similar to neurosyphilis. Adequate data from trials specifically addressing these issues are not available and definitive recommendations cannot as yet be made.

In HIV-infected patients with possible symptomatic neurosyphilis, unless contra-indicated, lumbar puncture should be performed as other diagnostic possibilities such as lymphoma need to be considered. This applies to patients with cranial nerve palsies, ocular or auditory symptoms and signs, behavioural and psychological abnormalities. Those patients with a clinical diagnosis compatible with neurosyphilis and positive serum or CSF VDRL should be treated for 10-14 days with aqueous crystalline penicillin G 2-4 mega units intravenously every 4 h. If hospitalisation is not possible, an alternative regimen is aqueous procaine penicillin G 2.4 mega units (2.4 g) i.m. daily for 10-14 days, together with probenicid 500 mg orally four times a day (Bolan 1992).

There is debate as to how neurologically asymptomatic HIV-positive patients with early syphilis should be managed. Although some workers recommend that lumbar puncture be performed in all cases of syphilis in HIV-infected individuals its value in this group of HIV-positive, neurologically asymptomatic, patients as an aid to diagnosis of neurosyphilis is uncertain for the reasons previously discussed. However, a reactive CSF VDRL would be strong evidence of active neurosyphilis. Treatment of CSF TPHA- or FTA-positive patients as cases of neurosyphilis may overdiagnose active neurosyphilis as these may remain positive after a previously treated episode or may appear to be positive due to contamination by blood during lumbar puncture. In cases with negative CSF serology, the cytochemical information obtained at lumbar puncture could nevertheless be used as a baseline for follow-up after therapy.

In view of the reports of treatment failures and relapses, together with documented inadequate CSF drug levels, it seems imprudent to treat this group of patients with a 10-day course of 600 mg procaine penicillin or a single 1800 mg dose of benzathine penicillin. Some authorities suggest that all patients infected with HIV who present with early syphilis should be treated with the regimen for symptomatic neurosyphilis. However, this is expensive, of unproven benefit, time consuming and unpleasant, which may result in non-compliance. An alternative is to prescribe a regimen intermediate between that used in routine therapy and neurosyphilis therapy. To date, no specific higher dose has been determined.

Until a consensus is reached regarding the management of this dually-infected group of neurologically asymptomatic patients, each case will have to be managed individually. What is clear is that careful follow-up is of paramount importance. Monthly rather than 3-monthly serological tests should be performed for at least the first 6 months after therapy.

Tuberculosis

Although there is no definite evidence that HIV infection predisposes to acquisition of new tuberculous infection, individuals with evidence of previous exposure are more likely to develop active tuberculosis if coinfected with HIV. Most of these cases are due to reactivation of latent infection rather than to new rapidly progressive disease. A retrospective study by Helbert et al. (1990) from St Mary's Hospital, London, UK, suggested that tuberculous infection occurred in up to 6% of AIDS patients.

In HIV-infected individuals tuberculosis usually occurs before other opportunistic infections such as pneumocystis carinii pneumonia which is indicative of its higher virulence. The mean CD4 count for disseminated tuberculosis was found to be $0.395 \times 10^9/l$ compared to $0.110 \times 10^9/l$ for pneumocystis carinii pneumonia and $0.130 \times 10^9/l$ for disseminated mycobacterium avium intracellulare infection (Crowe et al. 1991). Thus, tuberculous infection should be considered in the differential diagnosis of a relatively immunocompetent HIV-infected individual and conversely, HIV infection should be considered in a patient presenting with tuberculous disease.

A striking feature of *M. tuberculosis* infection in HIV is the high frequency of extra-pulmonary infection. In the less advanced stages this may occur in up to 45% of cases but rises to 70% in patients with AIDS (Barnes et al. 1991). In the central nervous system, this may present as tuberculous meningitis, spinal abscesses or intracerebral tuberculomas, which are indistinguishable from toxoplasma abscesses on CT scans. Stereotactic biopsy of patients who fail a trial of anti-toxoplasma treatment, or in whom such therapy results in resolution of some lesions but progression of others, is indicated.

Generally, the response rate to standard triple or quadruple therapy in all HIV groups is satisfactory, with few reported cases of treatment failures (Small et al. 1991). Recently, however, a nosocomial outbreak of multi-resistant tuberculosis has been reported in a group of AIDS patients in New York city (Edlin et al. 1992).

Lymphoma

Primary Central Nervous System Lymphoma

In the past, this rare tumour has been occasionally observed to occur spontaneously but was usually associated with immunodeficient states both congenital, as in ataxia telangiectasia, and acquired, as in transplant recipients. More recently, it is being observed increasingly frequently in AIDS, with an incidence of 2.6% (Levy et al. 1985). Post-mortem series document a prevalence of up to 7%. It is estimated that cases of AIDS-related primary cerebral lymphoma will be more common than low grade astrocytomas and will be almost as common as meningiomas (Baumgartner et al. 1990). Primary CNS lymphoma is the second most common cause of central nervous system mass lesions in adult AIDS patients and is the most common in cases of paediatric AIDS. Pathologically, these tumours are multicentric and derived from high grade B-cells (So et al. 1988a).

Although the pathogenesis has not been fully elucidated, it seems as if the following factors play an interdependent role: the CNS is an immunologically privileged site within which the normal regulatory restraints are lacking; immunosuppression results in defective oncogenic surveillance, and chronic infections, such as with the Epstein–Barr herpes virus (EBV), may be implicated as a trigger mechanism. Using refined RNA in-situ hybridisation techniques, MacMahon et al. (1991) found evidence of EBV infection of malignant lymphoma cells in all of 21 cases of AIDS associated primary CNS lymphoma.

The clinical presentation of primary CNS lymphoma may be non-specific, with confusion, lethargy, and memory loss. Alternatively, a focal presentation with, for example, hemiparesis or dysphasia may occur in up to 40%. Most patients will eventually demonstrate signs and symptoms suggestive of an intracranial mass lesion (So et al. 1986).

In non-AIDS cases, the prognosis is poor. In AIDS-related cases it is even worse. Most patients die within 2 months of presentation. However, recent data suggest that earlier diagnosis and treatment with radiotherapy result in improvement clinically and radiologically. Remissions of up to 12 months have been documented. Death in these treated cases is from the other complications of immunosuppression rather than tumour progression (Baumgartner et al. 1990).

Metastatic Non-Hodgkin's Lymphoma (NHL)

Since the beginning of the AIDS epidemic there has been a marked increase in the frequency of NHL. Furthermore, HIV-infected patients tend to present with high-grade tumours with widespread disease involving extranodal sites (Fig. 6.8a,b). Forty-two percent of patients in one study had evidence of CNS disease at presentation (Ziegler et al. 1984).

Clinically, leptomeningeal infiltration presents with cranial nerve palsies (the oculomotor and facial nerves most commonly) or spinal root dysfunction. Occasionally, extradural metastases may result in cord compression or the cauda equina syndrome. Parenchymal brain involvement may present with non-specific confusion, a deterioration in the level of consciousness and seizures. Treatment of the CNS complications is by the intrathecal or ventricular reservoir route with methotrexate and/or cytosine arabinoside. The acute compressive myelopathies are treated with radiotherapy. Since occult involvement of the CNS occurs commonly at presentation and particularly at relapse, prophylaxis with intrathecal methotrexate or cranial irradiation has been recommended (Krown 1990). However, in spite of these drug regimens the prognosis to date, is poor.

Cerebrovascular Disease

The incidence of cerebrovascular disease in clinical studies of AIDS patients is estimated at between 0.5% and 7% (McArthur 1987). In the general population, the incidence of stroke is 0.025% in the 35–45 year old age range.

In cases of ischaemic stroke, cardiac emboli due to bacterial endocarditis, especially in intravenous drug users (IVDU), and non-bacterial thrombotic endocarditis (marantic endocarditis) need to be excluded. Cerebral vasculitis causing strokes has been reported in association with herpes zoster (Fig. 6.9) (Eidelberg et al. 1986) and *Treponema pallidum* infections.

The presence of antiphospholipid antibodies such as lupus anticoagulant and anticardiolipin antibody is associated with arterial and venous thromboses. A high prevalence of the lupus anticoagulant has been documented in all stages of HIV infection (Boue et al. 1990). Anticardiolipin antibodies are also commonly found in HIV-infected groups of patients (Canoso et al. 1987). However, to date, only one case of thrombotic episodes in an HIV-infected patient with anticardiolipin antibodies, but not lupus anticoagulant, has been described (Keeling et al. 1990).

Neurological Complications due to HIV

As the AIDS epidemic has unfolded, it has became apparent that the most frequently seen complications in HIV are due to the virus itself. There is a substan-

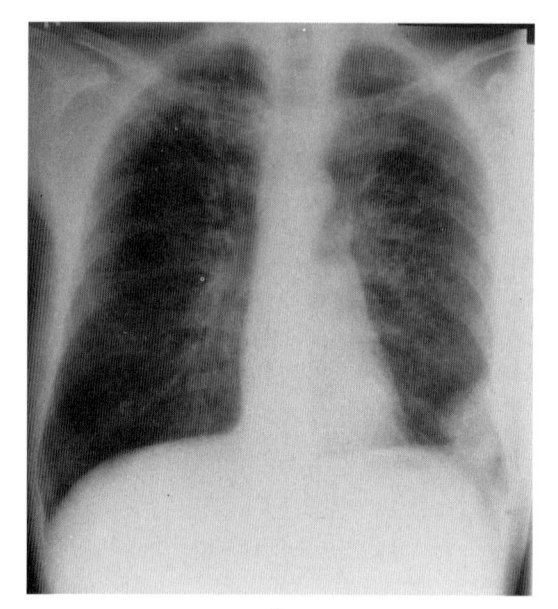

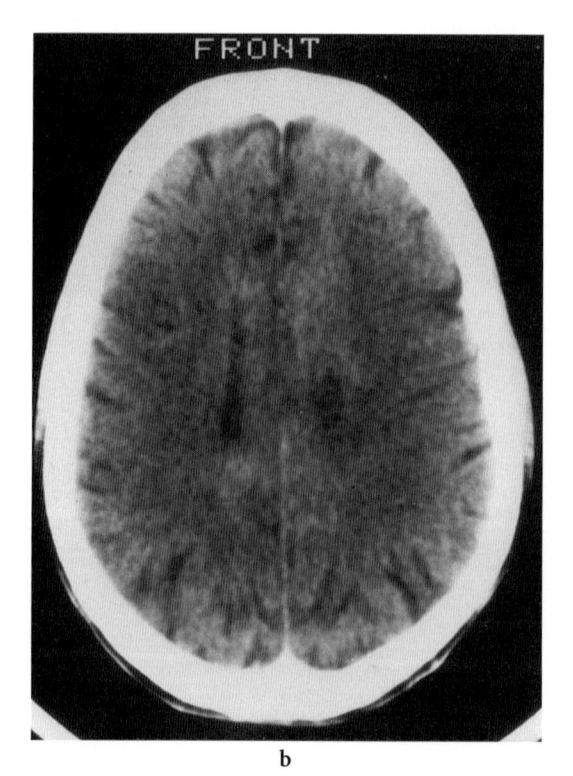

Fig. 6.8a. Chest x-ray showing a left pleural mass. Diagnosis: non-Hodgkin's lymphoma. b. CT scan, showing periventricular metastatic disease.

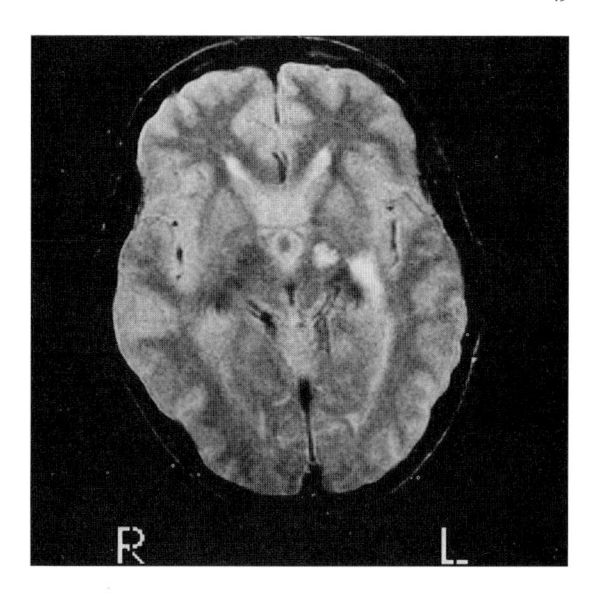

Fig. 6.9. MRI scan showing lesion in the internal capsule. Diagnosis: infarct due to herpes zoster vasculitis.

tive body of evidence, clinical and laboratory, to suggest that at least in some patients the virus enters the central nervous system early in the course of the disease. Seroconversion illnesses may include an aseptic meningitis (Ho et al. 1985b), a myelitis (Denning et al. 1987), a cauda equina syndrome (Zeman and Donaghy 1991) and an encephalitis (Carne et al. 1985). Lumbar puncture studies in asymptomatic patients reveal abnormalities in up to two-thirds. HIV can be cultured in up to one-third of these cases (McArthur et al. 1988). All areas of the neuraxis may be affected by the virus. To some extent the incidence of a particular complication varies with the stage of disease and hence the degree of immunosuppression. For example, the demyelinating neuropathy, which is postulated to have an autoimmune mechanism, tends to occur at the seroconversion or asymptomatic stages (Cornblath et al. 1987) when a polyclonal hypergammaglobulinaemia is evident. Other autoimmune phenomena manifesting at this stage include a thrombocytopenia and a polymyositis. Clinical evidence of the HIV encephalopathy occurs in the symptomatic stages of the disease.

HIV Meningitis

An acute monophasic aseptic meningitis may occur at the time of seroconversion. Although, initially, antibody tests for HIV may be negative, p24 antigen can usually be detected in the serum and CSF (Kessler et al. 1987; Stramer et al. 1989). Anecdotal reports suggest that occasionally HIV-I antibody may be detected in the CSF but not in the serum during the acute illness (Rolfs and Schumacher 1990).

Later on in the spectrum of HIV infection, recurrent episodes or a low-grade chronic meningitis may occur, occasionally with cranial nerve involvement (Hollander 1987). The trigeminal, facial and auditory nerves are most commonly affected. Cerebrospinal fluid examination is necessary to exclude the other potential causes of meningitis such as cryptococcus, lymphoma and syphilis.

Whether this group of patients with clinical evidence of a chronic HIV meningitis is more prone to developing HIV encephalopathy or whether there is a role of zidovudine at this stage has not been determined.

Vacuolar Myelopathy

Up to 30% of AIDS patients have evidence of spinal cord abnormalities at autopsy (Petito et al. 1985). The spinal cord dysfunction presents as a progressive paraparesis with sensory ataxia and sphincter involvement evolving over weeks or a few months. A sensory level is not usually detected. However, this myelopathy can be difficult to detect clinically in debilitated patients who are often in the terminal stages of their disease. HIV encephalopathy clinically and pathologically has been reported to be a frequent accompanying feature (Navia et al. 1986a,b).

Neuropathologically, there is white matter spongy vacuolation due to swelling within myelin sheaths most extensive in the cervical and thoracic cord. The vacuoles, most numerous in the lateral and dorsal columns, are associated with lipid-laden macrophages. Although pathologically there are similarities to subacute combined degeneration of the cord due to vitamin B_{12} and folate deficiency this has not been documented in HIV-infected patients with spinal cord disease. Despite the successful isolation of HIV from the spinal cord, the role of HIV in the pathogenesis remains controversial as the virus has not been demonstrated in the areas with vacuolar change. The association of another human retrovirus, human T lymphotropic virus type I (HTLV-I), with myelopathy suggests that HIV-I can itself affect the spinal cord directly. Anecdotal reports have documented patients dually-infected with both HIV-I and HTLV-I. It has been suggested that patients whose symptoms are primarily due to HTLV-I may improve with steroid therapy (Aboulafia et al. 1990; McArthur et al. 1990).

Peripheral Neuropathy

Peripheral neuropathy accounts for up to 20% of all the clinical neurological complications seen in HIV infection. A subclinical neuropathy has been reported in 50%–90% of all AIDS patients. However, within the context of HIV infection there is a wide spectrum of clinicopathological entities that may be encountered (Connolly and Manji 1991). Although there is doubt about the pathogenesis of some of these peripheral nerve syndromes, HIV has been isolated occasionally from the peripheral nerve, suggesting that direct viral infection can occur. Some authorities suggest that CMV may play an important role in some cases.

Inflammatory Demyelinating Neuropathies

Inflammatory neuropathies may occur at any stage of HIV infection. Although well documented in the literature, in practice they occur rarely (Fuller 1991). Most reported cases have been described at the seroconversion and early symptomatic stages. Clinically, the presentation may be acute, subacute or chronic. Distal muscle weakness, which may progress proximally, is associated with progressive areflexia. Sensory signs and symptoms are variable in severity. Nerve conduction tests show a demyelinating pattern, with slowing of motor and sensory conduction velocities and evidence of conduction block and prolonged distal motor latencies. The cerebrospinal fluid may reveal an elevated protein level. In contrast to demyelinating neuropathies (Guillain-Barre syndrome and chronic inflammatory demyelinating polyneuropathy) in non-HIV practice, the cell count may be elevated. Sural nerve biopsies, if performed, show axonal loss, areas of demyelination and an infiltrate of mononuclear cells (Cornblath et al. 1987).

A number of factors suggest that these demyelinating neuropathies result from autoimmune mechanisms. Most reported cases have occurred early in the course of HIV disease when a hypergammaglobulinaemia due to polyclonal B cell stimulation has been identified. Associated autoimmune phenomena described at this stage include thrombocytopenia and polymyositis. Anecdotal reports of treatment with plasmapheresis and corticosteroids have been shown to be successful.

The clinical course is variable. Progression is often slow, and spontaneous improvement can occur, making it difficult to assess the various treatments without a prospective randomised study. The therapeutic options lie between plasmapheresis and corticosteroids (Cornblath et al. 1987). Each form of therapy has advantages and disadvantages. Practically, there may be difficulties in obtaining the use of HIV-dedicated plasmapharesis equipment and the procedure has its own complications with the necessity of central lines and the risk of infection. High-dose steroid therapy may result in further immunosuppression. Recent evidence in non-AIDS related cases of the Guillain-Barre syndrome and chronic inflammatory demyelinating polyneuropathy (CIDP) suggests that intravenous immunoglobulin is effective (van der Meche et al. 1992; Cornblath et al. 1991). However, it is unclear whether this can be extrapolated to patients with HIV disease, but is another option to be considered.

Mononeuritis Multiplex

Mononeuritis multiplex has been described most commonly in the early symptomatic (ARC) stages of HIV infection (Lipkin et al. 1985). It is characterised by the abrupt onset of mononeuropathies occurring periodically in various distributions e.g. sensory loss over the trunk, face or limbs, or weakness in the distribution of any peripheral nerve or root. Cranial neuropathies may occur simultaneously.

The largest series of 9 patients in the literature collected by Lipkin et al. showed evidence, on EMG studies, of a multifocal axonal and demyelinating neuropathy. Sural nerve biopsy confirmed these neurophysiological findings but in addition showed evidence of epineural and endoneurial perivascular inflammation (Lipkin et al. 1985). Other workers have reported a necrotising vasculitis evident on biopsy (Dalakas and Pereshkpour 1988). In some patients, the mononeuritis progressed with the multifocal lesions coalescing into a distal symmetrical neuropathy. Treatment with steroids seemed to have little effect but one patient stabilised after plasmapharesis.

Distal Symmetrical Peripheral Neuropathy (DSPN)

This is the commonest type of neuropathy encountered in patients with AIDS. Clinical prevalence rates have been estimated between 10% and 35% (Cornblath and McArthur 1988; So et al. 1988b). However, these may be underestimates since patients over the age of 50 years, those with a history of excessive alcohol use, diabetes or exposure to a known neurotoxic drug such as isoniazid were excluded. Such individuals might well be much more sensitive to any HIV-related neurotoxic effect. Histopathological abnormalities were found in 19/20 (95%) of one autopsy series of patients dying with AIDS (de la Monte et al. 1988). This included some with no symptoms suggestive of peripheral nervous disease.

DSPN has been described in all HIV risk groups including homosexual and bisexual men, intravenous drug users and those infected through contaminated blood products. Although it is usually found in the later stages of AIDS, nevertheless some of the patients in the series by Cornblath et al. had ARC only.

Clinically, this is now a well-described entity with patients presenting with paraesthesias on the dorsum and soles of both feet but with complaints of weakness occurring only rarely. Painful dysaesthesias and hyperpathia occur 25%–62% of these patients. Some workers suggest that this group of painful polyneuropathy may represent a separate subgroup with cytomegalovirus playing an important role in the pathogenesis (Fuller and Jacobs 1989). In some cases the polyneuropathy is asymptomatic. The upper limbs and hands are usually symptom-free.

The most consistent signs on examination are absent or depressed ankle reflexes, the latter particularly when compared to brisk knee jerks, perhaps as a result of a vacuolar myelopathy. Impaired vibration sense is also a common finding whereas joint position and pinprick are less impaired. Muscle wasting and weakness of the small muscles of the feet are found in less than half of the patients with DSPN.

Neurophysiological studies have shown abnormalities in both motor and sensory components. The most consistent finding has been of reduced amplitude of the sensory action potential, particularly of the sural nerve. Conduction velocities are normal or only slightly reduced to a degree compatible with the degree of axonal loss (Cornblath and McArthur 1988; So et al. 1988b). Similar neurophysiological results are described by Fuller when studying AIDS patients with no symptoms or signs of a peripheral neuropathy (Fuller et al. 1991). Follow-up of these patients has produced disparate results, with some suggesting progression of the neuropathy with a decrease in ankle reflexes and the subsequent development of slowed conduction velocities and conduction block suggesting a secondary demyelinative process (Cornblath and McArthur 1988; Bailey et al. 1988). Others have described a fairly non-progressive course to the disease.

Thus, clinically and neurophysiologically, the underlying mechanism would seem to be one of a length-dependent dying-back axonopathy with perhaps the development, secondarily, of an associated demyelinative process.

Aetiological factors that have been studied have produced no clear-cut relationships. These have induced measurements of the following: glucose, vitamin B12, folate, ESR and immunoglobulin levels (So et al. 1988b). Immunological parameters such as CD4 and B2 microglobulin levels have also failed to be correlated with the development of this neuropathy. There have, however, been some correlations with factors which may be considered markers for generalised systemic disease such as severity of weight loss and the duration of systemic symptoms such as unexplained fevers; lymphadenopathy and recurrent cutaneous herpetic infections have been present (So et al. 1988b). Some workers have defined a specific painful peripheral neuropathy in AIDS and because of a temporal relationship with active CMV infection have ascribed a causal role to the CMV virus (Fuller et al. 1989). Furthermore, it is speculated that the anatomical localisation of pathology lies within the dorsal root ganglia although these ganglia have rarely been studied because of the technical difficulties in removing them at post mortem. However, against this argument, CMV infection is very common in end-stage AIDS; there are no data to suggest that this painful neuropathy improves on anti CMV therapy and CMV has not been isolated from the peripheral nerves of these patients.

Histopathological studies of nerves from cases of DSPN show evidence of axonal loss with some demyelination. An associated feature is the finding of mononuclear inflammatory cells around the endoneurial blood vessels and within the endoneurium. Multinucleated giant cells which are the hallmark of HIV encephalitis have not been described (de la Monte et al. 1988). An intriguing finding by de la Monte has been that these mononuclear cells stain intensely for HLA class I and class II antigens, implying activated cells associated with a cell mediated response. The induction of these major HLA antigens may be related to the release of lymphokines, which could result in axonal and myelin damage. This is particularly attractive in trying to propose any pathological mechanisms involved, since HIV has only been cultured from the sural nerve in 2 patients (Ho et al. 1985a), and retroviral-like particles isolated in one (Bailey et al. 1988).

A detailed study of the sural nerve in AIDS patients with no evidence of peripheral neuropathy found a non-specific low-grade axonal loss with no inflammation. These changes are similar to those found in normal ageing, lung cancer and chronic respiratory insufficiency. These findings did not correlate with the duration of AIDS, the degree of immunosuppression as indicated by the CD4 count, the body mass index, vitamin B12 levels or the albumin levels (Fuller et al. 1991).

To date, treatment has been symptomatic rather than curative. Anecdotally, 3 patients did not improve with zidovudine in one study (Cornblath and McArthur 1988), whereas one patient's symptoms have been reported to have improved with the drug (Yarchoan et al. 1987). Simple analgesics, tricyclic antidepressants, carbamazepine or clonazepam may relieve neuropathic pain. Transcutaneous nerve stimulation may provide some relief for some patients. Marked distal weakness may be helped by ankle-foot orthoses.

Myopathy

In the early years of the AIDS epidemic there were occasional reports of a steroid-responsive polymyositic illness (Dalakas et al. 1986). The reported cases occurred during both the symptomatic (ARC/AIDS) and asymptomatic phases of HIV infection (Dalakas and Pereshkpour 1988). Subsequent reports noted a paucity of inflammatory cells in some biopsy specimens (Lange et al. 1988), and other workers described the presence of nemaline (rod) bodies (Dalakas et al. 1987; Gonzales et al. 1988), microvesicular degeneration of muscle fibres and type II fibre atrophy in association with myofibre degeneration (Panegyres et al. 1988). HIV antigens were found in OKT4 antibody-positive lymphocytes but not within the muscle cells (Dalakas et al. 1986). The unusual features led to the use of the term "HIV myopathy". The largest series of patients with "HIV myopathy" studied reported some improvement in all patients treated with steroids

(Simpson 1988). However, 3 other patients improved spontaneously. Another study described one patient who was successfully treated with plasmapheresis (Gonzales et al. 1988). Although drug trials of zidovudine in animal models had not predicted muscle-related side effects, the first clinical trials of zidovudine in ARC/AIDS patients reported myalgia occurring significantly more frequently in the zidovudine group (Richman et al. 1987). In 1988, Bessen reported 4 cases of myopathy implicating zidovudine (Bessen et al. 1988). Clinically, there was little to differentiate these cases from those due to HIV myopathy. The biopsy specimens showed dissolution of muscle fibres but little evidence of inflammation, again making it difficult to differentiate histologically this presumed drug-induced myopathy from that due to HIV itself. Thus, although a distinct clinico-pathological syndrome was not delineated, zidovudine was incriminated in these and subsequently-reported cases because the patients were on the drug at the time of the development of the myopathy. However, there were inconsistencies. Some patients improved on drug withdrawal (Bessen et al. 1988; Gorard et al. 1988; Panegyres et al. 1988), but others who seemed similar in all other respects did not (Till and MacDonell 1990). Similarly, some (Gertner et al. 1989), but not all (Fischl et al. 1989; Simpson et al. 1989), had a recurrence of their myopathic symptoms on rechallenge.

Panegyres first described ultrastructural differences in the muscle biopsies of the zidovudine-exposed and non-exposed groups in a small study of subjects presenting with muscle symptoms (Panegyres et al. 1990). Vesicular changes present on light microscopy in the former were due to enlargement of mitochondria and cristae abnormalities. In the non-exposed group, vesicular changes were due to dilatation of the sarcoplasmic reticulum. Dalakas et al. 1990 confirmed this finding of a toxic mitochondrial myopathy in a zidovudine-treated group with the description of ragged red fibres in the treated, but not in the untreated group. The associated inflammatory myopathy was indistinguishable between the two groups. More recently, the same workers documented a decrease of up to 80% in the mitochondrial DNA content of patients with myopathy attributed to zidovudine (Arnaudo et al. 1991). Since zidovudine is readily incorporated into mitochondrial DNA by gamma-DNA polymerase, resulting in the termination of DNA replication, these are not unexpected findings. Thus, although there is evidence that zidovudine treatment is associated with ultrastructural changes, the clinicopathological correlates remain unclear. Whether zidovudine causes a toxic mitochondrial myopathy is still a question that is not resolved. For example, in the Dalakas study although 47% (7/15) of the drug-induced myopathy group improved on drug withdrawal, 27% (4/15) showed no change or even worsened. Twenty percent (3/15) improved on steroid therapy. Muscle biopsy findings did not predict these differing clinical responses. Rechallenge with zidovudine caused a recurrence of the myopathic problems in one case but not in two others. Simpson et al. (1992) studying similar patients has been unable to characterise a zidovudine-induced myopathy using the presence of ragged red fibres as a feature. The reasons for this discrepancy are still not clear.

The management of a patient presenting with symptoms of muscle disease can be difficult. Stopping zidovudine is not a decision to be undertaken lightly since it has been shown to slow down disease progression. Most strategies at present are based on anecdotal experience, and prospective, controlled trials are clearly needed. A suggested plan of management is outlined below. In patients with mild symptoms and little or no evidence of proximal muscle weakness a non-steroidal anti-inflammatory drug may alleviate the symptoms. In cases where the muscle biopsy shows significant inflammatory changes, corticosteroids are indicated without cessation of zidovudine therapy. Otherwise, or in cases where a muscle biopsy has not been performed, a trial of stopping the zidovudine for 2–4 weeks should be considered. If improvement occurs, then a lower dose of the drug can be gradually introduced at a later date. In cases where there is no improvement or there is continued deterioration, a course of corticosteroids should be tried, with the continuation of zidovudine. The dose of corticosteroid should be reduced to the lowest effective dose since the risks of prolonged therapy in this clinical setting are, as yet, unknown.

HIV Encephalopathy (HIV Encephalitis: AIDS Dementia Complex (ADC))

HIV Encephalitis or AIDS Dementia Complex (ADC) is often the most dreaded complication of HIV disease. It is characterised by a progressive deterioration in motor function, behaviour and cognition. The prevalence in AIDS patients has been estimated as between 6% and 66%. This reflects variables such as patient selection bias, the criteria used for diagnosis and the stage of disease (Maj 1990).

In 1987, Grant et al., using a battery of neuropsychological tests, suggested that 44% of a small group of HIV seropositive asymptomatic patients performed abnormally. However, this study has been criticised on methodological grounds. Subsequent larger cohort studies with appropriate seronegative controls showed the prevalence of neurological and neuropsychological abnormalities to be no higher in the asymptomatic group than in the seronegatives (McArthur et al. 1989; McAllister et al. 1992). MRI scans, similarly, have shown no evidence of the development of subclinical lesions suggestive of HIV encephalopathy in this asymptomatic group (Manji et al. 1991). Furthermore, longitudinal studies for periods up to 18 months showed no evidence of deterioration. Although most of these studies have concentrated on homosexual/bisexual men, similar results have been found in other HIV risk groups such as haemophiliacs. The issue of a subclinical encephalopathy in asymptomatic HIV infected individuals, however, remains controversial. In 1990, Wilkie et al. found significant abnormalities of information processing and certain memory tests in an asymptomatic HIV-positive group when compared to matched seronegative controls.

Clinical Features

In HIV encephalopathy the clinical and neuropsychological picture conforms to the pattern of dementia termed "subcortical". This is characterised by a diffuse slowing of psychomotor functioning. In non-HIV practice this is found in conditions such as progressive supranuclear palsy, Huntington's chorea and Parkinson's disease. The symptoms in the early stages may be non-specific with complaints of poor memory and concentration. Friends or family members may notice subtle personality changes. The differential diagnosis of these vague symptoms include depression, anxiety, recreational drug abuse, coincidental infection and metabolic disturbances. Neurological examination at this stage may show some clumsiness and difficulty with rapid alternating movements. If no physical cause can be found, a neuropsychiatric assessment is invaluable. It may, for example, reveal a pseudodementia due to depression. As the disease progresses, the severe cognitive dysfunction is associated with apathy, withdrawal or even complete mutism. Drowsiness is not a feature and should alert one to the possibility of infection or increased sensitivity to any one of a number of drugs such as narcotics and sedatives. At this late stage physical examination may reveal bilateral pyramidal signs, frontal lobe release sign (grasp and snout reflexes), impaired smooth eye movements and myoclonus. A spastic paraparesis, bladder and bowel problems are not uncommon, due to an associated vacuolar myelopathy. Seizures occur in 10% of cases. Death usually supervenes from the complications of immobility or the severe immunosuppression (Navia et al. 1986b; UCLA conference 1989).

Diagnosis

A diagnosis of HIV encephalopathy is made on the basis of a compatible history and examination together with the exclusion of other causes of dementia and confusion. This implies a thorough metabolic and radiological investigation, including a CT or MRI brain scan and examination of the cerebrospinal fluid. The CSF parameters in HIV encephalopathy are non-specific and cannot be used to substantiate a diagnosis of HIV encephalopathy. CSF examination serves rather to exclude other possible complications such as meningitis due to cryptococcus or lymphoma. Similarly, a normal brain scan does not rule out the diagnosis but helps to exclude space-occupying lesions such as toxoplasmosis, lymphoma and PML which may present with confusion, behavioural changes or dementia.

CT and MRI brain scans may, especially in the later stages, show evidence of progressive cerebral atrophy. Additionally, T_2-weighted images on MRI may reveal diffuse white matter abnormalities, usually starting in the frontal regions (Fig. 6.10).

Pathology

There is a spectrum of histopathological changes to be found in the brains of patients with HIV encephalopathy. Generally, there is poor correlation between the pathological findings and the clinical severity of the disease.

Macroscopically, cerebral atrophy and white matter pallor are common findings. Microscopically, this pallor correlates with a reactive astrocytosis and demyelination. This may represent the earliest pathological changes of HIV encephalopathy. Gray et al. (1992) recently described myelin pallor and a reactive astrocytosis in a small group of asymptomatic HIV-infected individuals who died of causes unrelated to HIV.

In the advanced stages of the disease, the pathological features include multinucleated giant cells (Navia et al. 1986a). These are syncytia of HIV-infected macrophages and are considered pathognomonic of HIV encephalitis. Microglial nodules are also commonly found in the cortex and in the basal ganglia. However, these are non-specific since they may be caused by CMV or HIV infection. There are increasing reports of pathological evidence of both cortical grey matter involvement in cases of HIV encephalopathy and neuronal loss (Scaravilli et al. 1990; Everall et al. 1991).

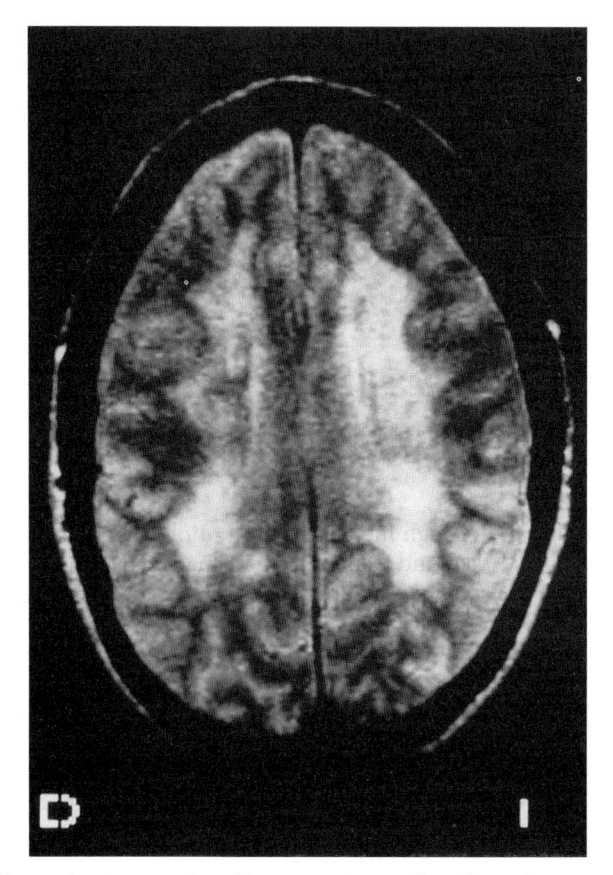

Fig. 6.10. MRI scan showing extensive white matter abnormality. Diagnosis: HIV encephalopathy.

Inflammatory changes with multinucleated giant cells may occasionally be found in the spinal cord. A vacuolar myelopathy is however a more common finding and seems to correlate with the degree of HIV encephalopathy (Navia et al. 1986a).

In cases of paediatric AIDS, HIV encephalopathy presents within the first 2 years of life. In addition to the neuropathological changes already described, a calcific vasculopathy results in calcium deposition in the basal ganglia and in the white matter (Belman et al. 1986).

Management

Zidovudine penetrates the cerebrospinal fluid and hence it has been postulated that it may have a beneficial effect on the course of HIV encephalopathy. A retrospective study suggested that the incidence of the condition has been reduced since the introduction of the drug (Portegies et al. 1989). However, an important confounding factor in the few studies that have claimed benefit with zidovudine has been the improvement in the patient's general wellbeing which could account for the changes reported (Schmitt et al. 1988). Until the results of further prospective trials are available no definite conclusions can be made.

Supportive measures are crucial in the management of this group of patients. This requires close cooperation between the medical, nursing, social work and home care teams. Minor infections may result in a dramatic deterioration. Drug regimens need to be regularly reviewed since these patients may be sensitive to sedatives and antidepressants.

Pathogenesis of HIV Encephalopathy

There is now substantial evidence that HIV enters the central nervous system and may cause an encephalopathy or a subacute encephalitis. HIV has been isolated from the cerebrospinal fluid, brain, spinal cord and sural nerve of AIDS patients with neurological complications (Ho et al. 1985a). Specifically, viral antigens have been localised within macrophages, the multinucleated giant cells which are pathognomonic for HIV encephalitis, and within capillary endothelial cells. In contrast, neuronal cells, oligodendrocytes and astrocytes have been shown to contain viral particles only rarely (Koenig et al. 1986; Pumarola-Sune et al. 1987; Vazeux et al. 1987; Wiley et al. 1986). This may simply reflect the insensitivity of current investigative techniques. Further evidence of central nervous system infection by HIV is provided by the transmission of HIV infection to chimpanzees by inoculation of brain tissue taken from AIDS patients (Gajdusek et al. 1985). Finally, HIV is very similar to visna virus, the prototype lentivirus which causes a chronic debilitative disorder in sheep.

Little is known at present concerning the mechanisms by which HIV gains access to the central nervous system. To date, most support has been given to the "Trojan Horse theory" whereby the virus is transported across the blood–brain barrier in lymphocytes and monocytes which have become infected in the peripheral tissues (Haase 1986). Other mechanisms postulated include direct infection of capillary endothelial cells followed by transfer into adjacent glial, neuronal and microglial cells.

With the current available evidence, the concept that HIV is truly neurotropic seems exaggerated. More appropriate is the idea that macrophage tropism of the virus is tightly coupled to neurotropism of the latter. It seems clear that the CD4 protein which interacts with the HIV viral envelope protein, the gp 120 antigen, is the receptor for HIV in lymphocytes and macrophages (Lasky et al. 1987). Although direct infection of neurons, oligodendrocytes and astrocytes has been rarely documented, there is evidence that CD4 is present on neural tissue cells (Funke et al. 1987). However, it has been possible to infect human neural lines lacking in CD4 (Harouse et al. 1989). This raises the possibility of other receptor mechanisms being present.

The pathogenic mechanisms of HIV-induced damage are also unclear. Direct virus infection of neurons could result in cell death or altered cellular metabolism.

Other hypotheses under investigation currently include the possibility that neuronal dysfunction results indirectly from the release of toxic HIV-specific products such as gp 120 (Brenneman et al. 1988) or cytokines such as interleukins, tumour necrosis factor and interferons from the HIV-infected macrophages. In support of this indirect mechanism is Everall's finding of a 30%

neuronal cell loss in the frontal lobes of patients who have died of AIDS even in cases with no evidence of an HIV encephalitis (Everall et al. 1991). Autoimmune phenomena occur in HIV disease, particularly in the early stages. Examples include thrombocytopenia, polymyositis and a demyelinating neuropathy. The small foci of demyelination found in HIV encephalopathy resemble the lesions found in post-infectious encephalomyelitis and experimental autoimmune encephalomyelitis. It is postulated that similar immune-mediated mechanisms may play a similar role in HIV encephalopathy, raising the possibility of treatment with drugs such as steroids (Dal Canto 1989). As yet, that is no substantial proof for the validity of any of these theories. The role, if any, of co-infection with other viruses in HIV-associated neurologic dysfunction is attractive but uncertain. Cytomegalovirus has been most often implicated. Although the simultaneous presence of CMV and HIV with the same cell has been demonstrated in an AIDS brain, it is unclear if this implies that there is an important role for the CMV or that this is merely a fortuitous finding (Nelson et al. 1988).

The Future

The first decade of the AIDS epidemic has been dominated by the advances made in the management of pneumocystis carinii pneumonia and in the use of zidovudine. As patients live longer, the neurological complications due to both HIV itself and those resulting from opportunistic infections and tumours are poised to play an increasingly important role. These include cytomegalovirus retinitis and encephalitis, progressive multifocal leucoencephalopathy, primary CNS lymphoma and HIV encephalopathy.

At present, the diagnosis of even some of the commoner complications is difficult. A clinico-neuropathological correlation study showed that 68% of primary CNS lymphoma and 50% of PML cases were undiagnosed antemortem (Vago et al. 1991). The diagnosis of toxoplasmic encephalitis is based upon a clinical and radiological response to an empirical trial of therapy. As more effective treatment regimens are developed for the main differential diagnoses of primary CNS lymphoma and PML, their full impact on the current grim outlook can only be assessed after early diagnosis and treatment are implemented. Thus, rapid, non-invasive diagnostic tests are needed, particularly for toxoplasmosis and PML. Polymerase chain reaction (PCR) techniques on CSF would seem to be the way forward.

Although treatment protocols are now well established for toxoplasmosis there is a high incidence of side effects. Furthermore, a significant drawback of the present therapies is their inability to eradicate the latent encysted bradyzoites which chronically infect host tissue and is the source of reactivation in immunocompromised patients. Hence the need for life-long maintenance treatment. Currently, studies are in progress using the napthoquinolone drug C56680 which looks promising against the toxoplasma bradyzoite cysts as well as showing efficacy against *Pneumocystis carinii* (Araujo et al. 1991).

The prevalence of HIV encephalopathy in AIDS patients has been estimated at between 6% and 66%. There are no clear data on the effectiveness of zidovudine in this condition. Much more information is needed on its CNS pharmacokinetics and appropriate controlled trials are required to assess its therapeutic effectiveness and optimum dosages. The neuropathogenic mechanisms of HIV encephalopathy need further clarifying so that appropriate drug regimens can be developed. For example, Lipton has studied neuronal damage caused by the HIV-I viral envelope protein g 120. The rise of intracellular calcium which results in necrosis engendered by the protein was prevented by the use of calcium channel antagonists (Lipton 1991). this may have important therapeutic implications.

Thus, the success achieved in the clinical management of AIDS patients in the 1990s will, to a large extent, reflect the successes achieved in the treatment of the wide spectrum of neurological complications encountered in HIV infection.

References

Aboulafia DM, Saxton EH, Koga H, Diagne A, Rosenblatt JD (1990) A patient with progressive myelopathy and antibodies to human t-cell leukaemia virus type 1 and human immunodeficiency virus type 1 in serum and cerebrospinal fluid. Arch Neurol 47: 477-499

Araujo FG, Huskinson J, Remington JS (1991) Remarkable in vitro and in vivo activities in the hydronaph to quinone 566C80 against tachyzoites and cysts of Toxoplasma gondii. Antimicrob Agents Chemother 35: 293-299

Arnaudo E, Dalakas M, Shankske S, Moraes CT, DiMauro S, Schon EA (1991) Depletion of muscle mitochondrial DNA in AIDS patients with zidovudine-induced myopathy. Lancet 337: 508-510

Bailey RO, Baltch AL, Venkatesh R, Singh JK, Bishop MB (1988) Sensory motor neuropathy associated with AIDS. Neurology 38: 886-891

Barnes PF, Bloch AB, Davidson PT, Snider DEJ (1991) Tuberculosis in patients with human immunodeficiency virus infection. New Engl J Med 324: 1644-1650

Baumgartner JE, Rachlin JR, Beckstead JH et al. (1990) Primary central nervous system lymphomas: natural history and response to radiation therapy in 55 patients with acquired immunodeficiency syndrome. J Neurosurg 73: 206-211

Belman AL, Lantos G, Horoupian D et al. (1986) Calcification of the basal ganglia in infants and children. Neurology 36: 1192-1199

Berger JR, Kaszovitz B, Donovan PJ, Dickenson G (1987) Progressive multifocal leucoencephalopathy associated with human immunodeficiency syndrome. Ann Int Med 107: 78-87

Berry CD, Hooton TM, Collier AC, Lukehart SA (1987) Neurologic relapse after benzathine penicillin therapy for secondary syphilis in a patient with HIV infection. N Engl J Med 316: 1587-1589

Bessen LJ, Greene JB, Louie E, Seitzman P, Weinberg H (1988) Severe polymyositis-like syndrome associated with zidovudine therapy of AIDS and ARC. New Engl J Med 318: 708

Bloom J, Palestine A (1988) The diagnosis of cytomegalovirus retinitis. Ann Int Med 109: 963-969

Bolan M (1992) Management of syphilis in HIV infected persons. In: Sande M, Volberdig P (eds) Medical management of AIDS, 3rd edn. WB Saunders, New York, pp 383-398

Boue F, Bridley F, Deifrassey J, Dormont J, Tchernia G (1990) Lupus anticoagulant and HIV infection: a prospective study. AIDS 4: 467-471

Bozzette S, Larsen R, Chiu J et al. (1991) Fluconazole treatment of persistent Cryptococcus neoformans prostatic infection in AIDS. Ann Intern Med 115: 285-286

Brenneman DE, Westbrook GL, Fitzgerald SP et al. (1988) Neuronal cell killing by the envelope protein in HIV and its prevention by vasoactive intestinal peptide. Nature 335: 639-642

Britton CA, Romagnoli M, Sisti M, Powers JM (1992) PML: analysis of outcome and response to intrathecal ara-C in 26 patients. Neuroscience of HIV infection 1992. Amsterdam. abstract 40

Canoso RT, Zon LI, Groopman JE (1987) Anticardiolipin antibodies associated with HTLV-III infection. Br J Haematol 65: 495-498

Carne E, Smith A, Elkington SG et al. (1985) Acute encephalopathy coincident with seroconversion for anti-HTLV III. Lancet ii: 1206-1208

Catterall D (1975) A short textbook of venerology. The sexually transmitted diseases. 2nd edition. English University Press, London.

Chesney AM, Kemp JE (1924) Incidence of *Spirochaeta pallida* in cerebrospinal fluid during early state of syphilis. JAMA 83: 1725-1728

Chuck SL, Sande M (1989) Infections with cryptococcus neoformans in the acquired immunodeficiency syndrome. New Engl J Med 321: 794-799

Circillo J, Rosenblaum D (1991) Imaging of solitary lesions in AIDS (letter) J Neurosurg 74: 1029

Collart P, Poltevin M, Milovanovic A, Herlin A, Durel J (1980) Kinetic study of serum penicillin concentrations after single doses of benzathine and benethamine penicillins in young and old people. Br J Vener Dis 56: 355-362

Connolly S, Manji H (1991) AIDS and the peripheral nervous system. Hosp Update 17: 474-485

Conway B, Halliday W, Brunham R (1990) HIV associated PML: apparent response to 3'-azido-3'-deoxythymidine. Rev Infect Dis 12: 479-481

Cornblath DR, McArthur JC (1988) Predominantly sensory neuropathy in patients with AIDS and AIDS-related complex. Neurology 38: 794-796

Cornblath DR, McArthur JC, Kennedy PGE, Witte AS, Griffin JW (1987) Inflammatory demyelinating peripheral neuropathies associated with human T-cell lymphotropic virus infection. Ann Neurol 21: 32-40

Cornblath DR, Chaudhry V, Griffin JW (1991) Treatment of chronic inflammatory demyelinating polyneuropathy with intravenous immunoglobulin. Ann Neurol 30: 104-106

Crowe SM, Carlin JB, Stewart KI, Lucas CR, Hoy JF (1991) Predictive value of CD4 lymphocyte numbers for the development of opportunistic infections and malignancies in HIV infected persons. J AIDS 4: 770-776

Dal Canto MC (1989) AIDS and the nervous system: current status and future perspectives. Hum Pathol 20: 410-418

Dalakas MC, Pereshkpour GH (1988) Neuromuscular diseases associated with human immunodeficiency virus infection. Ann Neurol 23 (suppl): S38-S48

Dalakas MC, Pereshkpour GH, Gravell M, Sever JL (1986) Polymyositis associated with AIDS retrovirus. JAMA 256: 2381-2383

Dalakas MC, Pereshkpour GH, Flaherty M (1987) Progressive nemaline (rod) myopathy associated with HIV infection (letter). New Engl J Med 317: 1602-1603

Dalakas MC, Pereshkpour GH, Laukaitis JP, Cohen B, Griffin JJ (1990) Mitochondrial myopathy caused by long-term zidovudine therapy. New Engl J Med 322: 1098-1105

Dannemann B, McCuthan J, Israelski D et al. (1992) Treatment of toxoplasmic encephalitis in patients with AIDS. Ann Intern Med 116: 33-43

De Bouchier T, Schlienger M, Matheron S et al. (1990) PML in AIDS: treatment with radiotherapy. Second European conference on clinical aspects of HIV infection. Brussels. Abstract 64

De Gans J, Portegies P (1989) Neurological complications of infection with the human immunodeficiency virus type 1: a review. Clin Neurol Neurosurg 91: 197-217

de Gans J, Tiersens G, Portegies P, Tuturarina J, Troost D (1990) Predominance of polymorphonuclear leucocytes in the csf of AIDS patients with cytomegalovirus polyradiculopathy. J AIDS 3: 1155-1158

de la Monte SM, Gabuzda DH, Ho DD et al. (1988) Peripheral neuropathy in the acquired immunodeficiency syndrome. Ann Neurol 23: 485-492

De la Paz R, Enzman D (1988) Neuroradiology of acquired immunodeficiency syndrome. In: Rosenblum ML, Levy RM, Bredesen DE (eds) AIDS and the nervous system. Raven Press, New York, pp 121-153

Denning DW, Anderson B, Rudge P, Smith H (1987) Acute myelopathy associated with primary infection with human immunodeficiency virus. Br Med J 294: 143-144

Dismukes WE (1988) Cryptococcal meningitis in patients with AIDS. J Inf Dis 157: 624-628

Drabick JJ, Tramont EC (1990) Utility of the VDRL test in HIV seropositive patients (letter). N Engl J Med 322: 271

Edlin BR, Tokars JI, Grieco MH (1992) An outbreak of multi-drug resistant tuberculosis among hospitalised patients with the acquired immunodeficiency syndrome. N Engl J Med 326: 1514-1521

Eidelberg D, Sotrel A, Vogel H, Walker P, Kleefield J, Crumpacker CSI (1986) Progressive polyradiculopathy in acquired immune deficiency syndrome. Neurology 36: 912-916

Everall IP, Luthert PJ, Lantos PL (1991) Neuronal loss in the frontal cortex in HIV infection. Lancet 337: 1119-1121

Fanning M, Read S, Benson M, Vas S (1990) Foscarnet therapy of cytomegalovirus retinitis in AIDS. J AIDS 3: 472-477

Fischl M, Gagnon S, Uttamchandani R et al. (1989) Myopathy associated with long term zidovudine therapy. Fifth International Conference on AIDS, Montreal, Abs MBP 329

Fuller GN (1991) Neuropathies in AIDS (editorial). Br J Hosp Med 46: 137

Fuller GN, Jacobs JM (1989) Cytomembranous inclusions in the peripheral nerves in AIDS. Acta Neuropathol 79: 336-339

Fuller GN, Jacobs JM, Guiloff RJ (1989) Association of painful peripheral neuropathy in AIDS with cytomegalovirus infection. Lancet ii: 937-941

Fuller GN, Jacobs JM, Guiloff RJ (1991) Subclinical peripheral nerve involvement in AIDS: an electrophysiological and pathological study. JNNP 54: 318-324

Funke I, Hahn A, Rieber EP et al. (1987) The cellular receptor (CD4) of the human immunodeficiency virus is expressed on neurons and glial cells in human brain. J Exp Med 165: 1230-1235

Gajdusek DC, Amyx HL and Gibbs CJ (1985) Infection of chimpanzees by human T-lymphocyte retroviruses in brain and other tissues from AIDS patients. Lancet i: 55-56

Galgiani JN (1990) Fluconazole, a new antifungal agent (Editorial). Ann Int Med 113: 177-179

Gertner E, Thurn JR, Williams DN et al. (1989) Zidovudine-associated myopathy. Am J Med 86: 814-818

Goh BT, Smith GW, Samarsinghe L, Singh V, Lim KS (1984) Penicillin concentrations in serum and cerebrospinal fluid after intramuscular injection of aqueous procaine penicillin 0.6MU with and without probenicid. Br J Vener Dis 60: 371-373

Gonzales MF, Olney RK, So YT et al. (1988) Subacute structural myopathy associated with human immunodeficiency virus infection. Arch Neurol 45: 585-587

Gorard DA, Henry K, Guiloff RJ (1988) Necrotising myopathy and zidovudine (letter). Lancet i: 1050

Grant I, Atkinson JH, Hesselink JR et al. (1987) Evidence for early central nervous system involvement in the acquired immunodeficiency syndrome (AIDS) and other human immunodeficiency virus (HIV) infections. Studies with neuropsychologic testing and magnetic resonance imaging. Ann Intern Med 107: 828-836

Grant IH, Gold JW, Rosenblum M, Niedzwiecki D and Armstrong D (1990) Toxoplasma gondii serology in HIV infected patients: the development of central nervous system toxoplasmosis in AIDS. AIDS 4: 519-521

Graveleau P, Perol R, Chapman A (1989) Regression of caudina equina syndrome in AIDS patients being treated with ganciclovir. Lancet ii: 511-512

Gray F, Gherardi R, Wingate E et al. (1989) Diffuse encephalitis in toxoplasmosis. J Neurol 236: 273-277

Gray F, Lescs MC, Keohane C et al. (1992) Early brain changes in HIV infection: neuropathological study of 11 HIV seropositive, non-AIDS cases. J Neuropath Exp Neurol 2: 177-185

Haas J, Bolan G, Larsen S, Clement M, Bacchetti P, Moss A (1990) Sensitivity of treponemal tests for detecting prior treated syphilis during human immunodeficiency virus infection. 162: 862-866

Haase AT (1986) Pathogenesis of lentivirus infections. Nature 322: 130-136

Hahn RD, Clerk EG (1946) Asymptomatic neurosyphilis: a review of the literature. Am J Syph Gon Vener Dis 30: 305-316

Harouse JM, Kunsch C, Hartle HT et al. (1989) CD4 independent infection of human neural cells by human immunodeficiency virus type 1. J Virol 63: 2527-2533

Haverkos HW (1987) Assessment of therapy for toxoplasma encephalitis. AJM 82: 907

Helbert M, Robinson D, Buchanan D et al. (1990) Mycobacterial infection in patients infected with the human immunodeficiency virus. Thorax 45: 45-48

Hicks CB, Benson PM, Lupton GP, Tramont EC (1987) Seronegative secondary syphilis in a patient infected with HIV with Kaposi's sarcoma: a diagnostic dilemma. Ann Intern Med 107: 492-495

Ho DD, Rota TR, Schooley RT et al. (1985a) Isolation of HTLV-III from cerebrospinal fluid and neural tissues of patients with neurologic syndromes related to the acquired immunodeficiency syndrome. New Engl J Med 313: 1493-1497

Ho DD, Sarngadharan MG, Resnick L (1985b) Primary human T-lymphotrophic virus type III infection. Ann Int Med 103: 880-883

Hollander HS S (1987) Human immunodeficiency virus associated meningitis. AJM 83: 813-816

Holliman RE (1988) Toxoplasmosis and the acquired immune deficiency syndrome. J Inf 16: 121-128

Holtzman DM, Kaku DA, So YT (1989) New-onset seizures associated with human immunodeficiency virus infection: causation and clinical features in 100 cases. AJM 87: 173-177

Katz DA, Berger JR (1989) Neurosyphilis in acquired immunodeficiency syndrome. Arch Neurol 46: 895-898

Kayser A (1990) Cauda equina syndrome due to toxoplasmosis. J. Neurosurg 1: 999-999

Keeling DM, Birley H, Machin SJ (1990) Multiple transient ischaemic attacks and a mild stroke in a HIV positive patient with anticardiolipin antibodies. Blood Coagulation Fibrinolysis 1: 333-335

Kessler HA, Blaauw B, Spear J et al. (1987) Diagnosis of HIV infection in seronegative homosexuals presenting with an acute viral syndrome. JAMA 258: 1196-1199

Klein RS (1989) Prophylaxis of opportunistic infections in individuals infected with HIV. AIDS 3 (Suppl 1): S161-S173

Koenig S, Gendelman HE, Orenstein JM et al. (1986) Detection of the AIDS virus in macrophages in brain tissue from AIDS patients with encephalopathy. Science 233: 1089-1093

Krown SE (1990) Treatment of AIDS associated malignancy. Cancer Detection Prevention 14: 405–409

Lange DJ, Britton CB, Younger DS, Hays AP (1988) The neuromuscular manifestations of human immunodeficiency virus infections. Arch Neurol 45: 1084–1088

Lanska MJ, Lanska DJ, Schmidley JW (1988) Syphilitic polyradiculopathy in an HIV-positive man. Neurology 38: 1297–1301

Laskin O, Cederberg DM, Mills J, Eton CJ, Speltor SA (1987) Ganciclovir for the treatment and suppression of serious infections caused by cytomegalovirus. AJM 83: 201–207

Lasky LA, Nakamura G, Smith DH et al. (1987) Delineation of a region of the human immunodeficiency virus type 1 gp 120 glycoprotein critical for interaction with the CD4 receptor. Cell 50: 975–985

Leport C, Raffi F, Matheron S et al. (1988) Treatment of central nervous system toxoplasmosis with pyrimethamine/sulphadiazine combination in 35 patients with AIDS. AJM 84: 94

Levy RM, Bredesen DE, Rosenblum ML (1985) Neurological manifestations of the acquired immunodeficiency syndrome (AIDS): experience at UCSF and review of the literature. J Neurosurg 62: 475–495

Levy RM, Janssen RS, Bush TJ, Rosenblum ML (1988) Neuroepidemiology of acquired immunodeficiency syndrome. J AIDS 1: 31–40

Levy RM, Mills CM, Posin JP, Moore SG, Rosenblum ML, Bredesen DE (1990a) The efficacy and clinical impact of brain imaging in neurologically symptomatic AIDS patients: A prospective CT/MRI study. J. AIDS 3: 461–471

Levy RM, Russel E, Brody BA, Yungbluth M (1990b) The efficacy of stereotaxic brain biopsy in neurologically symptomatic AIDS patients. Neurological and neuropsychological complications of HIV infection, Monterey, California. Abstract Neu 7

Lipkin WI, Parry G, Kiprov D, Abrams D (1985) Inflammatory neuropathy in homosexual men with lymphadenopathy. Neurology 35: 1479–1483

Lipton SA (1991) Calcium channel antagonists and human immunodeficiency virus coat protein-mediated neuronal injury. Ann Neurol 30: 110–114

Luft BJ, Hafner R (1990) Toxoplasmic encephalitis. AIDS 4: 593–595

Lukehart SA, Hook EW, Baker-Zander SA, Collier AC, Critchlow CW, Handsfield HH (1988) Invasion of the central nervous system by *Treponema pallidum*: implications for diagnosis and treatment. Ann Intern Med 109: 855–862

Luxton L, Harrison M (1979) Chronic subdural haematoma. Q J Med 189: 43–53

MacMahon M, Glass J, Hayward D et al. (1991) Epstein Barr virus in AIDS related central nervous system lymphoma. Lancet 338: 969–973

Maj M (1990) Organic mental disorders in HIV-1 infection (editorial review). AIDS 4: 831–840

Manji H, Connolly S, McAllister RM et al. (1991) A longitudinal study of brain magnetic resonance imaging in HIV infection: the Middlesex/MRC cohort. Neuroscience of HIV infection, Padua Italy. Abstract 46

Manji H, Malin A, Connolly S (1992) CMV polyradiculopathy: suggestions for new strategies in treatment (letter). Genitourin Med 68: 192

Mark AS, Atlas SW (1989) Progressive multifocal leucoencephalopathy in patients with AIDS: appearance of MR images. Radiology 173: 517–520

Matlow AG, Rachlis AR (1990) Syphilis serology in HIV infected patients with symptomatic neurosyphilis: case report and review. Rev Infect Dis 12: 703–707

McAllister RH, Herns MV, Harrison MJG et al. (1992) Neurological and neuropsychological performance in HIV seropositive asymptomatic individuals. JNNP 55: 143–148

McArthur JC (1987) Neurologic manifestations of AIDS. Medicine 66: 407–437

McArthur JC, Cohen BA, Homayoun F, Cornblath DR, Selnes O (1988) Cerebrospinal fluid abnormalities in homosexual men with and without neuropsychiatric findings. Ann Neurol 23 (Suppl): 534–535

McArthur JC, Cohen BA, Selnes OA et al. (1989) Low prevalence of neurological and neuropsychological abnormalities in otherwise healthy HIV-1-infected individuals: results of the multicenter AIDS cohort study. Ann Neurol 26: 601–611

McArthur JC, Griffin JW, Cornblath DR et al. (1990) Steroid-responsive myeloneuropathy in a man dually infected with HIV-1 and HTLV-I. Neurology 40: 938–944

Mehren A, Burns P, Mamani M et al. (1988) Toxoplasmic myelitis mimicking intramedullary cord tumour. Neurology 38: 1648–1650

Merritt HH (1940) The early clinical and laboratory manifestations of syphilis of the central nervous system. N Engl J Med 223: 446–450

Miller RG, Storey JR, Greco CM (1990) Ganciclovir in the treatment of progressive AIDS-related polyradiculopathy. Neurology 40: 569-574

Muscher DM, Hamill RJ, Baughn RE (1990) Effect of HIV infection on the course of syphilis and on the response to treatment. Ann Intern Med 113: 872-881

Navia BA, Cho E-S, Petito CK, Price RW (1986a) The AIDS dementia complex: II. neuropathology. Ann Neurol 19: 525-535

Navia BA, Jordan BD, Price RW (1986b) The AIDS dementia complex: I. clinical features. Ann Neurol 19: 517-524

Navia BA, Petito CK, Gold JW, Cho ES (1986c) Cerebral toxoplasmosis complicating the acquired immune deficiency syndrome: clinical and neuropathological findings in 27 patients. Ann Neurol 19: 224-238

Nelson JA, Reynolds-Kohler C, Oldstone MB et al. (1988) HIV and HCMV coinfect brain cells in patients with AIDS. Virology 165: 286-290

Panegyres PK, Tan N, Kakulas BA, Armstrong JA and Hollingsworth P (1988) Necrotising myopathy and zidovudine (letter). Lancet i: 1050-1051

Panegyres PK, Papadimitriou JM, Hollingsworth PN, Armstrong JA, Kakulas BA (1990) Vesicular changes in the myopathies of AIDS. Ultrastructural observations and their relationship to zidovudine treatment. JNNP 53: 649-655

Petito CK, Navia BA, Cho E-S et al. (1985) Vacuolar myelopathy pathologically resembling subacute combined degeneration in patients with the acquired immunodeficiency syndrome. New Engl J Med 312: 874-879

Pons VG, Jacobs RA, Hollander H (1988) Nonviral infections of the central nervous system in patients with AIDS. In: Rosenblum ML, Levy RM, and Bredesen DE (eds) AIDS and the nervous system. Raven Press, New York, pp 263-283

Portegies P, de Gans J, Lange JMA et al. (1989) Declining incidence of AIDS dementia complex after introduction of zidovudine treatment. Br Med J 299: 819-821

Portegies P, Algra PR, Hollack CEM et al. (1991) Response to cytarabine in progressive multifocal leucoencephalopathy in AIDS. Lancet 337: 680-681

Porter SB, Sande MA (1992) Toxoplasmosis of the central nervous system in the acquired immunodeficiency syndrome. N Engl J Med 327: 1643-1648

Pumarola-Sune T, Navia BA, Cordon-Cardo C et al. (1987) HIV antigen in the brains of patients with the AIDS dementia complex. Ann Neurol 21: 490-496

Richardson EP (1988) Progressive multifocal leucoencephalopathy 30 years later (Editorial). New Engl J Med 318: 315-316

Richman DD, Fischl MA, Grieco MH et al. (1987) The toxicity of azidothymidine (AZT) in the treatment of patients with AIDS and AIDS-related complex. New Engl J Med 317: 192-197

Rolfs A, Schumacher HC (1990) Early findings in the cerebrospinal fluid of patients with HIV-1 infection of the central nervous system (letter). New Engl J Med 323: 419

Rosenblum ML, Levy RM, Bredesen DE (eds) (1988) AIDS and the nervous system. Raven Press, New York

Saag MA, Powderly WG, Cloud GA et al. (1992) Comparison of amphotericin B with fluconasole in the treatment of acute AIDS associated cryptococcal meningitis. New Engl J Med 326: 83-89

Said G, Lacroix C, Chemouilli P et al. (1991) Cytomegalovirus neuropathy in acquired immunodeficiency syndrome: A clinical and pathological study. Ann Neurol 29: 139-146

Scaravilli F, Ciardi A, Sinclair E, Harcourt Webster J, Lucas S (1990) Involvement of grey matter in HIV encephalitis. Neurological and neuropsychological complications of HIV infection, Monterey, California. Abstract

Schmitt F, Bigley J, McKinnis R (1988) Neuropsychological outcome of zidovudine treatment of patients with AIDS and AIDS-related complex. New Engl J Med 299: 819-821

Simpson D (1988) Myopathy associated with human immunodeficiency virus (HIV) but not zidovudine (letter). Ann Intern Med 109: 842

Simpson D, Wolfe D, Farraye J (1989) HIV associated myopathy: features in 21 patients and the role of AZT. Fifth International conference on AIDS. Montreal. Abstract MBP 330.

Simpson D, Citak K, Wolfe D et al. (1991) Myopathies associated with HIV and zidovudine. Neuroscience of HIV infection. Padua, Italy. Abstract 57.

Small PM, G.F. S, Goodman PC, Sande MA, Chaisson RE, Hopewell PC (1991) Treatment of tuberculosis in patients with advanced HIV infection. N Engl J Med 324: 289-294

So YT, Becksted JH, Davis RL (1986) Primary central nervous system lymphoma in AIDS: a clinical and pathological study. Ann Neurol 20: 566-572

So YT, Choucar A, Davies RL, Wara W, Ziegler JL (1988a) Neoplasms of the central nervous system in AIDS. In: Rosenblum ML, Levy RM, Bredesen DE (eds) AIDS and the nervous system. Raven Press, New York pp 285-300

So YT, Holtzman DM, Abrams DI, Olney RK (1988b) Peripheral neuropathy associated with acquired immunodeficiency syndrome. Arch Neurol 45: 945–948

Stramer SL, Heller JS, Coombs RW et al. (1989) Markers of HIV infection prior to IgG antibody seropositivity. JAMA 262: 64–69

Stansall and Sande M. (1992) Cryptococcal infection in AIDS. In: Sande M, Volberding P (eds) Medical management of AIDS, 3rd edn. W B Saunders, New York, pp 297–310

Taelman H, Clerinx J, Kagame A, Batungwanayo J, Nyirabareja A, Bogaerts J (1991) Cryptococcosis, another growing burden for central Africa (letter). Lancet 338: 761

Tennant-Flowers M, Boyle M, Carey D et al. (1990) Sulphadiasine in patients with AIDS and toxoplasmosis. Sixth International Conference on AIDS. San Francisco. Abstract Th: B: 480

Till M, MacDonell KB (1990) Myopathy with human immunodeficiency virus type 1 (HIV-1) infection: HIV-1 or zidovudine. Ann Intern Med 113: 492–494

UCLA conference (1989). The acquired immunodeficiency syndrome dementia complex. Ann Intern Med 111: 400–410

Vago L, D'Arminio A, Castagna A, Formenti T (1991) Opportunistic pathologies of the central nervous system: correlation between clinical and autoptical findings in 225 AIDS patients. HIV neuroscience, Padua, Italy. Abstract 64.

van der Meche FGA, Schmitz PIM and group DGBs (1992) A randomised trial comparing intravenous immune globulin and plasma exchange in Guillain Barre syndrome. New Engl J Med 326: 1123–1129

Vazeux R, Brousse N, Jarry A et al. (1987) AIDS subacute encephalitis: identification of HIV infected cells. Am J Path 126: 403–410

Wiley CA, Schreier RD, Nelson JA et al. (1986) Cellular localization of human immunodeficiency virus infection within the brains of acquired immunodeficiency syndrome. Proc Natl Acad Sci USA 83: 7089–7093

Wilkie FL, Eisdorfe C, Morgan R, Loewenstein DA, Szapocznik J (1990) Cognition in early human immunodeficiency virus infection. Arch Neurol 47: 433–440

Wong MC, Suite NDA, Labar DR (1990) Seizures in human immunodeficiency virus infection. Arch Neurol 47: 640–642

Yarchoan R, Berg G, Brouwers P et al. (1987) Response of human-immunodeficiency-virus-associated neurological disease to 3′-azido-3′-deoxythymidine. Lancet i: 132–135

Zeman A, Donaghy M (1991) Acute infection with human immunodeficiency virus presenting with neurogenic urinary retention. Genitourin Med 67: 345–347

Ziegler JL, Beckstead JA, Volberding PA, Abrams DI, Levine AM et al. (1984) Non-Hodgkin's lymphoma in 90 homosexual men. N Engl J Med 311: 565–570

Zuger A, Louie E, Holzman RS, Simberhoff MS, Rahal JJ (1986) Cryptococcal disease in patients with the acquired immunodeficiency syndrome. Ann Int Med 104: 234–240

7 Dermatological Problems in HIV Infection and AIDS

Chris Bunker

Introduction

HIV infection and AIDS have been associated with dermatological disease since the first accounts of initially cryptic acquired immunodeficiency illness in homosexual men in the early 1980s. Mucocutaneous involvement, for example with Kaposi's sarcoma, provides criteria for diagnosis and staging. HIV has been demonstrated in the dermis of infected individuals and may be present in the dermal Langerhans (antigen presenting) cells. The incidence of several cutaneous diseases is increased in patients who are HIV positive or who have AIDS. It is apparent that the percentage of patients with skin manifestations and the number of these manifestations increases as HIV infection progresses. The incidence of these diseases and their severity correlates in many instances with the absolute numbers of T-helper cells and the prognostic significance of some disorders (e.g. hairy leukoplakia and Kaposi's sarcoma) is well recognised. There remains debate about the effect HIV infection may have on some dermatological conditions such as psoriasis and atopic dermatitis. Appearing in the literature all the time are case reports of rarer dermatoses in HIV-positive patients where an association is speculative.

All of these skin diseases may be distressing and difficult to manage. But they are of further interest in that they may shed light on both the immunopathological natural history of HIV infection and on the aetiology of common and rarer dermatoses which happen to be found with a higher incidence in HIV than non-HIV patients. Their occurrence highlights the understated role of the skin as an immunological organ.

Clinical Features

Seroconversion

It is not known whether infection can occur through the skin in the absence of overt trauma such as needlestick injury. Where seroconversion has been well substantiated in the clinical context of fever, myalgia, a mononucleosis-like illness and/or an acute neurological episode, dermatological events have almost invariably been recorded (Berger and Greene 1991). Self-limiting urticaria, a macular-papular toxic erythema and erythema multiforme (Lewis and Brook 1992) have been described. These patterns of exanthemata may be accompanied by an enanthem with oropharygeal candidiasis.

Asymptomatic seroconversion probably occurs most often; or non-specific symptoms, including non-specific dermatological reaction patterns, may go unnoted, unreported or undiagnosed. The differential diagnosis includes that of a toxic erythema, other infectious illnesses, either obscure or substantiable, such as EBV, CMV or toxoplasmosis mononucleosis, HTLV-1 infection, secondary syphilis (Calza et al. 1991), a drug reaction or idiopathy.

Inflammatory Dermatoses

Seborrhoeic dermatitis is a common itchy, scaly, erythematous dermatosis with a particular predilection for the scalp, face, chest, back, axillae and groins. It is undoubtedly very common in the later stages of HIV infection when it can be very severe and generalised, even amounting to erythroderma (Duvic 1991). It is established that seborrhoeic dermatitis is more common in seropositive homosexual men than in seronegative homosexuals. Whilst a common diagnosis amongst seropositive individuals who are otherwise well its severity is increased with CD4 counts below 100/mm^3. Some clinicians have noticed an association of erythroderma, xerosis and seborrhoeic dermatitis with the development of dementia and spinal cord disease. Extensive refractory seborrhoeic dermatitis appears to occur in particular conjunction with pulmonary tuberculosis and AIDS in Zambia (Hira et al. 1988). The differential diagnosis depends upon the particular clinical presentation but usually comprises other causes of widespread dermatitis, erythroderma, psoriasis and tinea corporis, with all of which seborrhoeic dermatitis may co-exist.

Atopic dermatitis or an atopic dermatitis-like condition appears to be common, especially in children (Prose 1991). In adults there have been reports of patients whose atopic eczema recurred or worsened during the course of HIV infection (Ball and Harper 1987; Parkin et al. 1987) and a case of the hyper IgE syndrome has been described (Lin and Smith 1988). But other commentators have not agreed (Duvic 1991; Cockerell 1991; Staughton and Goldsmith, personal communication). Ring et al. (1986) found a decreased frequency of atopic diseases, fewer positive RAST tests and lower average levels of IgE in HIV positive compared to HIV negative homosexual individuals.

The atopic diathesis is present in any individual with a personal or first degree family history of asthma, hay fever or rhinitis, conjunctivitis or eczema. The typical clinical features of atopic dermatitis are red, scaly, papular often excoriated patches on the face and trunk and in the flexures on a background of dry or ichthyotic skin. Signs of chronic disease are hypo- or hyperpigmentation and lichenification. The differential diagnosis includes other eczematous dermatoses such as discoid eczema, seborrhoeic dermatitis and asteatotic eczema and psoriasis.

Psoriasis may worsen or appear for the first time in the HIV-infected patient (Duvic 1991). Often it is very severe but interestingly may regress in the preterminal phase (Colebunders et al. 1992). Psoriasis is characterised by red, silver-scaled lesions which can be guttate, nummular or plaques. The scalp is frequently involved as are the nails with signs of pitting, onycholysis, dystrophy, subungual hyperkeratosis and even complete shedding. Pustulosis may occur, particularly in the palms and soles, and occasionally psoriasis is the cause of an erythroderma. The differential diagnosis includes atopic dermatitis, seborrhoeic dermatitis and, acutely, pityriasis rosea.

Reiter's syndrome is part of the same continuum as psoriasis in genetically predisposed individuals. Reiter's syndrome is defined as arthritis, urethritis and conjunctivitis and has been reported in AIDS and AIDS-related complex in its classical or incomplete form (Duvic 1991). Skin lesions in Reiter's syndrome may be similar to those of psoriasis. Non-AIDS patients have been long-recognised with features of both psoriasis and Reiter's syndrome. Classically, Reiter's patients may have thickened yellow palms and soles with a cobblestone appearance with or without pustular lesions (keratoderma blenorrhagica) and severe involvement of the penis (balanitis xerotica obliterans or circinate balanitis); but they may also have any of the features of psoriasis described above.

Eosinophilic folliculitis (previously Ofuji's disease) is an unusual clinicopathological entity suggested by a truncal eruption of pruritic, erythematous perifollicular papules and pustules. The presentation usually mimics staphylococcal or pityrosporum folliculitis or acne vulgaris. It was proposed that it occurs as a early sign of HIV infection (Frentz et al. 1989) but it is now argued to be an unique HIV-associated dermatosis occurring at CD4 counts of 250–300/mm^3. It is an important cutaneous eruption in patients thought likely to develop opportunistic infections. It does not seem to be caused by a microorganism but does have an association with elevated serum IgE levels (Cockerell 1991; Ferrandiz et al. 1992).

Other inflammatory dermatoses that have been reported in HIV infection are listed in Table 7.1 (Bratzke et al. 1988; Penneys 1990; Duvic 1991; Cockerell 1991, 1993; Gherardi et al. 1993).

Table 7.1. Inflammatory dermatoses reported in HIV infection

Papular eruption of AIDS
Granuloma annulare
Pityriasis rosea
Erythroderma
Pityriasis rubra pilaris
Acquired ichthyosis
Keratoderma
Lichen spinulosus
Lichenoid granulomatous papular dermatosis
Acne vulgaris
Hidradenitis suppuritiva
Vasculitis
Erythema nodosum
Behcet's disease
Sweet's neutrophilic dermatosis
Anetoderma
Transient acantholytic dermatosis (Grover's disease)
Autoimmune bullous diseases
Acrodermatitis enteropathica
Papular mucinosis

Classical *granuloma annulare* is seen in HIV positive individuals but it is a relatively common dermatosis. Strikingly violaceous lesions may arouse suspicion of Kaposi's sarcoma: corroborative skin biopsy is advised. An atypical form of *generalised granuloma annulare* has also been described (Cohen et al. 1991).

A persistent *pityriasis rosea*-like eruption without the classical herald patch appears in the literature (Kaplan et al. 1987).

Dry skin, xeroderma and pruritus appear common. To the litany of the causes of *generalised pruritus* with excoriations (and in the absence of a primary dermatological diagnosis) must now be added HIV infection (Hoover and Lang 1991)

The association of porphyria cutanea tarda with HIV infection is intriguing (Blauvelt et al. 1992). Overt porphyria cutanea tarda is thought to occur when an already abnormal porphyrin biosynthetic pathway in the liver becomes further compromised by some exogenous factor. Porphyrin deposition in the skin results in skin fragility, blisters and erosions at sun-exposed sites; the lesions frequently heal with scarring and the formation of milia. The differential diagnosis includes a drug eruption, epidermolysis bullosa acquisita and pseudoporphyria cutanea tarda.

Some of the cases reported have been familial and some have been haemophiliacs. Some of the latter were hepatitis B antibody positive, but presumably also had repeated exposure to non-A non-B hepatitis agents in transfused blood (which are thought to be the cause of the abnormal liver function tests seen in many patients with haemophilia). One of them had also attended a tanning parlour for cosmetic courses of UVA. It is worth elaborating upon a further case of a bisexual, alcoholic, iv drug user with a past history of hepatitis B who also had chronic anaemia which had required numerous transfusions. He presented with small tense blisters on the cheeks, ears and the dorsum of the hands which healed with scarring, but investigation for malaise showed him to be HIV positive, have liver disease, Coombs positive haemolysis and thalassaemia as well as Pneumocystis carinii pneumonia and disseminated Mycobacterium avium-intracellulare (MAI) infection (cultured from blood and bone marrow). The inference is not that HIV can exacerbate porphyria cutanea tarda but that the clinical context in which HIV occurs and its consequences generate several factors which may contribute to this metabolic disease, as in this patient. The combined effect of thalassaemia, HIV and MAI infections led to anaemia which required transfusions. Transfusions led to haemolysis (which exacerbated the anaemia) and iron deposition in the liver (which was already damaged by alcohol and viral hepatitis) limiting hepatic uroporphyrinogen decarboxylase activity to the extent that porphyria cutanea tarda ensued.

Drug reactions are common in HIV dermatology (Coopman et al. 1993). It is said that that about 60% of patients with PCP and treated with cotrimoxazole (sulphmethoxazole-trimethoprim) experience adverse reactions including rash, fever, nausea and vomiting (Kovacs and Masur 1988). Amoxycillin-clavulanate has been implicated in a cutaneous eruption in 44% of all patients with HIV in one study and in 66% of patients with a low CD4 count. This compares with a frequency of rash as high as or greater than 90% in patients with acute lymphoblatic leukaemia or infectious mononucleosis and contrasts with a frequency of around 3–10% during the treatment of bacterial illness in otherwise normal individuals (Battegay et al. 1989).

A morbilliform toxic erythema is the usual reaction seen and other drugs, such as dapsone or pentamadine, may be the cause. However, more seriously, erythema multiforme, Stevens – Johnson syndrome or toxic epidermal necrolysis (Lyell's syndrome) may eventuate with a much higher incidence than seen when these drugs are exhibited to the HIV-negative population. The drugs that confer the most risk in this regard are cotrimoxazole (sulphmethoxazole-trimethoprim), pyrimethamine, sulphadoxine, sulphadiazine, thiacetazone, streptomycin, phenytoin, griseofulvin, fluconazole and vancomycin (Coopman and Stern 1991; Rustin et al. 1989; Penneys 1990; Gussehaven et al. 1991; Vidal et al. 1992; Rzany et al. 1993).

Fixed drug eruptions have been reported with pentamadine, which can also cause ulcers at the site of injection, (Jones et al. 1992; Penneys 1990) and foscarnet which can also cause penile ulceration (Fegeux et al. 1990).

Urticaria, pruritus, photodermatitis and vasculitis seem to be relatively uncommon reaction patterns to drugs used in HIV (Coopman et al. 1993; Gherardi et al. 1993). Glucan has been implicated in causing palmar keratoderma (Duvic et al. 1987) and the striking flagellate erythema due to bleomycin has been observed (Caumes et al. 1990) but this is not unknown in general oncological practice.

The cutaneous side effects of zidovudine (AZT) deserve separate mention (Cockerell 1991). Skin, mucosal and nail discoloration (similar to that seen with other chemotherapeutic agents) is often seen. There seems to be a tendency amongst blacks to develop distally spreading, progressive but reversible proximal melanonychia and also cutaneous hyperpigmentation during AZT therapy. Some patients on AZT have developed polymyositis (Bessen et al. 1988) and vasculitis (Torres et al. 1992).

The mechanisms of common drug reactions are not known. It is interesting that in HIV, problems due to cotrimoxazole may disappear with continued therapy and some patients will tolerate rechallenge with amoxycillin-clavulanate. Continued treatment or retreatment with these drugs is not therefore contraindicated when adverse reactions occur (Battegay et al. 1989).

Infections

Bacteria

Folliculitis is an extremely common eruption in HIV-infected patients (Berger and Greene 1991). The appearances are of widespread perifollicular papules and pustules which may be excoriated. Clinical differentiation between staphylococcal folliculitis and pityrosporum folliculitis may be impossible and often the two may coexist. Eosinophilic folliculitis enters the differential diagnosis. If the eruption occurs in intertriginous areas then staphylococcal folliculitis may mimic candidiasis.

Other staphylococcal infections that may correlate with HIV infection include *bullous impetigo* (Donovan et al. 1992), *ecthyma* (crusted eroded lesions) and *staphylococcal scalded skin syndrome* (Donohue et al. 1991; Cone et al. 1992). Subcutaneous *abscesses* due to staphylococci are common and may complicate injection or intravenous-line sites. Sometimes uncommon organisms are isolated.

Severe streptococcal *cellulitis* (erysipelas) with lymphadenitis has been observed (Janssen et al. 1991). *Pseudomonas aeruginosa* can cause *ecthyma gangrenosum* and *panniculitis* (El Baze et al. 1991): these signs may be markers of pseudomonas septicaemia. *Fournier's gangrene* may complicate chemotherapy in AIDS (Hughes-Davies et al. 1991).

But an important facet of cutaneous bacterial infection in HIV-positive individuals is that it may predispose to bacteraemia and systemic infection, especially when central lines and chemotherapy are being used, in intravenous drug users and in patients with other dermatoses such as psoriasis (Jaffe et al. 1991). Systemic bacterial infection can produce skin signs such as splinter haemorrhages and acral papulonecrotic lesions.

The unusual entity of cutaneous vascular endothelial proliferation originally entitled epithelioid (haem)angiomatosis is in fact due to the cat-scratch disease organism *Rochalimaea henselae* affecting the skin. The disorder is now known as *bacillary angiomatosis* (Berger and Greene 1991). This presents with papular and nodular vascular lesions resembling Kaposi's sarcoma, the differential diagnosis of which is discussed later.

It is now well established that *syphilis* behaves differently in the HIV-infected individual (Musher et al. 1990). This complicates and confuses the clinical recognition of the classical dermatological manifestations of the disease, for example chancre, classical palmar plantar paulosquamous eruption of secondary syphilis and gumma. Dermatologists should be suspicious of all genital, perianal and oral ulceration and any papulosquamous eruption. Keratoderma and lues maligna (necrotic red nodules) have been reported (Glover et al. 1992).

Increasingly we are discovering that other sexually transmitted and endemic bacterial diseases are affected by HIV. *Yaws* (Noordhoek and van Embden 1991) and *leprosy* (Meyers 1992) are two important examples where the skin is a primary organ of involvement. A case of an unusual presentation of chancroid has been reported (Quale et al. 1990).

Tuberculosis is discussed at length elsewhere but reinfection with or reactivation of *Mycobacterium tuberculosis* seems to occur early in HIV infection and extrapulmonary tuberculosis is common (Pitchenik et al. 1984). Tubercular lymphadenitis has been said to be a characteristic of HIV infected intravenous drug abusers (Aguado and Castrillo 1987). The clinical presentation is diverse including cervical lymphadenopathy (scrofula – Pedersen and Nielsen 1987), scattered violaceous papules (Penneys 1990) and what has been termed acute miliary tuberculosis of the skin (Rohatgi et al. 1992).

Atypical mycobacterial skin disease is usually due to *mycobacterium avium intracellulare*. This occurs as part of a disseminated infection in up to one-third of patients (Hawkins et al. 1986). Lesions described include violaceous papules, nodules and ulcers (Freed et al. 1987). Skin lesions have also been reported with *M. kansasii* (Penneys 1990), *M. haemophilium* (Holton et al. 1991), *M. fortuitum* (Sack 1990) and *M. marinum* (Kaplan et al. 1987). In these instances the eruption has probably occurred after primary infection of the skin by the organism but there is on record a fatal case of disseminated *M. marinum* (Tchornobay et al. 1992). Non-dermatologists may not be aware of the clinical pattern of involvement, called "spirotrichoid spread", where a chain of lesions, presumably emanating from the local lymphatics, is seen up a limb from a distal primary site (Zukervar et al. 1991).

Viruses

Herpes simplex virus (HSV) infection is extremely common during the course of HIV illness (Berger and Greene 1991); severe chronic ulcerative perianal HSV-2 lesions were one of the first features of AIDS to be reported (Siegal et al. 1981). Acute lesions are vesico-bullous but they may become eroded and crusted, vegetative or ulcerating and, of course, may not resolve and heal because in immunosuppression HSV infection may not be self-limiting as it is in normal individuals. Any site may be affected and the diagnosis must be suspected with eruptions with any of the clinical features mentioned above. Whitlow (Norris et al. 1988), persistent necrotic digits (Baden et al. 1991) and perioral, genital and perianal ulceration may be particularly unpleasant. Even if resolution occurs and treatments are successful the condition often recurs.

Likewise, dermatomal *Herpes zoster* virus (HZV) infection frequently accompanies HIV infection and can be severe (Berger and Greene 1991). The presentation is of variously sized vesicles and pustules (which may become confluent and denuded) on erythematous bases. Some lesions become ulcerated and form eschars. The distribution is characteristically dermatomal but differentiation from HSV is sometimes clinically difficult. Recurrences of HZV do occur in normal HIV-negative people and in up to 20% of HIV-negative immunocompromised patients. The frequency of recurrence in HIV positivity is unknown. It is controversial whether all patients presenting with dermatomal HZV should be counselled about HIV testing.

Some patients have been reported who have developed an *atypical disseminated HZV* infection characterised by relatively sparse but ecthymatous necrotic lesions with a prolonged course (greater than a year in a few patients) and a poor prognosis. There is usually an overt dermatomal Varicella Zoster Virus (VZV) recurrence. The appearance of such lesions evokes a differential diagnosis including ecthyma gangrenosum and disseminated infection with atypical mycobacteria, fungi, vaccinia or HSV. A quarter of these patients may have involvement of the CNS but interestingly this may appear some weeks or months after the skin lesions. Lung involvement has also been reported in the literature.

Cytomegalovirus (CMV) infection is common in HIV-related practice (with ocular, pulmonary and gastrointestinal involvement) but although about 95% of patients get active CMV involvement at some stage of their illness skin involvement is relatively uncommon. Thirty percent of normal healthy individuals develop a non-specific maculopapular rash (especially when there is concomitant antibiotic therapy) during CMV infection and occasionally papulovesicular eruptions, purpura and nodular or ulcerative lesions have been described (Cohen and Corey 1985). In the context of HIV infection, the spectrum of clinical presentation appears to range between purpura, papules nodules, verrucous plaques and ulcers (Toome et al. 1991; Berger and Greene 1991). The differential diagnosis of these clinical lesions is extensive and special investigations may be necessary to confirm the clinical possibility. HSV and CMV skin involvement may be seen concurrently (Smith et al. 1991a).

Viral warts due to the human papillomavirus (HPV) are found in about 5%–30% of HIV patients (Berger and Greene 1991). Anogenital warts (conylomata acuminata) may be a marker for HIV infection. HPV types 6 and 11 have been identified most often when sought at extragenital sites; these are not types associated with malignant potential. However Bowenoid papulosis (lesions with the clinical appearance of viral warts but with the histology of Bowen's disease – squamous cell carcinoma in situ) have been found (in association with HPV 16) in the anogenital area (Bradshaw et al. 1992) and HPV infection is thought to be linked to the incidence of anal carcinoma in AIDS.

The diagnosis of warts is usually straightforward when papillomatous lesions are found affecting the dorsum of the hands, the palmar surfaces of the feet, in a periungual distribution and around the genitalia and anus. The warts may be unusually exuberant and a pattern like the rare, inherited condition epidermodysplasia verruciformis has been cited (Berger et al. 1991).

Mollusca contagiosum also occur commonly in HIV infection (Petersen and Gerstoft 1992). There are usually several papular or even larger nodular lesions, particularly on the face and neck. In non-HIV infected individuals mollusca are common in childhood but have a propensity for the trunk. Often, in the context of HIV infection, the lesions are not domed in shape and lack the characteristic classical central umbilication. Mollusca are due to pox virus infection but the clinical differential diagnosis includes sebaceous hyperplasia, syringoma, warts due to HPV, cutaneous cryptococcosis and histoplasmosis and even basal cell carcinoma.

Fungi

Oral *candidiasis* has classically been associated with immunosuppressive states and was one of the first features to be described in the early days of the HIV epidemic before the syndrome was clearly defined and the causative agent identified (Gottlieb et al. 1981). But candida is also responsible for nail and nail-fold disease. Paronychia and onycholysis due to candida are present proportionate to absolute numbers of T-helper cells and thus are of prognostic significance (Kaplan et al. 1987). In addition, angular cheilitis and interiginous candidiasis with the physical signs of moist erythema, papules, small pustules and often erosions, are common findings. Practically all people with HIV infection will have candida as a pathogen at some stage in their disease (Berger and Greene 1991).

Generally, *dermatophytes* are rarely responsible for cutaneous infection in immunocompromised patients (Koranda et al. 1974). Homosexual men are very likely to have a superficial fungal infection, regardless of their HIV status. For example, in Sweden (Torssander et al. 1988), 35% of seropositive homosexual men have been shown to have mycologically proven toe cleft dermatophytosis (usually *Trichophytum rubrum*) compared to about 9% of seronegative heterosexual men: but this was not significantly different from seronegative homosexual men (30%). Clinical findings, for example interdigital scaling, similar to those of tinea pedis are very common (65% of heterosexual men, 75% of seropositive homosexual men). Dermatophytes were isolated from normal toe clefts in about 7% of homosexual men (regardless of HIV status) but from no clinically normal toe clefts in heterosexual men. Coexistent toe cleft scaling, maceration and fissuring, however, are reliable physical signs of dermatophytosis.

Widespread dermatophytosis is most uncommon. The Swedish group found dermatophytes only in the groins, toe clefts and toe nails. I have seen several patients with widespread tinea incognito (secondary to chronic potent topical steroid misusage for another dermatosis).

Nail dystrophy and discoloration are physical signs which are highly suggestive of *onychomycosis* and this is very common in AIDS. *T. rubrum* appears to be the commonest organism (Dompmartin et al. 1990). The yellow nail syndrome should be considered and mycological confirmation obtained.

Esoteric superficial fungal infections are reported. For example there is a description of a case where the patient presented with "dirty" brown spots on the scrotum from which were cocultured the dematiaceous fungi *Bipolaris* and *Curvularia* (Duvic and Lowe 1987).

Cryptococcosis occurs in the immunosuppressed, and up to 20% of patients with disseminated disease may have skin involvement. In HIV infection and AIDS cryptococcal skin involvement should be suspected when papulonodular skin lesions with central umbilication very similar to molluscum contagiosum are seen in the context of neurological or pulmonary disease. A herpetic appearance, violaceous lichenoid lesions, an acneiform papulopustular and nodular eruption on the chin, rhinophyma, a warty tumour on the foot and cryptococcus admixed with (and mimicking) Kaposi's sarcoma have also been described (Ricchi et al. 1991).

Disseminated histoplasmosis may produce skin involvement. This is very rare in the UK although commoner in the USA where histoplasmosis is endemic. An exanthem, lesions resembling molluscum contagiosum, acneiform and psoriasiform eruptions and depressed pits on the palms and soles have been described (Penneys 1990; Lindgren et al. 1991).

Numerous ulcers due to cutaneous *sporotrichosis* are recognised (Berger and Greene 1991). *Coccidiodomycosis* is endemic in the south west USA and may disseminate in AIDS; skin lesions seem rare. Other fungal infections reported to have involved the cutis include paracoccidioidomycosis (Bakos et al. 1989), micropsoridiosis (Eeftinck Schattenkerk et al. 1991), nocardiosis (Boixeda et al. 1991), primary cutaneous aspergillosis (Hunt et al. 1992) and *Penicillium marneffiei* mycosis (Chiewchanvit et al. 1991).

Protozoa

Pneumocystis carinii pneumonia is common in HIV infection but disseminated disease and cutaneous involvement is rare (Hennessey et al. 1991; Berger and Greene 1991). Two patients have been described with mass lesions in the external auditory canal. Spread from middle ear infection itself due to retrograde spread from the pharynx up the eustachian tube has been proposed as the mechanism. Lesions masquerading as Kaposi's sarcoma have been encountered (Litwin and Williams 1992).

Cases of disseminated *amoebiasis* and skin involvement (e.g. a single papule on the thigh and an abscess in the soleus muscle), including where the skin manifestation led to the diagnosis of the disseminated infection, have been published (Smith et al. 1991b; May et al. 1992).

Analogous to the situation with bacterial infections, endemic protozoal diseases such as leishmaniasis (Pialoux et al. 1990; Sabbatani et al. 1991) may behave differently and also mimic or complicate Kaposi's sarcoma (Romeu et al. 1991).

Infestations

The role, if any, of the ectoparasitic demodex mites in human cutaneous disease has been a subject of enduring controversy in dermatology. The balance of opinion currently is that they are normal non-pathogenic commensals. However, two patients with AIDS who developed a pruritic, papulonodular eruption on the face and neck were found to have abnormal *demodicosis* and the rash subsided with anti-mite treatment (Dominey et al. 1989). The clinical differential diagnosis would include bacterial folliculitis, eosinophilic pustular folliculitis, scabies, drug reaction, the papular eruption of AIDS, atypical HSV or syphilis infection and deep fungal infection, but all of these would be expected to be more widespread than the face and neck dermatosis which Dominey et al. have reported.

Scabies occurs frequently in HIV-infected patients (Orkin 1993; Funkhouser et al. 1993). Theoretically, immunosuppression is associated with widespread, itchy, hyperkeratotic lesions (Norwegian scabies) with a heavy infestation of the mite *Sarcoptes scabei*, and such cases have been reported. Certainly scabies may have unusual clinical features when it does occur in the context of HIV infection, for example the skin of the head and neck is often involved, which is highly unusual in non-HIV-infected adults. It is important to have a high index of suspicion. Classical pointers include severe pruritus that interferes with sleep, excoriated burrows in the web spaces of the digits and nodular lesions on the buttocks and genitalia. Scabies is endemic in the HIV population in London and there are occasional epidemic outbreaks on HIV wards, in the hospices and in the community. Transmission is by sexual intercourse, nursing, comforting and massage. Norwegian scabies is highly contagious because of the heavy superficial infestation that occurs.

Neoplasms

The prevalence of *Kaposi's sarcoma* (KS) amongst the first 1000 homosexual men with AIDS reported to the Centers for Disease Control in the USA was 45% whereas it was 23.5% in the fourteenth group. The prevalence amongst intravenous drug abusers has remained at about 5% and in haemophiliacs at 1% (Schwartz et al. 1991; Fine 1992; Tappero et al. 1993).

Classical KS occurs in elderly male central Europeans, Italians or Jews and is solitary and acral. Endemic KS occurs in black Africans and is florid and aggressive. There has been a report of a Greek form of KS with Peloponnese clustering (Rappersberger et al. 1989). A third group of KS occurs in patients with iatrogenic immunosuppression. AIDS-related KS is multicentric and often involves the face, oral mucosa, palate and genitalia.

The characteristic lesion is a purple nodule which may ulcerate (Schwartz et al. 1991). There may be diagnostic difficulty with morphologically banal or cryptic lesions in at-risk or worried individuals. It is important to have a high index of suspicion and do a skin biopsy if necessary. The common differential diagnosis includes naevi and histiocytoma but cryptococcosis (Blauvelt and Kerdel 1992), histoplasmosis (Cole et al. 1992), leishmaniasis (Romeu et al. 1991), lesions due to pneumocystis (Litwin and Williams 1992) and dermatophytosis (Crosby et al. 1991) may also mimic and/or complicate KS. Pyogenic granuloma masquerading as KS has become a well recognised "catch". *Epithelioid angiomatosis* (or haemangiomatosis) which has some clinical similarity to KS was first described in the context of HIV infection by Cockerell but this has been recognised now to be the consequence of infection with the cat scratch organism as already described.

Two papers have documented the appearance in HIV-positive men of multiple new moles (*eruptive naevi*) which appeared in crops as the patients became more symptomatic from HIV infection. These patients did not have the dysplastic naevi syndrome (familial melanoma) although biopsy confirmed the presence of dysplastic features (Duvic et al. 1989; Betlloch et al. 1991).

It is now felt that there is an increased incidence of non-melanoma *basal cell carcinomas* (Lobo et al. 1992), *squamous cell carcinomas* (de Boer and Danner 1990) and even *melanomas* (van Ginkel et al. 1991; McGregor et al. 1992) in HIV-positive individuals particularly in association with excessive previous sun exposure and actinic damage.

Hodgkin's and non-Hodgkin's B cell lymphoma, both found in HIV-infected individuals, can cause skin lesions (Schwartz et al. 1991; Cockerell 1993). The likelihood is increasing that cutaneous T cell lymphoma (Mycosis fungoides and Sezarry syndrome) is also an illness that can occur concomitantly with AIDS (Myskowski 1991).

Hair and Nails

Abnormalities of hair and nails found in HIV infection are listed in Table 7.2 (Prose et al. 1992).

Some of the African patients with the yellow-nail syndrome had AIDS and tuberculous pleural effusion or pneumonia (Hira et al. 1988) and such nail changes are recognised pointers to chronic pulmonary disease.

Acquired trichomegaly of the eyelashes may be an early marker of HIV infection (Kaplan et al. 1991).

The Mouth

Many mouth signs have been reported in acute HIV infection. Transient intraoral redness, erosions and ulcers and candidiasis are all described (Greenspan and Greenspan 1991).

Distressing mouth ulceration occurs frequently in HIV infection. The differential diagnosis includes malignancy (KS), herpes simplex, fungal infections and idiopathic aphthous ulceration.

Oral candidiasis is common in HIV-positive individuals and almost universal in AIDS. The extent and persistence of the disease are responsible for much morbidity in patients with HIV and AIDS. Sometimes the entire oropharynx, larynx and oesophagus may be involved but mild forms with just angular cheilitis and/or focal red or white patches on the oral mucosa, palate or tongue (Gottlieb et al. 1981; Greenspan and Greenspan 1991).

Table 7.2. Abnormalities of hair and nail found in HIV infection

Hair
  Patchy and generalised alopecia
  Hypertrichosis of the eyelashes
  Eyelash trichomegaly
  Yellow nail syndrome

Nail
  Transverse and longitudinal ridging
  Loss of the lunula
  Opaqueness
  Onycholysis
  Longitudinal melanonychia

Hairy leukoplakia (HL) is a new clinical entity which has emerged during the HIV epidemic probably associated with Epstein-Barr virus infection. It is particularly important because it is an early specific sign of HIV infection with the sinister implication that 75% of patients develop AIDS within 2-3 years. It is usually asymptomatic although patients have often noticed the appearance of a roughened patch along the lateral margin of the tongue. To the patient it may feel rough and to the physician it may look craggy but it is not truly "hairy". Other intraoral sites have been reported (Samaranayake and Pindberg 1989).

The differential diagnosis includes trauma, candida, leukoplakia, lichen planus and white sponge naevus. Traumatic changes occur along the line of occlusion and are uncommon on the tongue. Candida, if present may involve the oropharynx more extensively than HL which is usually more focal. Leukoplakia is the presentation of a non-specific common disturbance of oral mucosal keratinisation. The tongue is not as commonly involved as the buccal mucosa or the edentulous alveolar ridge, but more frequently than the labial mucosa, the palate and the gingiva. Smoking and poor dental hygiene are associated factors. Leukoplakia of the tongue may eventuate from a syphilitic atrophic glossitis, although small white mucous patches may occur anywhere in the oral cavity during secondary syphilis: classically, the patch can be scraped off to leave a raw erosion. Lichen planus is diagnosed in the presence of Wickham's striae and is commoner on the buccal mucosa than the tongue although all intraoral sites may be involved. About 30% of patients will have extraoral lichen planus. 10%-50% of all patients with lichen planus have oral lesions.

HL has not yet been shown to involve other mucosal or extramucosal sites. White sponge naevus may be familial and may occur on the tongue. Biopsy may be necessary. HL is now known to occur in other immunocompromised people and has even been reported in healthy individuals (Anonymous 1989; Greenspan and Greenspan 1991).

HSV infection is common in and around the mouth. Painful red eroded lesions are characteristic and the extent and chronicity or frequent recurrences cause much debility.

Gangrenous stomatitis has been reported in both adults and children where opportunistic anaerobic organisms as well as candida, pseudomonas and staphylococci contribute to severely symptomatic perioral ulceration complicated by pain, bleeding and inability to feed by the enteral route (Giovanni et al. 1989). Severe periodontal disease is also not unusual (Greenspan and Greenspan 1991).

Kaposi's sarcoma occurs frequently in the mouth and lesions are more apparent on the palate. It appears as red plaques or nodules. The diagnosis is usually apparent clinically but early red lesions may be mistaken for HSV or candida.

Other entities that have occurred in the mouth include disseminated *histoplasmosis* (Penneys 1990), pigmentary changes (Cohen and Callen, 1992) and complications of drug reactions.

Children

Paediatric HIV disease has some differences from that seen in adults. Vertical transmission from an infected mother is the usual mode of infection. Additionally, there is a difficult, broader differential diagnosis of immunosuppression in children including DiGeorge's syndrome, ataxia telangectasia, Wiskott-Aldrich syndrome, aggamaglobulinaemias, T and B cell immunodeficiencies, malnutrition, malignancies, congenital infections, iatrogenic immunosuppression and graft-versus-host disease; all of these conditions may have dermatological manifestations.

Cutaneous disease is common in children with AIDS (Prose 1991). An eruption resembling seborrhoeic dermatitis has been described. Atopic eczema is found with increased frequency but unclassified excematous eruptions are also seen. Widespread nappy dermatitis can occur. As in adults a macular-papular toxic erythema appears to be common after treatment with a trimethoprim/sulphonamide combination or after ampicillin.

About half of children with advanced HIV disease can be expected to suffer a serious bacterial infection and 20% of these involve the skin. The commonest organism is *Staphylococcus aureus* and the usual clinical patterns are of cellulitis, impetigo, folliculitis and abscess formation; a persistent staphylococcal folliculitis may also be seen. The most common fungal infection seen is with *Candida albicans*. Of 36 children in one study 75% had persistent mucocutaneous candidiasis. Dermatophytic infection can occur. *Herpes simplex* infection of the skin and mucosae is common and may be very serious and chronic, likewise disseminated zoster infection. Molluscum contagiosum are often seen in healthy childhood where the lesions commonly affect the trunk. In HIV infection the lesions have a predilection for the face. Perianal warts (condylomata acuminata) have been reported and it is likely that papillomavirus infection at other sites will become more widely seen although normal children are not immune from digital warts or verrucae.

KS is rare (about 5%) and often affects other organs with sparing of the skin. Non-Hodgkin's and other lymphomas with cutaneous involvement are even rarer.

Skin changes compatible with pellagra, acquired zinc deficiency (acrodermatitis enteropathica) and scurvy have all been reported and the appropriate nutritional deficit substantiated. Zinc deficiency, at least, has been attributed to malabsorption associated with chronic infectious diarrhoea caused by opportunistic organisms.

Non-specific findings in paediatric HIV practice include exanthematous rashes and cutis marmorata or livedo appearance (Penneys 1990). Cold urticaria and idiopathic urticaria and the unusual finding of long eyelashes requiring frequent trimming have been reported. Patchy alopecia seems to be common. One case of erythema dyschromium perstans (ashy dermatosis) has been described in a six-year-old child with haemophilia B who was HIV positive. This rash is characterised by multiple well-defined slate-grey macules on the trunk and limbs. Its cause is unknown but it has been linked to lichen planus. The association with HIV in this case may of course be coincidental. Finally there has been an account of an HIV positive child with the indolent ulceration of pyoderma gangrenosum (Paller et al. 1990).

Haemophiliacs

Atopic eczema, seborrhoeic dermatitis, candidiasis, dermatophyte infection and folliculitis occur with an increased prevalence in HIV positive compared to HIV negative haemophiliacs. It appears that these HIV-related dermatoses may develop earlier in haemophiliacs than in homosexuals (Ball and Harper 1987; Telfer et al. 1989).

Diagnostic Investigations

Introduction

When confronted with a patient with a common dermatosis which happens to be associated with HIV infection it is not always immediately appropriate to seek to establish HIV seropositivity. Nonetheless a high index of suspicion is essential especially in the classically identified high risk groups. More often the patient is referred to the dermatologist with HIV infection already established. Under these circumstances a rash or a lump may be the first symptoms to trouble the patient and they may be worried that they are complications of HIV. Some dermatoses can be diagnosed confidently on clinical grounds but experience has shown that it is easy to be caught out. Immunological mechanisms in the skin determine the symptoms and morphology of probably all skin diseases so it is not surprising that "things look different" in HIV: several conditions may coincide in the whole skin organ or in one lesion.

A very low threshold for undertaking investigations, especially a skin biopsy (Smith et al. 1991b), is recommended. The operator and assistants should wear gloves, gowns and eyeglasses (Roenigk and Crane 1991). A good sized sample of representative lesional skin is mandatory as is a properly completed histopathological request form with the patient's HIV status clearly recorded. Special stains may be needed and the dermatologist may suggest these specifically. Some skin may be required for culture.

Swabs for bacteria, viruses and fungi may be collected from lesions for microscopic examination and culture. Skin scrapings may be examined under the microscope in the clinic (after clearing with potassium hydroxide solution) for the presence of fungal hyphae or spores. This should be supplemented by formal submission of scrapings for laboratory microscopy and culture.

Some authors recommend a wider use of cutaneous cytology than just for the identification of superficial fungal infections by potassium hydroxide preparations. It has been used to diagnose cryptococcosis and histoplasmosis. Skin scrapings are smeared on a slide. It is air dried and stained with the May–Grunwald–Giemsa stain or fixed in absolute alcohol for methenamine silver or Papanicolaou staining (Jimenez-Acosta et al. 1988).

It is the responsibility of the clinician to pay scrupulous attention to the collection and submission of all material for laboratory investigation which may constitute a health hazard to other members of staff.

Seroconversion

The rash is non-specific and suggests a wide differential amongst which are many trivial causes for a relatively common dermatological presentation. A high index of suspicion is generated when there are other constitutional or systemic symptoms or signs (particularly neurological) in a high risk individual. A diagnosis is made by excluding other diseases (which are listed in the previous section) and, clearly, demonstrating HIV infection serologically. Patients may have two or more illnesses. It is possible that classical serological confirmation of secondary syphilis may be unreliable in HIV infection and a skin biopsy should be taken with the possibility of lues and/or HIV disease suggested to the pathologist on the request form.

Inflammatory Dermatoses

In *seborrhoeic dermatitis* scrapings should be examined for fungi to exclude tinea. *Pityrosporum sp* will be seen in large numbers. Biopsy shows hyperkeratosis, a thickened Malphigian layer (epidermal acanthosis), epidermal oedema (spongiosis) and accumulation of neutrophils under the stratum corneum: a deeper lymphocytic infiltration of sebaceous glands and a more perivascular neutrophilic infiltrate is seen in HIV patients than in classical seborrhoeic dermatitis (Kaplan et al. 1987). The findings may be very similar to psoriasis. However, Soeprono et al. (1986), describing 25 biopsied cases of seborrhoeic dermatitis, list the following features: spotty keratinocyte necrosis, leukoexocytosis and a superficial perivascular infiltrate of plasma cells and neutrophils with occasional leukocytoclasis which are not commonly found in non-HIV associated seborrhoeic dermatitis or psoriasis.

The histology of *atopic dermatitis* is of marked acanthosis, spongiosis, fusion of rete ridges and an upper dermal chronic perivascular infiltrate.

Psoriasis is characterised on histology by a pattern of epidermal thickening consisting of hyperkeratosis thickened rete ridges with thinning of the Malpighian layer over the dermal papillae. There is parkeratosis in the stratum corneum, loss of the granular layer and often collections of degenerating neutrophils just under the stratum corneum. Sometimes these neutrophils accumulate to form epidermal microabscesses. The dermal papillary capillaries are dilated and tortuous and there is a lymphohistiocytic infiltrate found in the dermis.

The eruption which has come to be called *papular eruption of HIV*, although clinically distinct and specific, has no specific histological features (Smith et al. 1991).

Eosinophilic pustular folliculitis (Smith et al. 1991b) is characterised by the perifollicular presence of degranulating eosinophils and mast cells. Patients may have an eosinophilia, elevated levels of IgE and usually low CD4 (250–300/mm^3) counts. The lesions are sterile.

Infections

All pustular lesions should be swabbed. It may be difficult to tell the difference clinically between Pityrosporum and staphylococcal folliculitis and they can coexist. Abscesses are drained as part of their management and so that pus can be collected for Gram staining, culture and antimicrobial sensitivity testing.

Whilst clinically similar to KS, *bacillary angiomatosis* is distinguished histologically by being a vascular proliferation where the abnormal endothelial cells are epithelioid rather than spindled and manifesting a prominent neutrophilic infiltrate. It is a cutaneous manifestation of cat scratch disease in HIV positive individuals. The organisms of R. *henselae* can be demonstrated by Warthin–Starry staining, by immunoperoxidase staining (using CSD antisera) of lesional tissue where the bacilli are found mainly within the abnormally proliferative cutaneous vasculature or by electron microscopy (Berger and Greene 1991).

The serodiagnosis of *syphilis* in HIV infection is discussed in Chapter 1. The problems with this compound are those of clinical recognition. Skin biopsy may prove helpful with appropriate staining for spirochaetes in the problematical cases (Smith et al. 1991).

The diagnosis of mycobacterial infection is complicated because characteristic histopathological features such as caseating granuloma may be absent due to diminished cell mediated immunity (Smith et al. 1991b). All lesions where tuberculosis and/or atypical mycobacterial infection are suspected should be stained for acid-fast bacilli (which may be very numerous because of diminished cell mediated immunity) and a separate portion sent for mycobacterial culture.

Herpes simplex infection may be diagnosed clinically with less precision in the immunocompromised patient because of the altered morphology which attends the state of immune paresis. Fresh specimens may be obtained from lesional skin for electron microscopy, DNA hybridisation testing, immunofluorescence and for viral culture, and acute and convalescent sera may be examined for HSV antibodies (IgM and IgG). Dermatologists in the USA enthuse over the use of the Tzanck cytological preparation of serum or crust from a lesion, which allows rapid identification of the multinucleate giant cell typical of the HSV cytopathic effect (Penneys 1990; Smith et al. 1991b).

The possibility of making a retrospective diagnosis of HSV (and other pathogens) from paraffin-embedded tissue utilising the polymerase chain reaction has attracted much interest in general medicine and microbiology. This has clear advantages in HIV infection where the cutaneous involvement may be important yet non-specific and cryptic. Obviously such diagnostic endeavours rely on the enthusiasms and facilities of the virology department.

CMV infection may be suspected by histological signs in the dermis consisting of capillary neoangiogenesis, fibrinoid thrombi and cytomegalic, necrotic endothelial cells (with inclusions characteristic of CMV) and in the dermis consisting of hyperplasia, acantholysis, degeneration of keratinocytes and epidermal inclusions (again characteristic of CMV). The electron microscope may further confirm the viral morphology. Skin biopsy material cocultured with human fibroblasts may demonstrate a cytopathic effect characteristic of CMV. Specific DNA hydridisation with a CMV cDNA probe may also prove confirmatory. Serological testing may be difficult to interpret but the demonstration of a CMV viraemia is possible by the cytopathic effect of culturing a patients leucocytes with human fibroblasts (Toome et al. 1991).

Molluscum contagiosum is diagnosed with the greatest confidence by a skin biopsy because the morphology in the HIV-positive patient may not be pathognomic. The classical histological features are usually present, namely a domeshaped predominantly-epidermal protuberance with multiple basophilic inclusion bodies in the horny layer and hypertrophy of the spinous layer with multiple eosinophilic inclusion bodies (Smith et al. 1991).

Where *dermatophytosis* or *onychomycosis* is suspected skin scrapings cleared with potassium hydroxide solution can be examined by microscopy in the clinic for the presence of fungal hyphae or spores. Skin scrapings and clippings may also be collected for formal mycological culture. *Cryptococci* can be identified on skin biopsy but the pathologist needs to know that the diagnosis is suspected so that special stains for the cryptococcal capsule (e.g. mucicarmine) can be employed. *Histoplasma capsulatum* can be demonstrated by Gomori methenamine silver stain of a skin biopsy section. Tzanck preparations have been successfully used to demonstrate the presence of *Cryptococcus neoformans* and *Histoplasma capsulatum* (Lesher and Knight 1986; Jimenez-Acosta et al. 1988).

Mineral oil examination of skin scrapings for the *demodex* mite or its histological demonstration may help in the diagnosis of itchy papulonodular dermatoses (Dominey et al. 1989). Scrapings of the contents of classical burrows after clearing the keratin with potassium hydroxide solution will reveal the female acarus and/or her eggs in *scabies*. In *Norwegian scabies* small portions of scale from the crusted areas similarly cleared, show very large numbers of mites and eggs.

Neoplastic Conditions

The histological features of Kaposi's sarcoma are well described (Smith et al. 1991b) and consist of dilated irregular-shaped vascular structures which are typically slit-like in a fully developed nodular lesion. The differential diagnosis may be clarified by immunohistochemical techniques which identify endothelial cells (immunostaining for factor VIII related antigen and *Ulex europeus* lectin) which have been thought to be the cell of origin of KS. A staging classification of KS is given by Tappero et al. (1993).

Management

Inflammatory Disorders

In the very common situation of *seborrhoeic dermatitis*, emollients, topical steroids and anti-fungals represent the cornerstone of management. Hydrocortisone with vioform or clotrimazole ointment is suitable for the milder cases. A stronger steroid component is frequently required, at least initially (e.g. Trimovate, Lotriderm etc). Sometimes an oral imidazole is indicated such as ketoconazole. The success of antifungals in this condition is accompanied, where it has been measured, with a dimunition in the numbers of *Pityrosporum* organisms and these observations attest to the role of yeasts in the causation of seborrhoeic dermatitis (Groisser et al. 1989).

Atopic dermatitis and similar eczematous eruptions are managed with emollients and topical tar and corticosteroid ointments and occasionally UVB. If there are bacterially superinfected lesions then a steroid cream with an added antibiotic such as clioquinol or neomycin is chosen. Often in this situation a systemic anti-staphlococcal antibiotic such as flucloxacillin or erythromycin is appropriate (Duvic 1991). Parkin et al. (1987) have used interferon gamma to control the atopic manifestations of AIDS.

Psoriasis is usually controlled with topical emollients, tar or anthralin preparations, topical steroids and UVB or psoralens plus UVA (P-UVA) phototherapy (Ranki et al. 1991; Meola et al. 1993). However in HIV infection psoriasis may be atypical, severe and difficult to treat. Methotrexate which has been the mainstay of the treatment of severe psoriasis for three decades is immunosuppressive and may be inappropriate: it has been implicated in serious complications such as leucopenia and fulminant KS.

The synthetic retinoid etretinate has been successful in psoriasis and Reiter's syndrome in non-HIV patients and its efficacy in severe Reiter's syndrome and psoriasis in AIDS is encouraging (Duvic 1991; Williams and du Vivier 1991). The mode of action of the retinoids is unknown but retinoic acid appears to play a major role in the orchestration of growth and development in ectoderm. In psoriasis, etretinate has been shown to replete the epidermis with Langerhans (antigen presenting) cells: these are depleted in both psoriasis (Ranki et al. 1984) and (contentiously) in HIV infection (Kalter et al. 1991).

Cyclosporin is effective in severe psoriasis but at present its use in HIV related psoriasis is regarded with caution (Allen 1992). Concomitant treatment with AZT improves psoriasis (Duvic 1991). There is an interesting observation that cimetidine has antipsoriatic efficacy (Stashower et al. 1993).

Eosinophilic pustular folliculitis appears to be characterised by the lesional presence of degranulating eosinophils and mast cells and it has been claimed that topical cromolyn sodium and UVB phototherapy (treatments known to affect mast cells) ameliorate symptoms and signs in this condition. Other cases have responded to dapsone. Other effective treatments are said to include the antihistamines astemizole and cetirizine, UVB and potent topical corticosteroids (Ferrandiz et al. 1992; Harris et al. 1992).

UVB phototherapy is additionally useful for generalised pruritus and the papular pruritic eruption of HIV (Pardo et al. 1992).

Infections

The concomitant treatment of the inflammatory conditions discussed above with antibiotics such as erythromycin or flucloxacillin often improves symptoms, presumably because they are secondarily infected with low grade staphylococcal pathogens.

Staphylococcal folliculitis, if localised, may be managed with an antibiotic cream (neomycin, gentamicin, fusidic acid) but more often, because the eruption is widespread and the risk of bacteraemia high (because of the presence of central lines), then systemic erythromycin or flucloxacillin are indicated depending upon sensitivities. Treatment is often long-term. *Pityrosporum folliculitis* usually responds to an imidazole cream but sometimes tetracyclines (including minocycline) are effective. Again treatment is often long-term. Many patients with folliculitis have a background dermatitis (either seborrhoeic dermatitis or atopic dermatitis) and will require emollients and topical steroids. I routinely recommend the addition of an antiseptic (chlorhexidene or iodine) solution to the bath water. *Abscesses* should be treated with surgical drainage and appropriate systemic antibiotics.

Bacillary angiomatois associated with the cat scratch disease organism responds to oral erythromycin in most patients; others have been treated with additional or alternative isoniazid, rifampacin, ethambutol or clofazamine (Berger and Greene 1991).

The treatment of *tuberculosis and atypical mycobacterial infection* is discussed in Chapter 4. In general if the systemic illness responds to appropriate antimicrobial therapy then this is associated with resolution of the skin lesions.

The mainstay of the treatment of *HSV* (Berger and Greene 1991) is oral and intravenous acyclovir and often intercurrent oral acyclovir prophylaxis. Treatment should be aggressive because HSV activates HIV replication. It is usual to treat topically and systemically for secondary bacterial infection. Intravenous vidarabine may be effective in acyclovir resistant HSV (resistance is usually due to HSV isolates which are spontaneous mutants partially or completely lacking thymidine kinase, but progressive HSV-2 infection has been reported despite acyclovir therapy where the isolates were HSV acyclovir sensitive). Trisodium phosphoformate (foscarnet – which is a direct inhibitor of HSV DNA polymerase) intravenously appears to be beneficial where acyclovir has failed in severe mucocutaneous herpes (HSV-2).

In *Varicella zoster* infection (Berger and Green 1991) mild analgesics control the pain of the prodrome and the illness. A topical antibiotic is often needed for secondary infection. Post-herpetic neuralgia is a consequence of the main lesion of zoster which is in the nerves and not the skin. It is deservedly notorious for its intractability. There is some support for a short course of oral prednisolone from the beginning of the disease because it may reduce the risk but this may not be appropriate in HIV infection.

When zoster affects the ophthalmic branch of the trigeminal nerve there may be conjunctivitis or rarely optic neuritis: ophthalmological advice should be sought. Zoster of S2 and below may present with acute retention of urine and constipation and be complicated by a haemorrhagic cystitis. In these instances, as in motor zoster, zoster encephalomyelitis, purpura fulminans and zoster in the most immunologically compromised, then systemic therapy with acyclovir is probably always indicated and may save sight, sphincter function, facial expression and even life.

Disseminated HZV requires systemic antiviral treatment in HIV because of its severity, poor prognosis and the risk of visceral complications. Intravenous acyclovir (30 mg/kg/day or 1500 mg/m^2/day) eight hourly in divided doses is the established regimen. Intercurrent intramuscular HZV immunoglobulin may prevent recurrences and may be used intravenously where acyclovir fails. Emergent acyclovir resistance may become a serious problem but alternative agents include vidarabine, recombinant alpha interferon and 2-fluoro-5-iodo-arabinosylcytosine (Cohen and Grossman 1989).

The treatment of systemic and ocular *CMV* infection is described in Chapters 4 and 6. There is no reported experience of the response of cutaneous CMV disease to such treatments presumably because skin involvement has hitherto been so uncommon or unrecognised.

Molluscum contagiosum (Berger and Greene 1991) varies widely in its response to treatment. Curettage or shave biopsy of one or two lesions may be curative (and provides tissue for histological evaluation). Topical salycylic acid (20%) or podophylin may help. Liquid nitrogen cryotherapy is probably the best treatment but increasingly laser treatment may play a role.

The above remarks are also true for the management of warts due to HPV.

Candidal paronychia and onycholysis will usually respond to nystatin or imidazole cream preparations. It is usually a good idea to treat also for concomitant bacterial infection in the nail fold with, for example, a topical neomycin preparation. Angular cheilitis, and intertriginous candida can be cleared with 1% hydrocortisone and vioform cream or Trimovate (which has a stronger steroidal component than 1% hydrocortisone and also contains oxytetracycline and nystatin) cream.

Superficial *dermatophytosis* will usually respond to an imidazole preparation which must necessarily contain some steroid if the lesion(s) are very inflammatory. Oral treatment with griseofulvin, ketoconazole (or one of the newer systemic imidazoles) or terbinafine may be indicated. Ketoconazole has a known profile of idiosyncractic hepatotoxicity. The risk is greater in patients on long-term (>14 days) treatment. It is probably not suitable for patients with prexisting hepatic dysfunction and should therefore be monitored with clinical and biochemical assessment of liver function if used long term. Onychomycosis may respond to long term griseofulvin, which is relatively safe. Ketoconazole is not appropriate. In the past, topical antifungals have not been a success but there is now enthusiasm for a new imidazole, tioconazole, in a lotion formulation. Onychomycosis should be proven by mycological examination of clippings before expensive long-term therapy is commenced. The treatment should be continued until mycological assessment is negative.

The treatment of disseminated *cryptococcosis* and *histoplasmosis* is discussed in Chapters 5 and 6. The response of mucocutaneous lesions, if present, mirrors the systemic response.

If a diagnosis of *demodicidosis* is sustained then 1% gamma benzene hexachloride lotion or 1% permethrin cream rinse is effective topically (Dominey et al. 1989).

Scabies usually responds to single applications (although most physicians would recommend two applications) of sulphur ointment, gamma benzene hexachloride, benzyl benzoate or malathion lotion overnight. The whole body *including* the head and neck should be treated and all contacts should use the treatment synchronously to prevent cycles of reinfection. The scabicides are contact irritants in their own right so eczematisation often occurs. This may be treated with a moderately potent topical steroid cream. My preference is for aqueous malathion lotion because it is the least irritant. The pruritus of scabies can persist for several weeks after the mite has been successfully killed. Severe crusted scabies may require prolonged treatment and the cyclical use of several agents (Funkhouser et al. 1993). There are reports that the oral filoricide ivermectin may have a role in the management of crusted scabies.

Neoplasms

There is no cure for KS (Tappero et al. 1993). The radiotherapeutic and chemotherapeutic attitude to Kaposi's sarcoma has been discussed in several chapters. The dermatologist has a role to play in the diagnosis of the clinically less overt, more banal lesion. In patients with scarce lesions or with focal, unsightly skin involvement then excision may be appropriate. Occasionally cryotherapy with liquid nitrogen is successful.

Most dermatologists in the UK have a beneficial working relationship with skilled cosmetic advice from the Red Cross and this has helped several of our patients: it is fortunate in this respect that Kaposi's lesions on the face tend to offend more by their coloration than their bulk or because they obtrude.

Treatments used in KS are listed in Table 7.3 (Tappero et al. 1993).

The Mouth

Thalidomide has been found to be effective in healing severe refractory *aphthous ulceration* in all seven patients in one reported series although the impression was that relapse occurred if treatment was stopped. The dose was 100 mg nocte for two weeks followed by a maintenance dose of 100 mg every fifth day. Apart from early drowsiness, responsive to a reduction in dose, no serious side effects occurred up to 6 months.

Oral candida is managed by topical nystatin and clotrimazole or systemic ketoconazole or fluconazole (Greenspan and Greenspan 1991)

HL has been reported to respond to antiviral agents, such as acyclovir, ganciclovir and trisodium phosphonoformate, as well as topical retinoic acid. Because the disease spontaneously remits and relapses, is relatively uncommon, occurs in people who are ill, or shortly to become so, and who therefore require other treatments for more pressing indications these agents are difficult to evaluate. Treatment has rarely been a problematic issue and the presence of HL is most significant from the prognostic view.

Gangrenous stomatitis will require broad spectrum antimicrobial treatment systemically and topically, local anaesthetic preparations, topical haemostatic agents containing tranexamic acid and total parenteral nutrition but may still be difficult to control. Debridement and tooth extraction, whilst useful in severe periodontal disease (Greenspan and Greenspan 1991), have been avoided to prevent further bleeding, functional damage or superinfection (Giovanni et al. 1989).

Science and Research

Inflammatory Disorders

The increased incidence of *seborrhoeic dermatitis* in AIDS and HIV infection is unexplained (Duvic 1991). Various mechanisms have been postulated

Table 7.3. Treatments used for Kaposi's sarcoma

Local
  Cryotherapy
  Radiotherapy
  Interlesional e.g. TNF α, IFN α, vinca alkaloids
  Surgery

Systemic
  Aggressive chemotherapy
  Isotretinoin (under trial)

whereby neuro-endocrine or sebotropic factors are influenced by HIV infection and some authors believe that the same mechanism underlies both the seborrhoeic dermatitis and the neurologic disease in those patients with dementia and spinal cord pathology who have coexistent seborrhoeic dermatitis. Seborrhoeic dermatitis is essentially a hyperproliferative dermatosis and Kaplan et al. (1987) have suggested that epidermal keratinocyte stimulation may result from HIV infection either through lymphokine release from monocytes or due to a direct effect of the virus itself.

However, with the balance of opinion that classical seborrhoeic dermatitis represents an aberrant cutaneous reaction to the commensal *Pityrosporum* species of yeasts it is attractive to consider that in HIV infection the genesis of a cutaneous immunological defect alters the host–organism relationship and the skin disorder ensues. On the basis of quantitative correlation between numbers of yeast cells adherent to and extruded from keratinocytes and the clinical severity of seborrhoeic dermatitis an association if not a causative role for *Pityrosporum* has been strongly suggested in seborrhoeic dermatitis in patients with AIDS (Wikler et al. 1992). This association is strengthened by improvement with ketoconazole which is accompanied by a decrease in the numbers of *Pityrosporum* organisms per keratinocyte (Groisser et al. 1989). Abnormalities of skin surface lipids are not associated with the development of seborrhoeic dermatitis but are associated with HIV infection itself (Vidal et al. 1990).

The pathogenesis of *psoriasis* is unknown (Camisa 1994). It has two main components – proliferative and inflammatory. Psoriasis may be essentially an immune disease with secondary dysfunction of the vascular endothelium and keratinocytes, or a primary disorder of hyperproliferation of the dermal vascular endothelium and keratinocyte which may result in immune activation. Evidence mustered to argue for a primary autoimmune mechanism is that (a) epidermal autoantibodies and autoreactive T cells may be found in the lesions, (b) there is an association with HLA phenotypes, (c) psoriasis responds to immunosuppressive therapy. However, the association of psoriasis with streptoccal and viral infections, AIDS and physical trauma argues against a single provocative antigen.

Aspects of the immunopathogenesis of HIV infection that may be of interest in the context of psoriasis are: the (contentious) decreased numbers of epidermal antigen presenting Langerhans cells (as in psoriasis); Langerhans cells are thought to harbour HIV (either increased viral burden per cell during infection or various gene products of HIV may alter the immune function of the cell); selective defect in soluble antigen recognition by CD4 T lymphocytes; (until pre-terminally) increased numbers of CD8 T lymphocytes; polyclonal B cell activation; elevated gamma-delta T lymphocytes; decreased natural killer cell function; defective reticuloendothelial cell function.

HIV gene products may have a role in the pathogenesis of proliferative epidermal disorders as shown by experiments with transgenic mice that have been engineered to express some HIV genes in skin and which then develop a psoriasiform diffuse epidermal hyperplasia (Kopp et al. 1993).

Untangling the relationship of HIV with psoriasis may help our understanding of both conditions.

Infections

Two groups discovered the Warthin–Starry staining bacteria (*R. henselae* which are gram-negative rods) of cat scratch disease in the abnormal microvasculature of tissue taken from patients with *bacillary angiomatosis*. Investigators were struck by the similarity of bacillary angiomatosis with the cutaneous stigmata of chronic infection with *Bartonella bacilliformis*, the "forma mular of verruga peruana". These lesions may occur in the chronic phase of Oroya fever and are, apparently, clinically and histologically very similar to those of epithelioid haemangiomatosis. The abnormal vascular spaces, lined with proliferating endothelium, are found to be stuffed with clumps of the gram-negative *B. bacilliformis*. However patients with epithelioid haemangiomatosis do not appear to have an overt acute febrile haemolytic illness. This analogous situation is food for thought concerning the pathogenesis of Kaposi's sarcoma that is so similar to bacillary angiomatosis.

Neoplasms

The differential frequency of occurrence of KS in risk groups for HIV has been mentioned (Schwartz et al. 1991; Tappero et al. 1993). The sex ratios for classical sporadic KS appear to have changed during this century from about 10:1 (male to female) to 2:1. KS was first observed in a renal transplant patient in 1968 after many such operations had been performed and after an increased risk of lymphoma was already evident in these patients; the incidence of KS in immunosuppressed patients post-transplant is about 4%. Previously KS in children was almost unheard of, but children with AIDS (non-haemophiliacs) have a prevalence of KS of about 4%. Congenital non-AIDS immunodeficiency states do not predispose to KS as they do to lymphoma. The incidence of KS in post-transfusion AIDS patients is about 3%. There are epidemiological studies which suggest that Kaposi's sarcoma is acquired during particular types of sexual activity (receptive fellatio and frequent anal douching) and susceptibility is determined by immunogenetics, being strongly associated with HLA-DR1 and DQw1 (Goedert 1990). A homosexual man with benign, long-standing (10 years) multicentric non-classical KS with evidence of multiple previous infections but *not* HIV has been reported in whom the only evidence of immune dysfunction was slight impairment of monocyte phagocytosis and evidence of cutaneous anergy (Archer et al. 1990).

Observations like those above have been used to put forward the idea that KS is caused by an infectious agent with a pattern of transmission that overlaps with HIV. A virus rarely present in infected blood could be responsible for KS in the presence of immunodeficiency in patients who abuse drugs intravenously or who have transfusions (renal patients have frequently had multiple transfusions), but could also, like HIV, be transmitted sexually. CMV and more recently human papilloma virus type 16 have been implicated.

The similarity of KS to avian haemangiomatosis has been noted; this condition is due to an avian retrovirus. That the unusual vascular proliferation of bacillary angiomatosis in HIV infected patients seems to result from cat scratch disease suggests also that the similar KS may be a consequence of a separate infection and that the organism may not be a virus but a bacterium. Recent evidence has implicated a herpes virus (human herpes virus 8-HHV8).

References

Aguado JM, Castrillo JM (1987) Lymphadenitis as a characteristic manifestation of disseminated tuberculosis in intravenous drug abusers infected with human immunodeficiency virus. J Infect 14: 191-193
Anonymous (1989) Oral hairy leukoplakia. Lancet 2: 1194
Allen BR (1992) Use of cyclosporin for psoriasis in HIV-positive patient. Lancet 339: 686
Archer CB, Spittle MF, Smith NP (1989) Kaposi's sarcoma in a homosexual – 10 years on. Clin Exp Dermatol 14: 233-236
Baden LA, Bigby M, Kwan T (1991) Persistent necrotic digits in a patient with the acquired immunodeficiency syndrome. Herpes simplex virus infection. Arch Dermatol 127: 113-116
Ball LM, Harper JI (1987) Atopic eczema in HIV seropositive haemophiliacs. Lancet 2: 627-628
Bakos L, Kronfeld M, Hampe S, Castro I, Zampese M (1989) Disseminated paracoccidioidomycosis with skin lesions in a patient with acquired immunodeficiency syndrome. J Am Acad Dermatol 20: 854-855
Battegay M, Opravil M, Wuthrich B, Luthy R (1989) Rash with amoxycillin-clavulanate therapy in HIV-infected patients. Lancet ii: 1100
Berger TG, Greene I (1991) Bacterial, viral, fungal, and parasitic infections in HIV disease and AIDS. Dermatologic Clinics 9: 465-492
Berger TG, Sawchuk WS, Leonardi C, Langenberg A, Tappero J, Leboit PE (1991) Epidermodysplasia verruciformis-associated papillomavirus infection complicating human immunodeficiency virus disease. Br J Dermatol 124: 79-83
Bessen LJ, Greene JB, Louie E et al. (1988) Severe polymyositis-like syndrome associated with zidovudine therapy or AIDS and ARC. N Engl J Med 311: 708
Betlloch I, Amador C, Chiner E, Pasquau F, Calpe JL, Vilar A (1991) Eruptive melanocytic nevi in human immunodeficiency virus infection. Int J Dermatol 30: 303
Blauvelt A, Harris HR, Hogan DJ, Jimenez-Acosta F, Ponce I, Pardo RJ (1992) Porphyria cutanea tarda and human immunodeficiency virus infection. Int J Dermatol 31: 474-479
Blauvelt A, Kerdel FA (1992) Cutaneous cryptococcosis mimicking Kaposi's sarcoma as the initial manifestation of disseminated disease. Int J Dermatol 31: 279-280
Boixeda P, Espana A, Suarez J, Buzon L, Lado A (1991) Cutaneous nocardiosis and human immunodeficiency virus infection. Int J Dermatol 11: 804-805
Bradshaw BR, Nuovo GJ, DiCostanzo D, Cohen SR (1992) Human papillomavirus type 16 in a homosexual man. Association with perianal carcinoma in situ and condyloma acuminatum. Arch Dermatol 128: 949-952
Bratzke B. Eichhorn R, Hoffken G et al. (1988) Akute Primarphase als Indikator der HIV-1-Infektion. Dtsch Med Wschr 113: 1312-1316
Calza AM, Kinloch S, Mainetti C, Salomon D, Saurat JH (1991) Primary human immunodeficiency virus infection mimicking syphilis. J Infect Dis 164: 615-616
Camisa C (1994) Psoriasis. Blackwell Scientific Publications, Boston
Caumes E, Katlama C, Guermonprez G, Bournerias I, Danis M, Gentilini M (1990) Cutaneous side-effects of bleomycin in AIDS patients with Kaposi's sarcoma. Lancet 336: 1593
Chiewchanvit S, Mahanupab P, Hirunsri P, Vanittanakow N (1991) Cutaneous manifestations of disseminated Penicillium marneffei mycosis in five HIV-infected patients. Mycoses 34: 245-249
Cockerell CJ (1991) Noninfectious inflammatory skin diseases in HIV-infected individuals. In: William James LTC (Ed) Dermatologic Clinics AIDS: A Ten-Year Perspective. Saunders, pp 531-542
Cockerell CJ (1993) Organ-specific manifestations of HIV infection. II. Update on cutaneous manifestations of HIV infection. Aids 7 Suppl 1: S213-S218
Cohen JI, Corey GR (1985) Cytomegalovirus infection in the normal host. Medicine 64: 100-114
Cohen LM, Callen JP (1992) Oral and labial melanotic macules in a patient infected with human immunodeficiency virus. J Am Acad Dermatol 26: 653-654
Cohen PR, Grossman ME (1989) Clinical features of human immunodeficiency virus-associated disseminated herpes zoster infection – a review of the literature. Clin Exp Dermatol 14: 273-276
Cohen PR, Grossman ME, Silvers DN, DeLeo VA (1991) Human immunodeficiency virus-associated granuloma annulare. Int J STD AIDS 2: 168-171
Cole MC, Cohen PR, Satra KH, Grossman ME (1992) The concurrent presence of systemic disease pathogens and cutaneous Kaposi's sarcoma in the same lesion: Histoplasma capsulatum and

Kaposi's sarcoma coexisting in a single skin lesion in a patient with AIDS. J Am Acad Dermatol 26: 285–287

Colebunders R, Blot K, Meriens V, Dock P (1992) Psoriasis regression in terminal AIDS. Lancet 339: 1110

Cone LA, Woodard DR, Byrd RG, Schulz K, Kopp SM, Schlievert PM (1992) A recalcitrant, erythematous, desquamating disorder associated with toxin-producing staphylococci in patients with AIDS. J Infect Dis 165: 638–643

Coopman SA, Johnson RA, Platt R, Stern RS (1993) Cutaneous disease and drug reactions in HIV infection. New Engl J Med 328: 1670–1674

Coopman SA, Stern RS (1991) Cutaneous drug reactions in human immunodeficiency virus infection. Arch Dermatol 127: 714–717

Crosby DL, Berger TG, Woosley JT, Resnick SD (1991) Dermatophytosis mimicking Kaposi's sarcoma in human immunodeficiency virus disease. Dermatologica 182: 135–137

De Boer WA, Danner SA (1990) HIV infection and squamous cell carcinoma of sun-exposed skin. Aids 4: 91

Dominey A, Rosen T, Fschen J (1989) Papulonodular demodicidosis associated with the acquired immunodeficiency syndrome. J Am Acad Dermatol 20: 197–201

Dompmartin D et al. (1990) Onychomycosis and AIDS: clinical and laboratory findings in 62 patients. Int J Dermatol 29: 337–339

Donohue D, Robinson B, Goldberg NS (1991) Staphylococcal scalded skin syndrome in a woman with chronic renal failure exposed to human immunodeficiency virus. Cutis 47: 317–318

Donovan B, Rohrsteim R, Bassett I, Mulhall BP (1992) Bullous impetigo in homosexual men – a risk factor for HIV infection. Genitourin Med 68: 159–161

Duvic M (1991) Papulosquamous disorders associated with human immunodeficiency virus infection. In: William James LTC (Ed) Dermatologic Clinics AIDS: A Ten-Year Perspective. Saunders, pp 523–530

Duvic M, Lowe L (1987) Superficial phaeohyphomycosis of the scrotum in a patient with acquired immunodeficiency syndrome. Arch Dermatol 123: 1597–1599

Duvic M et al. (1989) Eruptive dysplastic naevi associated with human immunodeficiency virus infection. Arch Dermatol 125: 397–401

Duvic M, Reisman M, Finley V et al. (1987) Glucan-induced keratoderma in acquired immunodeficiency syndrome. Arch Dermatol 123: 751–756

Eeftinck Schattenkerk JK, van Gool T, van Ketel RJ, Bartelsman JF (1991) Microsporidiosis in HIV1 infected individuals. Lancet 338: 323

El Baze P, Thyss A, Vinti H, Deville A, Dellawonica P, Ortonne JP (1991) A study of nineteen immunocompromised patients with extensive skin lesions caused by *Pseudomonas aeruginosa* with and without bacteremia. Acta Derm Venereol (Stockh) 71: 411–415

Fegeux S, Salmon D, Picard C et al. (1990) Penile ulcerations with foscarnet. Lancet 335: 547

Ferrandiz C, Ribera M, Barranco JC, Clotet B, Lorenzo JC (1992) Eosinophilic pustular filliculitis in patients with acquired immunodeficiency syndrome. Int J Dermatol 31: 193–195

Fine RM (1992) AIDS-related Kaposi's sarcoma. Int J Dermatol 31: 471

Freed JA, Pervez NK, Chen V et al. (1987) Cutaneous mycobacteriosis: occurrence and significance in two patients with the acquired immunodeficiency syndrome. Arch Dermatol 123: 1601–1603

Frentz G, Niordson A-M, Thomsen K (1989) Eosinophilic pustular dermatosis: an early skin marker of infection with human immunodeficiency virus? Br J Dermatol 121: 271–274

Funkhouser ME, Omohundro C, Ross A, Berger TG (1993) Management of scabies in patients with human immunodeficiency virus disease. Arch Dermatol 129: 911–913

Gherardi R, Belec L, Mhiri C et al. (1993) The spectrum of vasculitis in human immunodeficiency virus-infected patients: a clinicopathological evaluation. Arthritis Rheum 36: 1164–1174

Giovannini M, Zucotti GV, and Fiocchi A (1989) Gangrenous stomatitis in a child with AIDS. Lancet 2: 1400

Glover RA, Piaquadio DJ, Kern S, Cockerell CJ (1992) An unusual presentation of secondary syphilis in a patient with human immunodeficiency virus infection. A case report and review of the literature. Arch Dermatol 128: 530–534

Goedert JJ (1990) Infectious and genetic factors in AIDS-associated Kaposi's sarcoma. Lancet 335: 547

Gottlieb MS, Schroff R, Schanker HM et al. (1981) Pneumocystis carinii pneumonia and mucosal candidiasis in previously healthy homosexual men. N Engl J Med 305: 1425–1430

Greenspan D, Greenspan JS (1991) Oral manifestations of HIV infection. In: William James LTC (Ed) Dermatologic Clinics AIDS: A Ten-Year Perspective. Saunders, pp 517–522

Groisser D, Bottone EJ, Lebwohl M (1989) Association of Pityrosporum orbiculare (Malassezia furfur) with seborrhoeic dermatitis in patients with acquired immunodeficiency syndrome (AIDS). J Am Acad Dermatol 20: 770-773

Gussenhoven MJ, Haak A, Peereboom-Wynia JD, van't Wout JW (1991) Stevens-Johnson syndrome after fluconazole. Lancet 338: 120

Harris DW, Ostlere L, Buckley C, Johnson M, Rustin MH (1992) Eosinophilic pustular folliculitis in an HIV-positive man: response to cetirizine. Br J Dermatol 126: 392-394

Hawkins CC, Gold JWM, Whimbey E et al. (1986) Mycobacterium avium complex infections in patients with the acquired immunodeficiency syndrome. Ann Intern Med 105: 184-188

Hennessey NP, Parro EL, Cockerell CJ (1991) Cutaneous Pneumocystis carinii infection in patients with acquired immunodeficiency syndrome. Arch Dermatol 127: 1699-1701

Hicks CB (1991) Syphilis and HIV infection. In: William James LTC (Ed) Dermatologic Clinics AIDS: A Ten-Year Perspective. Saunders, pp 493-502

Hira SK, Wadhawan D, Kamanga J. et al. (1988) Cutaneous manifestations of human immunodeficiency virus in Lusaka, Zambia. J Am Acad Dermatol 19: 451-457

Holton J, Nye P, Miller R (1991) Mycobacterium haemophilum infection in a patient with AIDS. J Infect 23: 303-306

Hoover WD Jr, Lang PG (1991) Pruritus in HIV infection. J Am Acad Dermatol 24: 1020-1021

Hughes-Davies L, Spittle M (1991) Cancer and HIV infection. Br Med J 302: 673-674

Hunt SJ, Nagi C, Gross KG, Wong DS, Mathews WC (1992) Primary cutaneous aspergillosis near central venous catheters in patients with the acquired immunodeficiency syndrome. Arch Dermatol 128: 1229-1232

Janssen F, Zelinsky-Guning A, Caumer E, Decares JM (1991) Group A streptoccocal cellulitis-adenitis in a patient with acquired immunodeficiency syndrome. J Am Acad Dermatol 24: 363-365

Jimenez-Acosta FJ, Vicandim B, Viguer JM et al. (1988) Diagnostic value of cutaneous cytology in opportunistic fungal infections of patients with acquired immunodeficiency syndrome. J Am Acad Dermatol 18: 383-384

Jones RS Jr, Collier-Brown C, Suh B (1992) Localized cutaneous reaction to intravenous pentamidine. Clin Infect Dis 15: 561-562

Kalter DC, Gendelman HE, Meltzer MS (1991) Monocytes, dendritic cells, and Langerhans cells in human immunodeficiency virus infection. In: William James LTC (Ed) Dermatologic Clinics AIDS: A Ten-Year Perspective. Saunders, pp 415-428

Kaplan MH, Sadick N, McNutt NS et al. (1987) Dermatologic findings and manifestations of acquired immunodeficiency syndrome (AIDS). J Am Acad Dermatol 16: 485-506

Kaplan MH, Dadick NS, Talmor M (1991) Acquired trichomegaly of the eyelashes: a cutaneous marker of acquired immunodeficiency syndrome. J Am Acad Dermatol 25: 801-804

Kopp JB, Rooney JF, Wohlenberg C et al. (1993) Cutaneous disorders and viral gene expression in HIV-1 transgenic mice. AIDS Res Hum Retrovirus 9: 267-275

Koranda FC et al. (1974) Cutaneous complications in immunosuppressed renal homograft recipients. JAMA 229: 419-424

Kovacs JA, and Masur H (1988) Pneumocystis carinii pneumonia: therapy and prophylaxis. J Infect Dis 158: 254-259

Lesher JL and Knight FJ (1986) Tzanck preparation as a diagnostic aid in disseminated histoplasmosis. J Am Acad Dermatol 15: 534-535

Lewis DA, Brook MG (1992) Erythema multiforme as a presentation of human immunodeficiency virus seroconversion illness. Int J STD AIDS 3: 56-57

Lin RY, Smith JK (1988) IgE and human immunodeficiency virus infection. Ann Allergy 61: 269-272

Lindgren AM, Fallon JD, Horan RF (1991) Psoriasiform papules in the acquired immunodeficiency syndrome. Disseminated histoplasmosis in AIDS. Arch Dermatol 127: 722-723

Litwin MA, Williams CM (1992) Cutaneous Pneumocystis carinii infection mimicking Kaposi sarcoma. Ann Intern Med 117: 45-49

Lobo DV, Chu P, Grekin RC, Berger TG (1992) Non-melanoma skin cancers and infection with the human immunodeficiency virus. Arch Dermatol 128: 623-627

Matis WL, Triana A, Shapiro R et al. (1987) Dermatologic findings associated with human immunodeficiency virus infection. J Am Acad Dermatol 17: 746-751

May LP, Sidhu GS, Buchness MR (1992) Diagnosis of Acanthamoeba infection by cutaneous manifestations in a man seropositive to HIV. J Am Acad Dermatol 26: 352-355

McGregor JM, Newell M, Ross J, Kirkham N, McGibbon DH, Darley C (1992) Cutaneous malignant melanoma and human immunodeficiency virus H(HIV) infections: a report of three cases. Br J Dermatol 126: 516-519

Meola T, Soter NA, Ostreicher R, Sanchez M, Moy JA (1993) The safety of UVB phototherapy in patients with HIV infection. Journal of the American Academy of Dermatology. 29: 216-20

Meyers WM (1992) Leprosy. Dermatologic Clinics 10: 73-96

Musher DM, Hamill RJ, and Baughn RE (1990) Effect of human immunodeficiency virus (HIV) infection on the course of syphilis and on the response to treatment. Ann Intern Med 113: 872-881

Myskowski PL (1991) Cutaneous T-cell lymphoma and human immunodeficiency virus. The spectrum broadens. Arch Dermatol 127: 1045-1047

Noordhoek GT, van Embden JD (1991) Yaws, an endemic treponematosis reconsidered in the HIV era. Eur J Clin Microbiol 10: 4-5

Norris SA, Kessler HA, and Fife KH (1988) Severe, progressive herpetic whitlow caused by an acyclovir-resistant virus in a patient with AIDS. J Infect Dis 157: 209-210

Orkin M (1993) Scabies in AIDS. Semin Dermatol 12: 9-14

Paller AS, Sahn EE, Garen PD, Dobson RL, Chadwick EG (1990) Pyoderma gangrenosum in pediatric acquired immunodeficiency syndrome. J Pediat 117: 63-66

Pardo RJ, Bogaert MA, Penneys NS, Byrene GE Jr, Ruiz P (1992) UVB phototherapy of the pruritic papular eruption of the acquired immunodeficiency syndrome. J Am Acad Dermatol 26: 423-428

Parkin JM, Eales LJ, Galazka AR, Pinching AJ (1987) Atopic manifestations of the acquired immunodeficiency syndrome: response to recombinant interferon gamma. Br Med J 294: 1185-1186

Pedersen C, Nielsen JO (1987) Tuberculosis in homosexual men with HIV disease. Scand J Infect Dis 19: 289-290

Penneys NS (1990) Skin manifestations of AIDS. Martin Dunitz, London

Petersen CS, Gerstoft J (1992) Molluscum contagiosum in HIV-infected patients. Dermatology 184: 19-21

Pialoux G, Hannequin C, Dupont B, Ravisse P (1990) Cutaneous leishmaniasis in an AIDS patient: cure with itraconazole. J Infect Dis 162: 1221-1222

Pitchenik AE, Cole C, Russell BW et al. (1984) Tuberculosis, atypical mycobacteriosis, and the acquired immunodeficiency syndrome among Haitian and non-Haitian patients in South Florida. Ann Int Med 101: 641-645

Prose NS (1991) Cutaneous manifestations of HIV infection in children. Dermatologic Clinics 9: 543-550

Prose NS, Abson KG, Scher RK (1992) Disorders of the nails and hair associated with human immunodeficiency virus infection. Int J Dermatol 31: 453-457

Quale J, Teplitz E, Augenbraun M (1990) Atypical presentation of chancroid in a patient infected with the human immunodeficiency virus. A J M 88: 43-44

Ranki A, Puska P, Mattinen S, Lagerstedt A, Krohn K (1991) Effect of PUVA on immunologic and virologic findings in HIV-infected patients. J Am Acad Dermatol 24: 404-410

Ranki A, Lauharanta J, Kanerva L (1984) Effect of etretinate on the distribution of Langerhans cells and T lymphocytes in psoriatic skin. Arch Dermatol Res 276: 102-104

Rao GG, Lock SH, Maddocks AC, Pinching AJ (1991) Listeriosis in AIDS: consequence and cofactor. Int J STD AIDS 2: 291-292

Rappersberger K, Hatzakis A, Zonitza E, Tschachler E et al. (1989) J Invest Dermatol 92: 503

Ricchi E, Manfredi R, Scarani P, Costigliola P, Chiodo F (1991) Cutaneous cryptococcosis and AIDS. J Am Acad Dermatol 25: 335-336

Ring J, Froschl M, Brunner R, Braun-Falco O (1986) LAV/HTLV III infection and atopy; serum IgE and specific IgE antibodies to environmental allergens Acta Derm Venereol (Stockh) 66: 530-532

Roenigk Jr HH, Crane G (1991) AIDS and infection control in dermatologic surgery. In: William James LTC (Ed) Dermatologic Clinics AIDS: A Ten-Year Perspective. Saunders, pp 579-584

Rohatgi PK, Palazzolo JV, Saini NB (1992) acute miliary tuberculosi of the skin in acquired immunodeficiency syndrome. J Am Acad Dermatol 26: 356-359

Romeu J, Milla F, Batlle M et al. (1991) Visceral leishmaniasis involving lung and a cutaneous Kaposi's sarcoma lesion. AIDS 5: 1272

Rosen T (1991) Pruritic papular eruption of AIDS. J Am Acad Dermatol 25: 866-867

Rustin MHA, Bunker CB, Dowd PM, Robinson TWE (1989) Erythema multiforme due to griseofulvin. Br J Dermatol 120: 455-458

Rzany B, Mockenhaupt M, Stocker U, Hamouda O, Schopf E (1993) Incidence of Stevens-Johnson syndrome and toxic epidermal necrolysis in patients with the acquired immunodeficiency syndrome in Germany. Arch Dermatol 129: 1059

Sabbatani S, Isuierdo Calzado A, Ferro A et al. (1991) Atypical leishmaniasis in an HIV-2-seropositive patient from Guinea-Bissau. Aids 5: 899-901

Sack JB (1990) Disseminated infection due to *Mycobacterium fortuitum* in a patient with AIDS. Rev Infect Dis 12: 961-963

Samaranayake LP, Pindborg JJ (1989) Hairy leucoplakia. Br Med J 298: 270-271

Schwartz JJ, Dias BM, Safai B (1991) HIV-related malignancy. In: William James LTC (Ed) Dermatologic Clinics AIDS: A Ten-Year Perspective. Saunders, pp 503-516

Siegal FP, Lopez C, Hammer GS et al. (1981) Severe acquired immunodeficiency in male homosexuals manifested by chronic perianal ulcerative herpes simplex lesions. N Engl J Med 305: 1439-1444

Smith KJ, Skelton III HG, James WD, Angritt P (1991a) Concurrent epidermal involvement of cytomegalovirus and herpes simplex virus in two HIV-infected patients. Military Medical Consortium for Applied Retroviral Research (MMCARR). J Am Acad Dermatol 25: 500-506

Smith KJ, Skelton III HG, Angritt P (1991b) Histopathologic features of HIV-associated skin disease. Dermatologic Clinics 9: 551-578

Soeprono FF, Schinella RA, Cockerell CJ, Comite SL (1986) Seborrheic-like dermatitis of acquired immunodeficiency syndrome. J Am Acad Dermatol 14: 242-248

Stashower ME, Yeager JK, Smith KJ, Skelton HG, Wagner KF (1993) Cimetidine as therapy for treatment-resistant psoriasis in a patient with acquired immunodeficiency syndrome. Arch Dermatol 129: 848-850

Tappero JW, Conant MA, Wolfe SF, Berger TG (1993) Kaposi's sarcoma. J Am Acad Dermatol 28: 371-395

Tchornobay AM, Claudy AL, Perrot JL, Levigne V, Denis M (1992) Fatal disseminated *Mycobacterium marinum* infection. Int J Dermatol 31: 286-287

Telfer NR, Mathews JM, Wojnarowska F (1989) Skin diseases in haemophiliacs with and without antibodies to the human immunodeficiency virus (HIV): further evidence of altered disease behaviour in different risk groups? Br J Dermatol 120: 795-799

Toome BK, Bowers KE, Scott GA (1991) Diagnosis of cutaneous cytomegalovirus infection: a review and report of a case. J Am Acad Dermatol 24: 857-863

Torres RA, Lin RV, Lee M, Barr MR (1992) Zidovudine-induced leukocytoclastic vasculitis. Arch Intern Med 152: 850-851

Torssander J, Karlsson A, Morfeldt-Manson L et al. (1988) Dermatophytosis and HIV infection: A study in homosexual men. Acta Derm Venereol (Stockh) 68: 53-56

van Ginkel CJ, Sang RT, Blaauwgeers JL, Schattenkerk JK, Mooi WJ, Hulsebosch HJ (1991) Multiple primary malignant melanomas in an HIV-positive man. J Am Acad Dermatol 24: 284-285

Vidal C, Girard P-M, Dompmartin D et al. (1990) Seborrheic dermatitis and HIV infection: qualitative analysis of skin surface lipids in men seropositive and seronegative for HIV. J Am Acad Dermatol 23: 1106-1110

Vidal C, Gonzalez Quintela A, Fuente R (1992) Toxic epidermal necrolysis due to vancomycin. Ann Allergy 68: 345-347

Wikler JR, Nieboer C, Willesze R (1992) Quantitative skin cultures of Pityrosporum yeasts in patients seropositive for the human immunodeficiency virus with and without seborrheic dermatitis. J Am Acad Dermatol 27: 37-39

Williams HC, Du Vivier AW (1991) Etretinate and AIDS-related Reiter's disease. Br J Dermatol 124: 389-392

Zukervar P, Canillot S, Gayrard L, Perrot H (1991) Sporotrichoid Mycobacterium marinum infection in a patient infected with human immunodeficiency virus. Ann Dermatol Venereol 118: 111-113

8 Haematological Complications of HIV Infection, AIDS and HIV-associated Lymphoma

Sally E. Kinsey

Introduction

At about the same time that Kaposi's sarcoma was recognised in homosexual men (Hymes et al. 1981) it emerged that there was a high incidence in the same population group of thrombocytopenia which was indistinguishable from immune thrombocytopenic purpura (ITP) seen in young women (Morris et al. 1982). Since the early 1980s the numbers of cases of HIV infection and AIDS have escalated both in groups at risk of infection (homosexualmen, haemophiliacs, intravenous drug abusers), in their sexual partners and offspring (in the case of females) and increasingly in the heterosexual population. It has gradually become obvious that haematological manifestations and complications of HIV infection are manifold.

Haematological complications of HIV infection may be related to: (a) HIV infection directly, i.e. virus mediated problems; (b) Secondary superadded and opportunistic infection, i.e. immunosuppression and bone marrow failure; (c) The treatment of HIV or other intercurrent complications with myelotoxic agents further compromising immune system and bone marrow function.

This chapter describes the peripheral blood and bone marrow abnormalities of HIV infection and other specific haematological disorders associated with HIV infection; in addition, a discussion of HIV-related lymphomas is included. The presentation, diagnosis and management of these conditions is reviewed.

Peripheral Blood Presentation

Primary Infection

Primary HIV infection is usually asymptomatic but may be associated with an acute "infectious mononucleosis-like" illness, although the symptoms of an acute viral illness are usually only recognised retrospectively on specific questioning. Clark et al. (1991) and Daar et al. (1991) have described groups of individuals in high risk groups presenting with severe mononucleosis-like illnesses who later became seropositive. Busch et al. (1991) suggest that the intensity of symptoms associated with primary infection may be proportional to the level of viraemia. As a consequence of this, HIV infection should be included in the differential diagnosis of such an infection. A peripheral blood smear examined at the time may contain "atypical" lymphocytes (Fig. 8.1). These large lymphoid cells are identified on May–Grunwald–Giemsa stained smears by their abundant basophilic (blue) cytoplasm which tends to adhere to adjacent red cells, large nucleus with open chromatin pattern and often a prominent nucleolus. These cells are CD8 positive on immunophenotyping. Levy et al. (1991) have identified a high level of antiviral activity by CD8 positive lymphocytes in HIV infected people. Progressive disease and a decline in CD8 positive cell numbers correlates with re-emergence of HIV viraemia. This suggests that CD8-positive lymphocytes are of major importance to host immune defence in HIV infection. Usually the identification/recognition of HIV infection is at a much later date in the course of its disease. In haemophiliacs the timing of seroconversion has been well documented from stored sera. Tucker and colleagues (1985) observed that there was a higher incidence of neurological disease in a group of haemophiliacs experiencing an infectious mononucleosis-like illness at time of seroconversion, which again may reflect high level viraemia.

Peripheral Blood Features

HIV infects cells via the CD4 receptor (Dalgleish et al. 1984) and is cytotoxic, thus causing lysis of CD4 positive cells with a consequent fall in the number of CD4-positive lymphocytes. This leads inevitably to the reversal of the CD4 : CD8 lymphocyte ratio. Other cells which express the CD4 receptor include monocyte/macrophages (Klatzmann et al. 1984; Ho et al. 1986), myeloid cells (Cortes et al. 1986), microglial cells (Maddon et al. 1986) and Langhans'

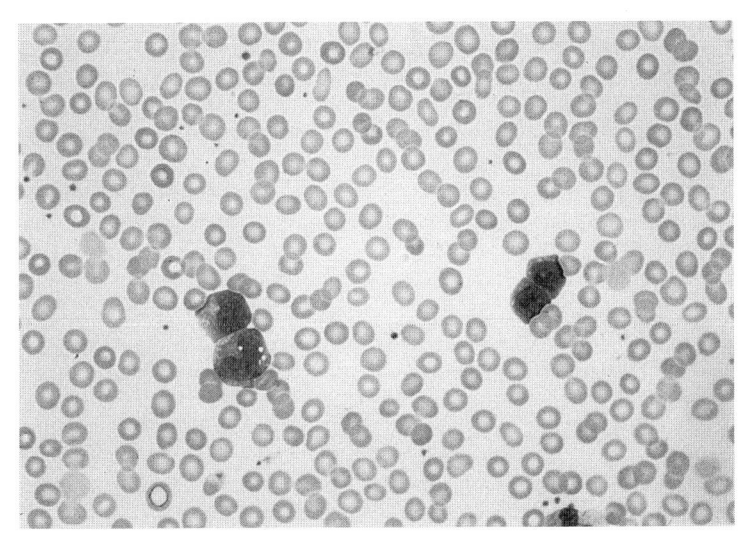

Fig. 8.1. Peripheral blood smear with atypical lymphocytes. Abundant cytoplasm with vacuolation and increased cytoplasmic basophilia where the cytoplasmic membrane impinges upon adjacent red cells.

dendritic cells (antigen presenting cells) (Gartner et al. 1986). Thus, with wide expression of the CD4 antigen throughout, the haemopoietic system is vulnerable to HIV infection.

Lymphopenia

Lysis of CD4 positive cells will reduce total lymphocyte numbers. But the fall in the peripheral lymphocyte count cannot only be due to this. HIV infection stimulates CD4 positive cell syncytial formation in combination with non-infected CD4 cells; the subsequent formation of non-functioning giant cells causes both a reduction in cell numbers and death of cells (Lifson et al. 1986). Part of the host response to HIV infection is manifest in the development of lymphocytotoxic auto-antibodies directed against CD4-positive cells reducing lymphocyte numbers still further (Kloster et al. 1984; Dorsett et al. 1985; Stricker et al. 1988). Additionally, impaired IL-2 production reduces the normal reconstitution of T cell numbers and their proliferation in response to alloantigens (Siegel et al. 1985). Progressive HIV disease is associated with decreasing peripheral CD4 cell numbers; a poorer survival is seen in those patients presenting with low CD4 counts despite therapy with zidovudine (Moore et al. 1991a).

Morphologically lymphocytes are often atypical and plasmacytoid in appearance, frequently with abundant cytoplasm with or without cleaved or cerebriform nuclei.

Neutropenia

A reduction in the numbers of circulating neutrophils occurs due to the development of specific granulocyte antibodies (Murphy et al. 1987) which shorten peripheral neutrophil survival. Also a reduction in numbers of bone marrow myeloid precursor colonies occurs as a result of a cross-reacting antibody directed towards part of the HIV glycoprotein causing inhibition of marrow proliferation (Leiderman et al. 1987). In addition there is an element of ineffective myelopoiesis.

Many authors describe abnormal neutrophil/granulocyte morphological features, but the only consistent feature in peripheral blood is that of "left shift" (i.e. more immature, less well lobulated forms, Fig. 8.2) (Spivak et al. 1983, 1984; Castella et al. 1985; Treacy et al. 1987; Zon et al. 1987).

Thrombocytopenia

The thrombocytopenia seen in HIV infection cannot be distinguished from classical immune thrombocytopenic purpura (ITP), that is, reduced platelet numbers in the face of normal or elevated numbers of bone marrow megakaryocytes and a shortened platelet lifespan (Morris et al. 1982).

The mechanism of ITP is thought to be due to platelet auto-antibody formation or to immune complex formation: The management of ITP is discussed in greater detail below.

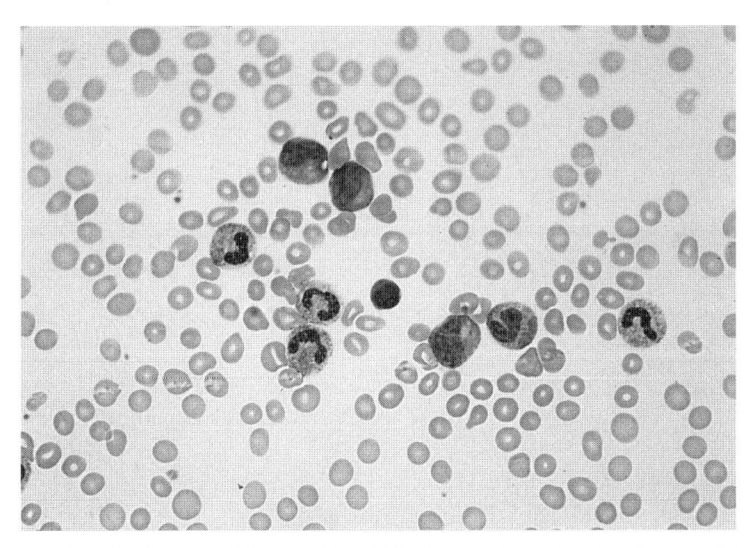

Fig. 8.2. "Left-shifted" neutrophils in peripheral blood smear. There is reduced nuclear lobulation. Additionally there is "toxic" cytoplasmic granulation and Döhle bodies (cytoplasmic remnants of denatured RNA).

Progressive HIV infection is associated with thrombocytopenia as a result of bone marrow failure. An improvement in peripheral platelet counts (Hirschel et al. 1988; Hymes et al. 1988) and bone marrow thrombopoiesis (Ballem et al. 1988) is seen following commencement of treatment with zidovudine, suggesting a direct effect of HIV on megakaryocyte activity. A more recent study of ^{111}In-labelled platelets (Ballem et al. 1992) identified reduced platelet survival in HIV-infected homosexual men regardless of platelet count or zidovudine therapy, compared with normal controls, although no increased uptake was seen in liver or spleen. Reduced platelet production was also seen in untreated thrombocytopenic individuals compared with normal controls. However, those on zidovudine therapy or non-thrombocytopenic had increased platelet production. This suggests that there seems to be a direct effect of HIV on thrombopoiesis. Landonio et al. (1993), in a study of HIV-related thrombocytopenia in drug abusers, showed a similar reduction in platelet survival and platelet turnover but with splenic or hepatic pooling of platelets. This may be accounted for by the known association of immune-complex disease and viral hepatitis (common in drug abusers) thus implicating an ITP mechanism. Landonio and colleagues suggest that HIV-related thrombocytopenia is multifactorial comprising megakaryocyte hypoplasia or impaired maturation, ITP and splenic/hepatic pooling.

Pechere et al. (1993) comment that the improvement in thrombopoiesis by zidovudine treatment is important and that the use of other anti-HIV agents may not (or do not) have the same effect. This is particularly important if patients are switched from zidovudine to another agent.

Louache et al. (1991) have shown the presence of HIV in megakaryocytes by in situ hybridisation in HIV-positive symptomatic and asymptomatic patients. Interestingly HIV transcripts could not be detected in cultured megakaryocyte colony units suggesting that either infection of megakaryocytes occurs late in differentiation or that infected megakaryocyte colony units are unable to differentiate in vitro. Thrombocytopenia may also be a manifestation of drug-induced myelotoxicity.

Anaemia

Anaemia is seen in the majority of patients with AIDS; the cause is not clear but is almost certainly multifactorial. Likely contributing factors must be

(a) ineffective erythropoiesis (identified as bone marrow erythroid hyperplasia with peripheral anaemia);
(b) reduced erythroid precursor numbers directly due to HIV infection;
(c) direct blood loss from Kaposi's sarcoma lesions and from cytomegalovirus colitis;
(d) the consequence of direct drug toxicity on bone marrow function. (There appears to be a group of patients with an increased sensitivity of erythroid precursors to zidovudine with resultant reticulocytopenia (Miles et al. 1991). Moore et al. (1991a) demonstrated an increase in haemoglobin in 52% of patients on cessation of zidovudine);
(e) bone marrow suppression due to infection (e.g. atypical mycobacteria), infiltration (e.g. by lymphoma) or down regulation of erythropoiesis by TNF released as a consequence of infection/inflammation elsewhere;
(f) destruction of red cells by haemolysis (e.g. in auto-immune haemolytic anaemia) or sequestration of red cells within an enlarged spleen (hypersplenism).

There is no appropriate rise in erythropoietin levels for the degree of anaemia, but an increase may be seen following commencement of zidovudine (Spivak et al. 1989). A recently reported study of the role of recombinant human erythropoietin (r-HuEPO) in anaemic AIDS patients treated with zidovudine, indicated that patient response could be predicted on the basis of the baseline endogenous EPO level (Epo study group; Rudnick 1989). Those patients with a low baseline level (<500 mU/ml) had a clear response to r-HuEPO with a statistically significant reduction in transfusion requirement when compared with controls. Those with higher baseline values (>500 mU/ml) did not respond.

In a cohort of AIDS patients treated with zidovudine, Moore et al. (1991a) identified that the development of anaemia (haematocrit 0.29) was the most significant prognostic indicator of early death.

The combined administration of bone marrow colony stimulating factors with erythropoietin may improve the neutropenia and anaemia of AIDS and simultaneously allow full-dose zidovudine in patients in whom the haematological effects of zidovudine had limited its dosage (Groopman 1990; Miles et al. 1991).

Positive direct antiglobulin tests (DAT) (Coomb's Test) have been reported in as many as 18% HIV-positive patients (Toy et al. 1985). The role of auto-haemolysis in the pathogenesis of anaemia is probably minimal; frank haemolysis is, in fact, quite rare. A positive DAT may be a non-specific phenomenon secondary to increased serum globulins in association with intercurrent infections (McGinnis et al. 1986).

Red cell morphological features are non-specific, often with aniso-poikilocytosis and reticulocytopenia. Marrow erythroid precursors often appear dysplastic and megaloblastic (with normal serum vitamin B_{12} and folate levels). Erythrophagocytosis has been reported. However the significance of this is not clear, as this is not infrequent in viral infection (Spivak et al. 1983; Castella et al. 1985; Treacy et al. 1987; Zon et al. 1987).

Low levels of serum vitamin B_{12} have been reported in AIDS patients, a finding which does not correlate with low serum cobalamin levels. Remacha et al. (1991) studied 60 consecutive HIV patients for vitamin B_{12} abnormalities. Low serum vitamin B_{12} levels were found in 16.7% of patients and in the majority of these impaired absorption was detected. Those with low B_{12} had lower haemoglobin, white cells, lymphocytes and CD4 lymphocytes compared to those with normal B_{12} levels. However only a minority of patients with low B_{12} had megaloblastic bone marrow features. Hansen et al. (1992) studied cobalamin-binding proteins in HIV infection and showed no decrease in cobalamin-binding proteins. Therefore this is not the explanation for low serum B_{12} in some individuals. Low serum B_{12} may contribute to neurological symptoms in HIV infection, e.g. neuropathy or myelopathy.

Bone Marrow Features

A number of reports have described the bone marrow features associated with HIV infection and AIDS. These changes include hypercellularity, hypocellularity (Fig. 8.3), myelodysplastic features (of all three cell lines) (Fig. 8.4), marrow fibrosis, lymphoid granulomata (Fig. 8.5), evidence of infection and infiltration (Osborne et al. 1984; Spivak et al. 1984; Castella et al. 1985; Geller et al. 1985; Schneider and Picker 1985; Shenoy and Lin 1986; Treacy et al. 1987; Zon et al. 1987; Holland and Spivak 1990; Karcher and Frost 1991). The reports show a

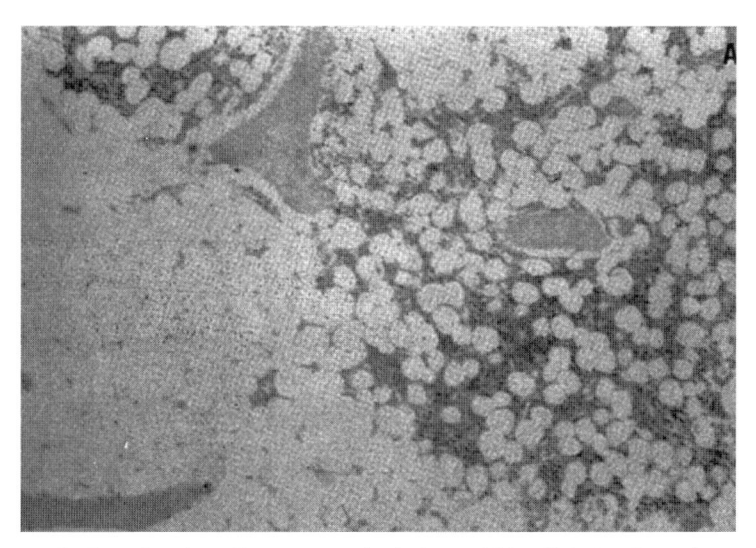

Fig. 8.3. Histological section of bone marrow displaying variable cellularity of a patchy nature. The area to the right is normocellular and that on the left is hypocellular.

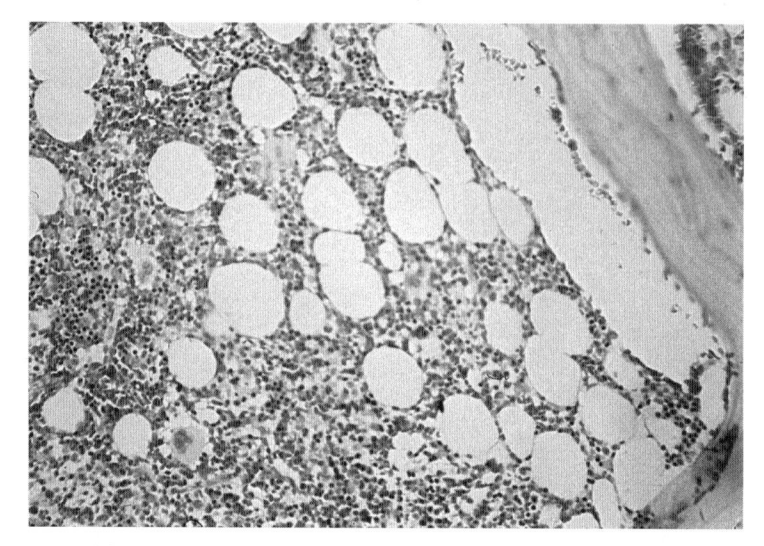

Fig. 8.4. Bone marrow histology with evidence of myelodysplasia.

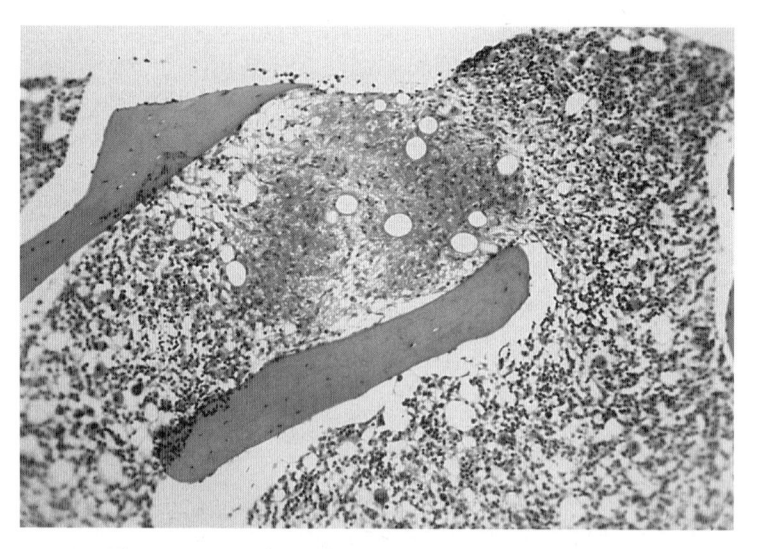

Fig. 8.5. Bone marrow histology with granuloma formation.

wide variation in the extent of the abnormalities identified; it remains unclear how much the contribution of the stage of HIV disease, intercurrent infections and therapeutic agents employed affects the bone marrow abnormalities seen.

A further bone marrow feature which has been widely reported is that of reticuloendothelial iron blockade, which is characteristic of the so-called anaemia of chronic disease and is usually associated with chronic infection, inflammation and neoplasia. This is likely to be another major factor in the aetiology of HIV associated anaemia. Karcher and Frost (1991) were able to correlate the degree of reticuloendothelial iron blockade with CDC class IV disease; the correlation was particularly strong in those with a history of opportunistic infection.

Bone marrow reticulin fibrosis is a common feature in HIV infection, identified in 20%–91% of cases. The cause of marrow fibrosis is not clear, but it is likely that it is a non-specific response to systemic disease rather than a primary bone marrow abnormality. Bone marrow fibrosis has been identified in many non-HIV related conditions and may be related to immune complex deposition in some cases (Lewis and Pegrum 1978; McCarthy 1985). A bone marrow trephine biopsy is necessary to assess cellularity and fibrosis.

Dysplastic features of erythroid and myeloid precursors and of megakaryocytes is reported to occur in 30%–50% of AIDS patients. Dyserythropoietic changes consist of multinucleate erythroid precursors with irregular nuclear membranes and internuclear bridge formation. Micromegakaryocytes, nuclear hyposegmentation and nuclear fragmentation are features of megakaryocyte dysplasia. Myeloid dysplasia is manifest as asynchronous nuclear and cytoplasmic maturation, abnormal nuclear condensation and hypogranularity of the cytoplasm (Fig. 8.6).

Haemophagocytosis and increased marrow macrophages may be a prominent bone marrow feature, as a response to HIV or to viral, fungal, bacterial opportunistic infections (Spivak et al. 1984).

Careful marrow scrutiny can reveal the presence of opportunistic infections, particularly atypical mycobacterium (with granuloma formation), or of malignancy, Kaposi's sarcoma (Little et al. 1986) or lymphoma (Knowles et al. 1988). Karcher and Frost (1991) suggest that although opportunistic micro-organisms may be found unexpectedly in bone marrow specimens on histological grounds, (i.e. in the absence of granuloma formation) this occurrence is uncommon (approximately 10%). In the same marrow series a significant number of the marrow specimens showing Burkitt-like lymphoma or Hodgkin's disease was the first evidence of malignancy in the individuals concerned.

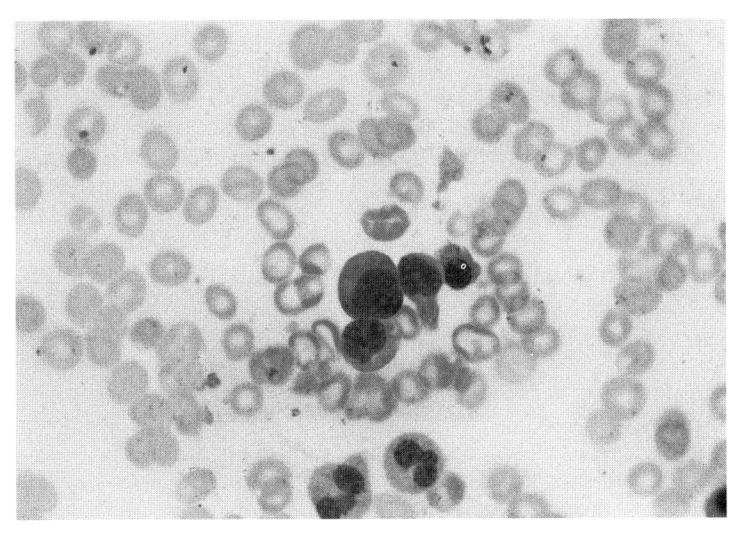

Fig. 8.6. Bone marrow aspirate with features of myeloid dysplasia. Abnormal nuclear condensation and reduced cytoplasmic granulation.

There are obviously profound effects of HIV infection upon haematopoiesis, and some of these are directly due to involvement by opportunistic organisms and the effect of chronic disease/debility. Nevertheless many of the effects are due directly to HIV itself via infection of haemopoietic precursors and interference with differentiation and maturation. As the processes of haematological damage are elucidated the indication for bone marrow examination will diminish. However there will still remain clinical situations when bone marrow examination will be invaluable, e.g. in the identification and staging of lymphoma.

In addition to the rather non-specific nature of the bone marrow abnormalities associated with HIV infection, and bearing in mind that there are attendant operator risks in performing the procedure, the indications for marrow examination should probably be restricted to those cases in which there is a high suspicion of malignancy or of unusual infection where the relevant tissue cannot be obtained by other means.

Effect of Drugs Used in the Management of HIV Infection

Many drugs used in the treatment of HIV and opportunistic infections are associated with haemopoietic toxicity. Myelotoxicity is most frequently seen in association with the administration of zidovudine and co-trimoxazole, however with increasing intensity of management and the necessity to treat HIV-associated malignancies, awareness of the potential myelotoxic side effects of combined therapeutic agents must be considered.

The use of zidovudine is associated with a fall in haemoglobin (often necessitating blood transfusion), an increase in the MCV (to the region of 110 fl), erythroid hypoplasia (Walker et al. 1988), leucopenia – particularly neutropenia (Richman et al. 1987), which is reversible – and equivocally increased or decreased platelet numbers. It is important to note that cytopenia associated with zidovudine administration is only seen in symptomatic AIDS patients; HIV-positive asymptomatic patients have a much lower incidence of haemopoietic toxicity (de Wolf et al. 1988). It thus becomes clear that haematological tolerance of therapy (particularly with zidovudine) is important with respect to successful treatment of HIV infection. The anaemia and neutropenia associated with the use of zidovudine requires dose reduction (Richman et al. 1987) and may prevent or limit the simultaneous use of other agents, e.g. co-trimoxazole, ganciclovir, α-interferon or pentamidine (Miles et al. 1991). As with all treatment, reduced doses of effective agents or the use of alternative therapies may result in the development of resistant HIV disease (Larder et al. 1989) or early relapse of the condition (Goldie and Coldman 1979). As far as HIV infection is concerned this may actually mean early death due to an inability to treat adequately the complications of the disease. However Fischl et al. (1990) reported that a reduced dose of zidovudine was at least as effective as conventional dose therapy with significantly reduced toxicity.

Co-trimoxazole used for the treatment of *Pneumocystis carinii* pneumonia causes a pancytopenia which is not reversed by folinic acid (bone marrow suppression is rare in non-AIDS patients and is reversed by folinic acid). In 1986 Jaffe reported the development of pancytopenia in 50% of AIDS patients on co-trimoxazole, often preceded by fever with subsequent neutropenia, thrombocytopenia and anaemia. These effects were reversible on discontinuation of co-trimoxazole. In 1987 Anderson et al. identified that pentamidine is also associated with neutropenia.

Management of Treatment Induced Cytopenias

As discussed above, haematological toxicity is the major dose-limiting effect of zidovudine therapy in patients with AIDS. However as treatment with zidovudine is associated with increased survival there is an impetus to ameliorate the haematological toxicity induced. There are broadly two ways in which to overcome this problem, either by reducing the dosage of myelotoxic drugs or attempting to limit toxicity with marrow colony stimulating factors (CSF). Fischl *et al.* (1990) have presented data suggesting that low dose zidovudine is at least as effective and less toxic than conventional high dose zidovudine in those with advanced HIV disease.

The use of erythropoietin to ameliorate HIV/zidovudine-associated anaemia has been discussed above, response to which appears to be dependent upon the initial endogenous EPO level. Granulocyte-macrophage colony stimulating factor (GM-CSF) and other growth factors may improve peripheral white counts (particularly neutrophil numbers), but may not necessarily improve immune function. Some in vitro work has shown that M-CSF, GM-CSF and IL3, but not G-CSF may actually increase viral production from within HIV-infected macrophages (Koyanangi et al. 1988). Obviously it is of paramount importance to ascertain whether this phenomenon also occurs in vivo. Other studies have suggested that zidovudine inhibits viral infection of macrophages and in combination with GM-CSF gave a corresponding increase in viral suppression. The suggestion is that GM-CSF augments macrophage uptake and activity of zidovudine (Perno et al. 1989). In clinical studies, GM-CSF overcomes the haematological toxic effects of zidovudine, and in zidovudine-intolerant patients allowed re-introduction of zidovudine in the face of documented increased bone marrow cellularity (Groopman 1990).

There is no doubt that CSFs improve the tolerance of drugs necessary for AIDS management. It is unclear whether they will increase the duration of antiretroviral therapy and hence survival. CSFs will not reconstitute the immune system; indeed some patients have developed opportunistic infections during CSF therapy (Groopman 1990). Almost certainly the main role of cytokines will be as adjunctive agents to facilitate other treatment modalities.

The combination of subcutaneous, self-administered EPO and GM-CSF improved the neutropenia and anaemia associated with AIDS in a recent study (Miles et al. 1991), and allowed reinstitution of zidovudine in most zidovudine-intolerant individuals with no increase in HIV expression. Recombinant GM-CSF has been used during chemotherapy for HIV associated NHL and resulted in a reduction in the severity and duration of chemotherapy induced neutropenia, which decreased length of hospital stay (Kaplan et al. 1991) and allowed maximal chemotherapy. The same authors noted an increase in p24 antigen concentration in the treated group compared with controls, but this effect was seemingly short lived. However it does suggest that concurrent antiretroviral therapy should be considered with CSFs.

Lupus Anticoagulant

Lupus anticoagulants are anti-phospholipid antibodies which cause in vitro phenomena and are so named as they were first recognised in patients with SLE (Conley and Hartmann 1952). Circulating IgG or IgM antibodies with antiphospholipid characteristics interfere with phospholipid dependent coagulation tests (i.e. activated partial thromboplastin time (APTT) and prothrombin time (PT). The biologically false positive test for syphilis is also an associated feature. The consequence of this interference results in an abnormally prolonged APTT (less frequently PT) in the absence of bleeding problems. Paradoxically there is an increased incidence of thrombotic events associated with lupus anticoagulant (Bowie et al. 1963). The mechanism of the thrombotic tendency has not been demonstrated and is probably multifactorial, but may be due to a reduction in vascular endothelial prostacylin synthesis (Lindsey et al. 1992), or endothelial cell damage (Holt et al. 1989), possibly mediated immunologically, which may increase local tissue factor procoagulant activity or impair fibrinolysis (Angeles-Cano et al. 1979).

In a study by Bloom et al. (1986) 63% of AIDS patients had an identifiable lupus anticoagulant, there were no cases of bleeding and only one of thrombosis. In a longitudinal study of 50 homosexual males with AIDS, lupus anticoagulant appeared in 10 (20%) during a period of 2 years. These tended to be coincident with acute infection and the lupus anticoagulant effect diminished following treatment (Cohen et al. 1986). In another report 26 in a group of 52 AIDS patients were positive for lupus anticoagulant; almost all were associated with the onset of *Pneumocystis carinii* and resolved following successful treatment of the infection (Gold et al. 1986).

Anticardiolipin antibodies are also antiphospholipid antibodies and are associated with a thrombotic tendency and the so called "antiphospholipid syndrome" (Stricker 1991). Anticardiolipin antibodies have been identified in HIV-negative homosexual men, in addition to those who were HIV positive, suggesting that the presence of anticardiolipin antibodies may be induced by factors other than HIV in people at risk for HIV infection.

Thrombotic thrombocytopenic purpura (TTP) has been reported in association with HIV infection (reviewed by Stricker 1991). TTP is characterised by microangiopathic haemolysis, thrombocytopenia, renal impairment, neurological signs and fever. Anti-endothelial antibodies have been implicated in the pathogenesis of this disorder.

Protein S Deficiency

Protein S deficiency is well recognised as a prothrombotic state (Dolan et al. 1989). Lafeuillade et al. (1991) reported two cases of thrombosis associated with protein S deficiency and followed this up by a prospective study revealing 31% of 71 HIV-positive patients with protein S levels below the normal range. The underlying cause may be abnormal endothelial cell function in HIV infection.

HIV-related Immune Thrombocytopenia

The immune thrombocytopenia (ITP) seen in relation to HIV infection is indistinguishable from classical ITP (Morris et al. 1982); i.e. with reduced peripheral platelet numbers, plentiful marrow megakaryocytes and a reduced platelet lifespan. However HIV associated ITP is associated with a higher level of platelet associated IgG (Karpatkin 1990) and circulating immune complexes (Walsh et al. 1985) than usually seen in non-HIV-infected patients with ITP. However unlike the situation in classical ITP, platelet counts are not inversely related to platelet-bound IgG in HIV-positive patients (Karpatkin 1988).

Almost all (87%–93%) patients in high risk groups presenting with ITP are seropositive for HIV antibody (Hymes et al. 1981). At the time of presentation with ITP patients may already have symptomatic AIDS, may be asymptomatic and progress to frank AIDS within months, or may be asymptomatic and not progress to AIDS, in some cases, for up to 5 years (Karpatkin 1990).

The AIDS-free survival of HIV-seropositive individuals presenting with ITP is no different from HIV-seropositive individuals not developing ITP. Therefore thrombocytopenia should not be considered to be a stage in the progression of asymptomatic HIV infection to AIDS (Karpatkin 1990). Recent follow-up data on a cohort of HIV-positive intravenous drug users from Edinburgh suggest that 12% have severe thrombocytopenia (platelet count $<50 \times 10^9/l$) during the asymptomatic phase of their infection (Cameron and Flegg 1991). The same authors have shown that there is no statistical significance in the time to progression to symptomatic HIV disease between those with severe thrombocytopenia (platelet count $<50 \times 10^9/l$) and those with mild thrombocytopenia (platelet count $>50 \times 10^9/l$).

Importantly, HIV-related ITP must be included in the differential diagnosis of unexplained thrombocytopenia.

ITP rarely results in clinical bleeding in homosexuals and drug abusers. However, in haemophiliacs who are already at risk of bleeding as a consequence of their factor deficiency, thrombocytopenia compounds this tendency. In a series published by Ragni et al. (1990), 82% of haemophiliacs with HIV-related ITP had serious bleeding episodes, including 4 cases of intracranial haemorrhage (fatal in three).

Pathogenesis

There are two major mechanisms of thrombocytopenia in HIV infection:

1. Reticuloendothelial system destruction secondary to platelet bound IgG and circulating immune complexes
2. Ineffective thrombopoiesis, identified by a rapid rise in peripheral platelet numbers following commencement of zidovudine, suggesting that HIV inhibits megakaryocyte function (Ballem et al. 1988; Hirschel et al. 1988; Hymes et al. 1988).

Circulating immune complexes are higher in homosexuals and drug abusers than in haemophiliacs; this is felt to be due to increased immune system stimulation in association with other infections and in the case of intravenous drug abusers, with the associated contaminants injected (Karpatkin and Nardi 1988; Karpatkin 1990).

Management

As in the management of non-HIV related ITP, there are three main therapeutic approaches: (i) corticosteroids; (ii) splenectomy; (iii) intravenous immunoglobulins.

The use of corticosteroids in patients already immunocompromised by HIV infection may theoretically be of concern. Corticosteroids have been shown to improve platelet counts (Rosenfelt et al. 1984; Walsh et al. 1985; Karpatkin 1988; Ratner 1989); however, the response is often of limited duration.

A prompt response in the peripheral count following the administration of intravenous immunoglobulin is thought to be due to reticuloendothelial blockade, with increased platelet survival. The response is often rapid, but again is of short duration (Beard and Savidge 1988; Pollak et al. 1988). However this is sufficient to allow an elevation in the platelet count prior to splenectomy (or any other surgical procedure).

Not all those patients with HIV-related ITP require treatment intervention, and some will achieve spontaneous remission (Abrams et al. 1986).

HIV-related Lymphoma

Non-Hodgkin's Lymphoma

It is well recognised that there is an increased incidence of non-Hodgkin's lymphoma (NHL) in individuals with either inherited or acquired abnormalities of cellular immune function compared with the general population. These were identified originally in patients with primary immunodeficiency, e.g. ataxia telangiectasia or Wiscott–Aldrich syndromes (Frizzera et al. 1980) and in acquired cases post allogeneic transplant procedures (Penn 1975, 1983) secondary to iatrogenic immunosuppression. Thus it came as no great surprise that due to their immunosuppression HIV-infected individuals had a similarly increased incidence of NHL and are at risk from developing high grade B-cell malignancies (Levine et al. 1984). The development of high grade NHL in HIV-positive patients was first recognised as being associated with AIDS in 1985 (Centers for Disease Control 1985).

An outbreak of NHL in homosexual men was observed in 1982 soon after AIDS was first described (Doll and List 1982; Zeigler 1982). Interestingly there was a high incidence of Burkitt's lymphoma in these patients. Biggar et al. (1987) reported an increase in the incidence of NHL in males aged 20–49 years in San Francisco.

Beral et al. (1991) have published an epidemiological study of cases reported to the Centers of Disease Control, Atlanta, USA, up to June 1989 which included 97,258 AIDS patients of whom 2824 (2.9%) developed NHL. The majority of these cases were high grade, large cell immunoblastic type. Twenty percent were primary central nervous system (CNS) NHL and a surprisingly high 20% were

Burkitt's lymphoma. The Burkitt's cases were "true" with c-myc oncogene chromosomal translocations. The numbers of Burkitt's lymphoma cases is unusually high compared with those seen in Epstein–Barr virus (EBV) associated NHL in other immunosuppressed patient groups. From the same epidemiological study the authors identified that NHL was 360 times more common in AIDS sufferers under 20 years of age compared with the general population and in AIDS patients 60 years or older it was 20 times more common. Overall the incidence was 60 times higher than in the general population. This figure is similar to that seen in immunosuppressed transplant recipients. A higher incidence of NHL was seen in the homosexual and haemophiliac groups of AIDS patients compared with drug abusers. This may be partly explained by the increased likelihood of zidovudine therapy in the former groups, prolonging survival sufficiently long for NHL to develop (Pluda et al. 1990), in contrast to the drug abusers group.

In addition, Biggar et al. (1987) have reported an incidence of 2.5% NHL in primary AIDS cases. The majority of these tumours are aggressive B cell malignancies, often widespread and at unusual sites at presentation (Hanto et al. 1981; Penn 1983). Other authors have seen a higher incidence of large cell lymphoma (LCL) and immunoblastic lymphoma (IL) with few Burkitt's type (a distribution more similar to the NHL subtypes seen in immunoincompetent non-AIDS patients (Roithmann et al. 1991). The development of LCL or IL often appears relatively late in the course of HIV disease and may therefore have been underestimated in the Atlanta study (Beral et al. 1991).

Ragni et al. (1993) report an incidence of NHL of 5.5% in HIV positive haemophiliac patients with symptomatic AIDS, 29 times the incidence in the general population: 71% were high grade, and 21% intermediate grade NHL.

Lymphoma in AIDS patients is becoming an increasing cause of death largely due to the reduction in mortality from pneumocystis pneumonia and the decline in the incidence of Kaposi's sarcoma (Peters et al. 1991; Tirelli et al. 1994). Increased survival of AIDS patients due to reduced intercurrent infection-related deaths and zidovudine therapy prolongs the duration of immunosuppression with an increased emergence of malignancies.

Most adults have been infected by Epstein–Barr virus (EBV) which remains latent in B lymphocytes in the nasopharynx. Epstein–Barr virus has been implicated in the pathogenesis of lymphoma in immunocompromised individuals (Harrington et al. 1988), presumably due to an emerging imbalance between viral replication and host immunity. EBV-DNA genome has been identified within the tumour tissue in some patients, and reactivation of EBV infection often occurs in transplant patients receiving immunosuppressive therapy (Crawford et al. 1980; Purtilo et al. 1981). Interestingly the tumours are often polyclonal in nature (malignant transformation is usually monoclonal in nature) but despite this they are clinically aggressive (high grade) tumours frequently causing death of the individual (Hanto et al. 1981).

The aetiology of NHL in HIV-infected patients is less well defined. Unlike other immunosuppressed groups, up until the late 1980s, EBV genomic sequences had only been identified in the minority of peripheral systemic lymphomas (Subar et al. 1988; Kaplan et al. 1989a,b,c), but the incidence of EBV-derived tissue was much higher in primary CNS lymphomas (Kaplan et al. 1989c). Data more recently published (Shibata et al. 1991) have revealed the presence of EBV-derived DNA, by polymerase chain reaction (PCR) and in situ DNA hybridisation techniques in 37% of benign lymph node biopsies in 35 HIV-infected men. This finding had a significant association with concurrent or subsequent EBV-positive NHL, suggesting that the presence of EBV infected cells precedes or is associated with the development of NHL in HIV-infected patients. The exact pathogenesis of EBV-positive lymphomas in uncertain, but may relate to immune deficiency allowing the development of genetic aberrations, e.g. the chromosomal translocation t(8;14) or activation of the c-myc oncogene giving rise to malignant proliferation. Thus far HIV has not been identified in any tumour derived tissue (Subar et al. 1988).

In the majority (50%–70%) of AIDS related systemic lymphoma tissue biopsy specimens EBV-genomic material can be identified (Subar et al. 1988). However MacMahon et al. (1991) have demonstrated a consistent 100% association of EBV protein in tissue from AIDS-related CNS lymphoma specimens. All tumours were high grade LCL. This contrasts with the absence of EBV from most cases of CNS lymphoma in non-immunosuppressed individuals. The difference in the rate of EBV protein identification between systemic and CNS lymphomas may suggest that the pathogenesis of primary CNS lymphomas may be different from other AIDS-related lymphomas.

Several groups (Pluda et al. 1990; 1993; Kaplan et al. 1989a; Levine et al. 1991a) have identified that the development of lymphoma and poor outlook is highly correlated with low numbers of CD4 positive cells (those with CNS lymphomas having the lowest peripheral blood CD4 count), Karnofsky score <70% and marrow involvement by lymphoma. In a prospective study of patients treated with zidovudine (Moore et al. 1991b), the incidence of NHL was 3.2% by 24 months of therapy (1.6 per 100 person years). The same authors noted an increased risk of developing NHL in those patients with a prior history of Kaposi's sarcoma, *Herpes simplex* virus infection or a low mean neutrophil count ($2.1 \times 10^9/l$).

Clinical Features

Most patients have advanced NHL disease at presentation which is associated with a poor prognosis. Extranodal disease is seen in the majority (55%–90%; Zeigler et al. 1984; Knowles et al. 1988; Raphael et al. 1991; Kaplan et al. 1989a; Levine 1991a). The main sites are bone marrow and liver. Primary CNS NHL is common (18%–20%) and frequently seen in those with more severe underlying HIV disease (Levine 1991a; Beral et al. 1991).

Boyle and colleagues (Boyle et al. 1990) reported two distinct types of AIDS-associated NHL which can be distinguished by histology, CD4 count and site of disease. Poor survival (median 96 days) is associated with large cell immunoblastic NHL (LCI), severe immunodeficiency (CD4 $<0.2 \times 10^9/l$) and widespread extranodal disease, compared with better survival (median 130 days) in those with small non-cleaved cell NHL (SNCC), CD4 $>0.2 \times 10^9/l$ and predominantly nodal disease. Poor survival also correlates with poor performance status, prior AIDS and marrow involvement (stage IV) disease (Levine 1991a). These features are also associated with early death from AIDS. Levine et al. (1991) have shown a statistically significant better survival with two risk factors compared with three, 11.3 months and 4 months respectively ($P = 0.0002$). The same group have also identified features with no predictive significance of survival, including leptomeningeal disease, pathological type, disease stage, mass size, LDH elevation, "B" symptoms and gastrointestinal involvement. As there is a high incidence of CNS involvement by NHL, Kaplan et al. (1989a) recommend a lumbar puncture as routine in staging investigations at presentation.

The clinical and radiographic presentation of CNS lymphoma is almost indistinguishable from CNS toxoplasmosis. Headaches are a common presenting symptom as are confusion, lethargy, poor memory etc. CT scanning reveals single or multiple contrast-enhancing lesions.

Lymphoma may present in many ways in HIV-infected individuals and a high index of suspicion must be maintained. NHL should be suspected in patients with rapidly enlarging or progressive lymphadenopathy or an enlarging mass at any site, unexplained gastrointestinal symptoms or bleeding, or with CNS signs and symptoms.

Radiographic imaging to assess extent of disease and tissue diagnosis is imperative.

Management

In non-HIV infected individuals intermediate or high grade NHLs are usually treated with combination chemotherapy. In HIV infected patients with a poorer prognosis disease there are added problems both with respect to worsening immunodeficiency following chemotherapy with the attendant increased risk of opportunistic infections, and compromised bone marrow with poor reserve to recover function following myelotoxic agents. Morbidity and mortality following chemotherapy can therefore be expected to be high. Less aggressive chemotherapeutic regimes may theoretically result in inadequate treatment of the malignant process (Goldie and Coldman 1979).

Since the recognition of HIV-related NHL, treatment strategies have altered. Management with combination chemotherapy was seen to be effective, but unfortunately 50% of complete responders relapsed (Ziegler et al. 1984). Factors predicting survival post-chemotherapy include; CD4 count ($>0.1 \times 10^9$/l) (the most important predictor), asymptomatic HIV infection, Karnofsky performance score >70% and absent extranodal disease (Kaplan et al. 1989a).

Kaplan et al. (1989a) present details of San Francisco patients with HIV-related lymphoma, the majority of whom had high grade stage III/IV disease treated with several standard chemotherapy regimes (CHOP, M-BACOD, PROMACE/MOPP, CVP) and a novel regime, COMET-A. This regime comprised aggressive combination chemotherapy including 1.4 g/m^2 cyclophosphamide, vincristine, methotrexate with folinic acid rescue, etoposide and cytarabine administered over 2-week period, then repeated. Overall response to all regimes was 54% complete response, although 58% were complete responders after COMET-A. Median survival for the group receiving standard chemotherapy was 11.3 months whilst those treated with COMET-A it was 5.3 months (P = 0.03). The authors felt that aggressive chemotherapy had increased the immunosuppressive state of these patients making them more susceptible to opportunistic infection, thereby reducing longer term survival.

Levine and colleagues (Levine et al. 1991a) report a group of 60 HIV-related lymphoma patients all treated with curative intent with BACOP type regimes (bleomycin, adriamycin, cyclophosphamide, vincristine and prednisolone) in which 41% achieved a complete response and 12% partial response. The median survival was 6 months. Of 40 deaths, 21 were due to an AIDS-related problem and 19 were NHL related. In their conclusions these authors point out that any patient attaining complete remission whether good or poor risk with respect to NHL is still at risk from death from AIDS whilst the lymphoma is in remission. They suggest that prolongation of survival in those with AIDS-related lymphoma has to be based upon effective chemotherapy for NHL and control of the underlying HIV infection.

In another study, Levine and colleagues (1991b) report results of the use of low-dose chemotherapy (M-BACOD) with central nervous system prophylaxis and continuing zidovudine therapy, the rationale being improved efficacy with decreased risk of intercurrent infection. There was a response in 51% patients with NHL, and in 46% a complete response. Opportunistic infections were seen in 21%. Median survival was 6.5 months; however, in the complete responders it was 15 months. This successfully demonstrated that combination of low-dose therapeutic regimes and continuing antiretroviral therapy can be associated with useful prolongation of survival.

Gisselbrecht et al. (1993) have published results of intensive combination chemotherapy in 141 HIV-positive patients with NHL, 93 high grade, 48 intermediate grade. Therapy consisted of three consecutive courses of ACVB (doxorubicin, cyclophosphamide, vindesine, bleomycin and prednisolone) followed by consolidation with high-dose methotrexate with folinic acid rescue, ifosfamide, etoposide, asparaginase and cytarabine (LNH 84). Intrathecal methotrexate was given as central nervous system prophylaxis. Zidovudine therapy was started after the chemotherapy was completed. Complete remission was achieved in 63% of patients, partial remission in 13.5% but 9% failed to respond. Fourteen percent died during ACVB, almost half of these dying from progressive disease. With a median follow up of 28 months, median survival was 9.3 months overall. Median disease-free survival is 16.7 months for those attaining complete remission, with a 42% probability of survival at 2 years. Twenty-three patients died of opportunistic infections whilst in complete remission. Patients with no response had a median survival of 5 months. The authors conclude that in a selected group intensive chemotherapy can achieve a high complete remission rate. Long-term remission can be attained in patients without adverse risks, but short survival is due to HIV-related infections.

Prognosis for HIV positive patients with primary CNS lymphoma is bleak. Following CNS radiotherapy, survival has been reported variously as less than 2 months (Gill et al. 1985), 2.7 months (So et al. 1986) and 5.5 months (Formenti et al. 1989).

Pneumocystis carinii pneumonia is the most frequently encountered opportunistic infection following chemotherapy of HIV associated NHL (Kaplan et al. 1989a), thus prophylaxis should be given during and following chemotherapy.

The treatment of HIV-related NHL must be based upon the characteristics of the lymphoma itself and upon the degree of immunosuppression of the patient. It is clear that combination chemotherapy of intermediate and high intensity does achieve a response in a majority of patients. Despite some encouraging signs of improvement in the outlook for HIV-associated lymphoma, HIV symptoms are relentless, therefore antiretroviral therapy needs to be a component of management. The combination of intensive chemotherapy with zidovudine may lead to unacceptable myelotoxicity with reduced survival due to intercurrent opportunistic infection or from thrombocytopenic bleeding. A balance between potential improved survival against increased immunosuppression has to be reached. Newer antiretroviral agents may be less myelotoxic than zidovudine when used in combination with chemotherapy.

Hodgkin's Disease

Previous studies of lymphoma developing in immunosuppressed groups have not shown any increase in the incidence of Hodgkin's disease (HD) compared with the general population (Hanto et al. 1981; Penn 1983). Unlike the incidence of NHL, there has not been any change in the incidence of HD in young males between the ages of 20 and 49 years in San Francisco since 1979 (Kaplan et al. 1987).

Despite the lack of causal association between HIV infection and HD, HIV infected patients tend to present with aggressive nodular sclerosing or mixed cellularity stage III or IV with very poor survival (Kaplan et al. 1987; Knowles et al. 1988; Italian Co-operative 1988). Interestingly Brousset et al. (1991) have identified the presence of EBV and mRNA by in situ hybridisation techniques in the pathognomonic Reed–Sternberg cells of Hodgkin's disease. This series included one patient who was HIV antibody positive. This represents the first demonstration of EBV in Hodgkin's disease diagnostic cells. The findings support the role of EBV in the aetiology of HD. If EBV plays a part in the pathogenesis of HD it is surprising that a greater incidence of HD has not been recognised in immunocompromised individuals (HIV-infected or otherwise).

Increasing numbers of patients with HIV-associated HD are being recognised (Tirelli et al. 1994), with a high frequency of lymphocyte depleted and mixed cellularity subtypes. It still remains unclear whether HD should be included as an AIDS defining tumour in HIV-infected people.

In the same way as with NHL, due to the presentation of HD late in the time course of HIV disease, individuals usually have a CD4 count circa $200 \times 10^6/l$ and therefore require antiretroviral treatment in addition to specific HD-directed chemotherapy.

Ames et al. (1991) present a series of HIV-related HD from New York in which the survival was 30% at 1 year, which compares with 80% at 9 years and >60% at 10 years in non-HIV associated HD. However death was often related to opportunistic infection. Interestingly of the cases discussed only 10% had a diagnosis of AIDS prior to diagnosis of aggressive HD. These patients were subsequently found to be HIV-positive and many had a rapid demise.

As with management of NHL the capacity to tolerate chemotherapy is reduced due to prior compromised bone marrow function and the risk of opportunistic infection. There may be a role in the future for combined intensive chemotherapy, antiretroviral therapy and growth factors to reduce to a minimum problems of myelotoxicity.

Conclusions

HIV infection and AIDS have many haematological manifestations, either as a presenting feature of the disease, or as a consequence of disease progression and its treatment. In watchful, anticipation of haematological complications arising, treatment of HIV associated problems and haematological disorders may be managed optimally.

It is anticipated that cytokines and growth factors will play a more important role in the management of HIV complications in the future, although much more work is still required both in clinical and laboratory settings before specific roles and agents are identified.

It should always be remembered that haematological disorders and lymphomas presenting in unusual circumstances may be a manifestation of HIV infection.

Acknowledgement. Many thanks to Mike Watts, Department of Haematology, University College Hospital, London, for providing the photomicrographs of and bone marrow sections, which are reproduced with his permission.

References

Abrams DI, Kiprov DD, Goedert JJ, Sarngadharan MG, Gallo RL, Volberding PA (1986). Antibodies to human T lymphotropic virus type III and development of the acquired immunodeficiency syndrome in homosexual men presenting with immune thrombocytopenia. Ann Int Med 104: 47–50

Ames ED, Conjalka MS, Goldberg AF, Hirschman R, Jain S, Distenfeld A, Metroka CE (1991) Hodgkin's Disease and AIDS. Hem/Onc Clinics North Am 5: 343–356

Anderson R, Boedecker M, Ma M, Goldstein EJC (1987). Adverse reactions with pentamidine isethionate in AIDS patients: Recommendations for monitoring therapy. Drug Intelligence and Clinical Pharmacology, 20: 862–866

Angeles-Cano E, Sultan Y, Clauvel JP (1979). Predisposing factors to thrombosis in systemic lupus erythematosus: possible relation to endothelial cell damage. J Lab Clin Med 94: 312–323

Ballem P, Belzberg A, Devine D, Buskard N (1988). Pathophysiology of HIV-ITP and the mechanism of the response to AZT. Blood 72 (Suppl 1): 261A

Ballem PJ, Belzberg A, Devine D, Lyster D, Sprusten B, Chambers H, Donbrott P, Mikulash K (1992). Kinetic studies of the mechanism of thrombocytopenia in patients with human immunodeficiency virus infection. New Engl J Med 327: 1779–1784

Beard J, Savidge GF (1988). High-dose intravenous immunglobulin and splenectomy for the treatment of HIV-related immune thrombocytopenia in patients with severe haemophilia. Br J Haematolo 68: 303–306

Beral V, Peterman T, Berkelman R, Jaffe H (1991). AIDS-associated non-Hodgkin lymphoma. Lancet 337: 805–809

Biggar RL, Horm J, Goedert JJ, Melbye M (1987). Cancer in the group at risk of acquired immunodeficiency syndrome (AIDS) through 1984. Am J Epidemiol 126: 578–586

Bloom EJ, Abrams DI, Rodgers G (1986). Lupus anticoagulant in the acquired immunodeficiency syndrome. JAMA 256: 491–493

Boyle MJ, Swanson CE, Turner JJ et al. (1990). Definition of two distinct types of AIDS-associated non-Hodgkin lymphoma. Br J Haematol 76: 506–512

Bowie WEJ, Thompson JH, Pascuzzi CA, Owen GA (1963). Thrombosis in systemic lupus erythematosus despite circulating anticoagulant. J Clin Invest 62: 416–430

Brousset P, Chittal S, Schlaifer D et al. (1991). Detection of Epstein-Barr virus messenger RNA in Reed-Sternberg cells of Hodgkin's Disease by in situ hybridization with biotinylated probes on specially processed modified acetone methyl benzoate xylene (ModAMeX) sections. Blood 77: 1781–1786

Busch MP, Arnad Z, Sheppard HW, Ascher MS, Lang W (1991). Primary HIV-1 infection. New Engl J Med 325: 733

Cameron DA, Flegg PJ (1991). The prognostic importance of thrombocytopenia. (Letter). AIDS 5: 1266–1267

Castella A, Croxson TS, Mildvan D, Witt DH, Zalusky R (1985). The bone marrow in AIDS: a histologic, hematologic and microbiologic study. Am J Clin Pathol 84: 425–432

Centers for Disease Control (1985). Revision of the case definition of AIDS for national reporting: United States. Ann Intern Med 103: 402–403

Clark SJ, Saag MS, Decker WD et al. (1991). High titres of cytopathic virus in plasma of patients with symptomatic primary HIV-1 infection. New Engl J Med 324: 954–960

Cohen AJ, Philips TM, Kessler CM (1986). Circulating coagulation inhibitors in the acquired immunodeficiency syndrome. Ann Intern Med 104: 175–180

Conley CL, Hartmann RC (1952). A hemorrhagic disorder caused by circulating anticoagulant in patients with disseminated lupus erythematosus. J Clin Invest 31: 621–622

Cortes E, Koeffler HP, Gaynor R et al. (1986). Infectivity and genetic regulation of human immunodeficiency virus (HIV) in myeloid cell lines. Blood 68: 123

Crawford DH, Thomas JA, Janossy G et al. (1980) Epstein-Barr virus nuclear antigen positive lymphoma after cyclosporine A treatment in patients with renal allograft. Lancet i: 1355–1356

Daar ES, Mondgil T, Meyer RD, Ho DD (1991). Transient high levels of viraemia in patients with primary human immunodeficiency virus type 1 infection. New Engl J Med 324: 961–964

Dalgleish AG, Beverley PCL, Clapham PR, Crawford DH, Greaves MF, Weiss RA (1984). The CD4(T4) antigen is an essential component of the receptor for the AIDS retrovirus. Nature 312: 763–767

de Wolf F, Goudsmit R, Lange J et al. (1988). Effect of zidovudine on serum human immunodeficiency virus antigen levels in symptom-free subjects. Lancet i: 373–376

Dolan G, Ball J, Preston FE (1989). Protein C and protein S. Baillière's Clin Haematol 2: 999–1042

Doll DC, List AF (1982). Burkitt's lymphoma in a homosexual. Lancet i: 1026–27

Dorsett B, Cronin W, Chuma W, Iaochim HL (1985). Anti-lymphocyte antibodies in patients with the acquired immune deficiency syndrome. Am Med 78: 621–626

Erythropoietin (EPO) Study Group, Rudnick SA (1989). Human recombinant erythropoietin (r-HuEPO): a double-blind, placebo-controlled study in acquired immunodeficiency syndrome (AIDS) patients with anaemia induced by disease and AZT [abstract no. 7]. Proc Am Soc Clin Oncol 8: 2

Fischl MA, Parker CB, Pettinelli C et al. (1990). A randomised trial of a reduced daily dose of zidovudine in patients with the acquired immunodeficiency syndrome. New Engl J Med 323: 1009–1014

Formenti S, Gill P, Lean E et al. (1989). Primary central nervous system lymphoma in AIDS. Cancer 63: 1101–1107

Frizzera G, Rosai J, Dehner LP, Spector BD, Kersey JH (1980). Lymphoreticular disorders in primary immunodeficiencies: new findings based on an up-to-date histologic classification of 35 cases. Cancer 46: 692–699

Gartner S, Markovits P, Markovitz DM, Kaplan MH, Gallo RC, Popovic M (1986). The role of mononuclear phagocytes in HTLV III/LAB infection. Science 233: 215–219

Geller SA, Muller R, Greenberg ML, Seigal FP (1985). Acquired immunodeficiency syndrome: distinctive features of bone marrow biopsies. Arch Path Lab Med 109, 138–141

Gill PS, Levine AM, Meyer PR et al. (1985). Primary central nervous system lymphoma in homosexual men. Am J Med 78: 742–748

Gisselbrecht C, Oksenhendler E, Tirelli U et al. (1993). Human immunodeficiency virus-related lymphoma treated with intensive combination chemotherapy. Am J Med 95: 188–196

Gold JE, Haubenstock A, Zalusky R (1986). Lupus anticoagulant and AIDS. New Engl J Med 314: 1252–1253

Goldie JH, Coldman AJ (1979). A mathematical model for relating the drug sensitivity of tumors to the spontaneous mutation rate. Cancer Treat Rep 63: 1727–1733

Groopman JE (1990). Management of the hematologic complications of Human Immunodeficiency Virus infection. Rev Infect Dis 12: 931–937

Hansen M, Gimsing P, Ingeberg S, Jans H, Nex E (1992). Cobalamin binding proteins in patients with HIV infection. Eur J Haematol 48: 228–231

Hanto DW, Frizzera G, Purtilo DT et al. (1981) Clinical spectrum of lymphoproliferative disorders in renal transplant recipients and evidence for the role of Epstein-Barr virus. Cancer Res 41: 4253–4261

Harrington DS, Weisenberger DD, Purtilo DT (1988). Epstein-Barr virus-associated lymphoproliferative lesions. Clin Lab Med 8: 97–118

Hirschel T, For the Swiss Group for clinical studies on Acquired Immunodeficiency Syndrome (AIDS) (1988) Zidovudine for the treatment of thrombocytopenia associated with Human Immunodeficiency Virus (HIV). Ann Int Med 109: 718–721

Ho DD, Rota TR, Hirsch MS (1986) Infection of monocyte/macrophages by human T-lymphotropic virus type III. J Clin Invest 77: 1712–1715

Holland HK, Spivak JL (1990). Haematological manifestations of AIDS. Baillière's Clin Haematol 3: 103–114

Holt CM, Lindsey N, Moult J et al. (1989). Antibody dependent cellular cytotoxicty of vascular endothelium; characterisation and pathogenic associations in systemic sclerosis. Clin Exp Immunol 78: 359–365

Hymes KB, Cheung T, Greene JB et al. (1981). Kaposi's sarcoma in homosexual men: a report of 8 cases. Lancet ii: 598–600

Hymes KB, Greene JB, Karpatkin S (1988). The effect of azidothymidine on HIV-related thrombocytopenia. New Engl J Med 318: 516–517

Italian Cooperative Group for AIDS-related tumours (1988). Malignant lymphomas in patients with or at risk for AIDS in Italy. J Nat Cancer Inst 80: 855–860

Jaffe IA (1986). Adverse effects of sulfhydryl compounds in man. Am J Med 80: 471–476

Kaplan LD, Abrams DA, Volberding PA (1987). Clinical course and epidemiology of Hodgkin's disease in homosexual men in San Francisco. Third International Conference on AIDS. P9

Kaplan LD, Abrams DI, Feigal E et al. (1989a). AIDS-associated Non-Hodgkin's Lymphoma in San Francisco. JAMA 261: 719–724

Kaplan LD, Meeker T, Feigal E et al. (1989b). Clonality of AIDS-associated non-Hodgkin's lymphoma predicts survival. Am Fed Clin Res Annual Meeting (Abstract)

Kaplan LD, Khan JO, Crowe S et al. (1991). Clinical and virologic effects of recombinant human granulocyte-macrophage colony-stimulating factor in patients receiving chemotherapy for human immunodeficiency virus-associated Non-Hodgkin's lymphomas: results of a randomised trial. J Clin Oncol 9: 929–940

Karcher DS, Frost AR (1991). The bone marrow in human immunodeficiency virus (HIV)-related disease. Morphology and clinical correlation. Am J Clin Pathol 95: 63–71

Karpatkin S (1988). Immunologic thrombocytopenic purpura in HIV-seropositive homosexuals, narcotic addicts and hemophiliacs. Semin Hematol 25: 219–229

Karpatkin S (1990) HIV-1-related thrombocytopenia. Baillière's Clin Haematol 3: 115–138

Karpatkin S, Nardi M (1988). On the mechanism of thrombocytopenia in haemophiliacs multiply transfused with AHF concentrates. J Lab Clin Med 111, 441–448

Klatzmann D, Champagne E, Chamaret S et al. (1984). T-lymphocyte T4 molecule behaves as the receptor for human retrovirus LAV. Nature 312: 767–768

Kloster BE, Tomar RH, Spira TJ (1984). Brief communication: lymphocytotoxic antibodies in the acquired immune deficiency syndrome (AIDS). Clin Immunol Immunopathol 30: 330–335

Knowles DM, Chamulak GA, Subar M et al. (1988). Lymphoid neoplasia of the acquired immunodeficiency syndrome (AIDS). The New York University Medical Center experience with 105 patients (1981–1986). Ann Intern Med 108: 744–753

Koyanagi Y, O'Brien WA, Zhao JQ, Golde DW, Gasson JC, Chen ISY (1988). Cytokines alter production of HIV-1 from primary mononuclear phagocytes. Science 241: 1673–1675

Lafeuillade A, Alessi M-C, Poizot-Martin I et al. (1991). Protein S deficiency and HIV infection. New Engl J Med 324: 1220

Landonio G, Nosari A, Spinelli F (1993). HIV-related thrombocytopenia. New Engl J Med 328: 1785

Larder BA, Darby G, Richman DD (1989). HIV with reduced sensitivity to zidovudine (AZT) isolated during prolonged therapy. Science 243: 1731–1734

Leiderman Z, Greenberg ML, Adelsberg BR, Siegel FP (1987). A glycoprotein inhibitor of in vitro granulopoiesis associated with AIDS. Blood 70: 1267–1272

Levine AM, Meyer PR, Begandy MK et al. (1984). Development of B-cell lymphoma in homosexual men. Ann Intern Med 100: 7–13

Levine A, Sullivan-Halley J, Pike MC et al. (1991a). Human immunodeficiency virus-related lymphoma, prognostic factors predictive of survival. Cancer, 68: 2466–2472

Levine AM, Wernz JC, Kaplan L et al. (1991b). Low-dose chemotherapy with central nervous system prophylaxis and zidovudine maintenance in AIDS-related lymphoma. JAMA 3266: 84–88

Levy JA, Mackwicz CE, Walker CM (1991). Primary HIV-1 infection. New Engl J Med 325: 734

Lewis CM, Pegrum GD (1978). Immune complexes in myelofibrosis. A possible guide to management. Br J Haematol 39: 233–239

Lifson JD, Reyes GR, McGrath MS, Stein BS, Engleman EG (1986). AIDS retrovirus induced cytopathology: giant cell formation and involvement of CD4 antigen. Science 232: 1123–1127

Lindsey N, Henderson F, Malia R, Greaves M, Hughes P (1992). Serum masks the inhibition of thrombin-induced prostacyclin release produced by anti-cardiolipin antibodies. Br J Rhematol 31: 179–183

Little BJ, Spivak JL, Quinn TC, Mann RB (1986) Case report: Kaposi's sarcoma with bone marrow involvement: occurrence in a patient with the acquired immunodeficiency syndrome. Am J Med Sci 292: 44–46

Louache F. Bettaiels A, Henri A et al. (1991). Infection of megakaryocytes by human immunodeficiency virus in seropositive patients with ITP. Blood 78: 1697–1705

MacMahon EME, Glass JD, Hayward SD et al. (1991). Epstein-Barr virus in AIDS-related primary central nervous system lymphoma. Lancet 338: 969–973

Maddon PJ, Dalgleish AG, McDougal JS, Clapham PR, Weiss RA, Axel R (1986). The T4 gene encodes the AIDS virus receptor and is expressed in the immune system and the brain. Cell 47: 333–348

McCarthy DM (1985). Fibrosis of the bone marrow. Content and causes. Br J Haematol 59: 1–7

McGinnis MH, Macher AM, Rook AH, Alter HJ (1986). Red cell autoantibodies in patients with acquired immune deficiency syndrome. Transfusion 26: 405–409

Miles SA, Mitsuyasu R, Moreno J et al. (1991). Combined treatment with recombinant granulocyte colony-stimulating factor and erythropoietin decreases haematologic toxicity from zidovudine. Blood 77: 2109–2117

Moore RD, Cregh-Kirk T, Keruly J (1991a). Long-term safety and efficacy of zidovudine in patients with advanced human immunodeficiency virus disease. Arch Intern Med 151: 981–986

Moore RD, Kessler H, Richman DD, Flexner C, Chaisson RE (1991b) Non-Hodgkin's lymphoma in patients with advanced HIV infection treated with zidovudine. JAMA 265: 2208–2211

Morris L, Distenfeld A, Amorosi E, Karpatkin S (1982). Autoimmune thrombocytopenic purpura in homosexual men. Ann Intern Med 96: 714–717

Murphy MF, Metcalfe P, Waters AH (1987). Incidence and mechanism of neutropenia and thrombocytopenia in patients with human immunodeficiency virus infection. Br J Haematol 66: 337–340

Osborne BM, Guarda LA, Butler JJ (1984). Bone marrow biopsies in patients with the acquired immunodeficiency syndrome. Hum Path 15: 1048–1053

Pechere M, Samii K, Hirschel B (1993). HIV-related thrombocytopenia. New Engl. J Med 328: 1785–86

Penn I (1975). The incidence of malignancies in transplant recipients. Transplant Proc 7: 323–326

Penn I (1983). Lymphomas complicating organ transplantation. Transplant 15: 2790–2797

Perno C-F, Yarchoan R, Cooney DA et al. (1989). Replication of human immunodeficiency virus in monocytes. Granulocyte/macrophage colony-stimulating factor (GM-CSF) potentiates viral production yet enhances the antiviral effect mediated by 3′-azido-2′3′ dideoxythymidine (AZT) and other dideoxynucleoside congeners of thymidine. J Exp Med 169: 933–951

Peters BS, Beck EJ, Coleman DG et al. (1991). Changing disease patterns in patients with AIDS in a referral centre in the United Kingdom: the changing face of AIDS. Br Med J 302: 203–207

Pluda JM, Yarchoan R, Jaffe ES et al. (1990). Development of non-Hodgkin's lymphoma in a cohort of patients with severe human immunodeficiency virus (HIV) infection on long-term antiretroviral therapy. Ann Intern Med 113: 276–282

Pluda JM, Venzon DJ, Tosato G, Lietzau J et al. (1993). Parameters affecting the development of non-Hodgkin's lymphoma in patients with severe human immunodeficiency virus infection receiving antiretroviral therapy. J Clin Oncol 11: 1099–1107

Pollak AN, Janinis J, Green D (1988). Successful intravenous immune globulin therapy for human immunodeficiency virus-associated thrombocytopenia. Arch Intern Med 148: 695–697

Purtilo DT, Sakamoto K, Saemundsen AK et al. (1981). Documentation of Epstein-Barr virus infection in immunodeficient patients with life-threatening lymphoproliferative diseases by clinical, virological and immunopathological studies. Cancer Res 41: 4226–4236

Ragni MV, Bontempo FA, Myers DJ, Kiss JE, Oral A (1990). Hemorrhagic sequelae of immune thrombocytopenic purpura in human immunodeficiency virus-infected hemophiliacs. Blood 75: 1267–1272

Ragni MV, Belle SH, Jaffe RA, Duerstein SL et al. (1993). Acquired immunodeficiency syndrome-associated non-Hodgkin's lymphomas and other malignancies in patients with haemophilia. Blood 81: 1889–1897

Rapheal M, Gentilhomme O, Tulliez M, Byron P-A, Diebold J (1991). Histopathologic features of high-grade non-Hodgkin's lymphomas in acquired immunodeficiency syndrome. Arch Pathol Lab Med 115: 15–20

Ratner L (1989). Human immunodeficiency virus-associated autoimmune thrombocytopenic purpura: a review. Am J Med 86: 194–198

Remacha AF, Riera A, Cadafalch J, Gimferrer E (1991). Vitamin B-12 abnormalities in HIV-infected patients. Eur J Haematol 47: 60–64

Richman DD, Fischl MA, Greico MH et al. (1987). The toxicity of azidothymidine (AZT) in the treatment of patients with AIDS and AIDS-related complex. New Engl J Med 317: 192–197

Roithmann S, Tourani J-M, Andrieu J-M. (1991). AIDS-associated non-Hodgkin's lymphoma. Lancet 338: 884–885

Rosenfelt FP, Rosenbloom BE, Weinstein IM (1984). Immune thrombocytopenia in homosexual men. Ann Intern Med 104: 583

Schneider DR, Picker LJ (1985). Myelodysplasia in the acquired immune deficiency syndrome. Am Clin Path 84: 144–152

Shenoy CM, Lin JH (1986). Bone marrow findings in acquired immunodeficiency syndrome (AIDS). Am J Med Sci 292: 372–375

Siegel JP, Djue JT, Masur H, Gelmann EP, Quinman GV (1985). Sera from patients with the acquired immunodeficiency syndrome inhibit production of interleukin-2 by normal lymphocytes. J Clin Invest 74: 1957–1964

Shibata D, Weiss LM, Nathwani BN, Brynes RK, Levine AM (1991). Epstein-Barr virus in benign lymph node biopsies from individuals infected with the human immunodeficiency virus is associated with concurrent or subsequent development of non-Hodgkin's lymphoma. Blood 77: 1527–1533

So YT, Beckstead JH, Davis RL (1986). Primary central nervous lymphoma in acquired immunodeficiency syndrome: a clinical and pathological study. Ann Neurol 20: 566–572

Spivak JL, Seloncik SE, Quinn TC (1983). Acquired immune deficiency syndrome and pancytopenia. JAMA 250: 3084–3087

Spivak JL, Bender BS, Quinn TC (1984). Hematologic abnormalities in the acquired immune deficiency syndrome. Am J Med 77: 224 228

Spivak JL, Barnes DC, Fuchs E, Quinn TC (1989). Serum immunoreactive erythropoietin in HIV-infected patients. JAMA 261: 3104–3107

Stricker RB, Blackwood LL, McHugh TM, Stites DP, Neyma PD (1988). Autoantibody-mediated cytotoxicity directed against a histone-like protein on CD4 and T-cells in the acquired immunodeficiency syndrome. Blood 72: 360

Striker RB (1991). Hemostatic abnormalities in HIV disease. Hemat Oncol Clinics North Am 5: 249–265

Subar M, Neri A, Inghirami G, Knowles DM, Dalla-Favera R (1988). Frequent c-myc oncogene activation and infrequent presence of Epstein-Barr virus genome in AIDS associated lymphoma. Blood 72: 667–671

Tirelli U, Franceschi S, Carbone A (1994). Malignant tumours in patients with HIV infection. Br Med J 308: 1148–1153

Toy PTCY, Reid ME, Burns M (1985). Positive direct antiglobulin test associated with hyperglobulinemia in acquired immunodeficiency syndrome (AIDS). Am J Hematol 19: 145–150

Treacy M, Lai L, Costello C, Clark A (1987). Peripheral blood and bone marrow abnormalities in patients with HIV related disease. Br J Haematol 65: 289–294

Tucker J, Ludlam CA, Craig A et al. (1985). HTLV-III infection associated with glandular fever-like illness in haemophiliacs. Lancet i: 585

Walker RE, Parker RI, Kovacs JA (1988). Anemia and erythropoiesis in patient with the acquired immunodeficiency syndrome (AIDS) and Kaposi's sarcoma treated with zidovudine. Ann Intern Med 108: 372–376

Walsh C, Krigel R, Lennette ET, Karpatkin S (1985). Thrombocytopenia in homosexual patients. Prognosis, response to therapy and prevalence of antibody to the retrovirus associated with the acquired immunodeficiency syndrome. Ann Intern Med 103: 542–545

Ziegler JL, Drew WL, Miner RC et al. (1982). Outbreak of Burkitt's-like NHL in homosexual men. Lancet ii: 631–633

Ziegler JL, Beckstead JA, Volberding PA et al. (1984). Non-Hodgkin's lymphoma in 90 homosexual men – relation to generalised lymphadenopathy and the acquired immunodeficiency syndrome. New Engl J Med 311: 565–570

Zon LI, Arkin C, Groopman JE (1987). Haematologic manifestations of the human immunodeficiency virus (HIV). Br J Haematol 66: 251–256

9 Clinical Manifestations of HIV Infection and AIDS in Injecting Drug Users

Christopher Sonnex

Introduction

In 1988, Welsby predicted that the "second phase" of epidemic HIV infection in developed countries would occur within the injecting drug using population. This has been borne out, with injecting drug users (IDUs) accounting for an increasing proportion of the cases of HIV infection and AIDS in the USA, North America and Europe (MMWR Update 1991; Salmaso et al. 1991; Des Jarlais et al. 1992). Although the clinical spectrum of HIV disease differs little between risk groups, there are a number of specific features relating to the HIV-infected injecting drug user which merit attention. However, before considering these clinical problems in more detail it is important to remember that IDUs are prone to a variety of medical conditions related to both drug abuse and the act of injecting. The subject of the narcotic addict as a medical patient has been well reviewed by Sapira (1968) and, more recently, by Novick (1992).

Symptoms

Pyrexia

There are a variety of conditions which may present as pyrexia in the drug user. Group G streptococcal bacteraemia, frequently secondary to soft tissue infection, has been previously reported in parenteral drug abusers (Craven et al. 1986) and cases in the USA appear to be increasing annually (McMeeking and Holzman 1988). Whether this increased incidence is related solely to HIV infection requires further study.

Disseminated candidiasis, often associated with acute hepatitis, has been reported in heroin addicts (Dupont and Drouhet 1985; Podzamczer and Guidol 1986; Collignon and Sorrell 1987). Although these cases were apparently unrelated to HIV infection some workers have predicted an increase in severe disseminated candidiasis amongst drug users (Collignon and Sorrell 1987). Osteoarticular infection caused by *Candida albicans* has recently been reported in HIV-infected IDUs (Munoz-Fernandez et al. 1993).

The injecting drug user is at increased risk for developing infective endocarditis (Luttgens 1949) and the diagnosis should be considered in all IDUs presenting with pyrexia. Studies comparing HIV-seropositive with seronegative drug users with endocarditis found a higher morbidity and mortality amongst seropositives, possibly related to persistence of infection in spite of seemingly adequate therapy (Slim et al. 1988; Ruggeri et al. 1988). Other important features of the HIV-seropositive groups were polybacteraemia, a greater diversity of unusual pathogens and a high rate of major emboli.

Constitutional Symptoms

Many drug users experience episodes of extreme lethargy or profuse sweating as part of drug use or withdrawal. These drug-related symptoms are often difficult to distinguish from the constitutional symptoms of HIV disease. In such cases an assessment of immunostatus, for example by measuring the CD4 lymphocyte count, may help to determine whether symptoms are likely to be HIV related.

Enlarged Lymph Nodes

Axillary and epitrochlear lymphadenopathy are frequently detected in IDUs, and may be asymmetrical if one arm is used predominantly for injecting. The nodes tend to be smaller than those found in persistent generalised lymphadenopathy and are usually firm and non-tender. In the absence of scalp lesions, enlargement of the posterior cervical lymph glands is unlikely to be secondary to skin and soft tissue infection associated with injecting and should raise the suspicion of HIV infection. Generalised hyperplasia of the entire lymphatic system has been previously reported in drug abusers with the lymph nodes at the hilum of the liver and around the head of the pancreas under the pylorus being particularly affected (Helpern and Rho 1966; Siegel et al. 1966).

Cough and Shortness of Breath

Pulmonary disease is common in both HIV infected and non-infected IDUs. Shortness of breath may be the result of pulmonary complications arising directly from drug injection. These include talc granuloma, vasculitis, interstitial fibrosis, obstructive lung disease, pulmonary oedema and angiomatoid malformation of the pulmonary arteries (Butz 1969; Hahn et al. 1969; Johnston et al. 1969; Zientara and Moore 1970; Hopkins 1972; Siegel 1972; Stern and Subbarao 1983; Glassroth et al. 1987).

Although a diagnosis of pneumocystis carinii pneumonia should always be considered in the HIV infected patient with chest symptoms, bacterial pneumonia is a significant cause of morbidity in the IDU. Reports suggest that bacterial pneumonia may be more severe in the HIV-infected IDU. Clinicians working in New York have reported an increase in the number of non-AIDS pneumonia deaths amongst HIV-seropositive drug users.

A prospective study of 433 IDUs documented a fivefold increased risk of hospitalisation for bacterial pneumonia amongst HIV-seropositives without AIDS compared to seronegative subjects (Selwyn et al. 1988). It was of interest that over two-thirds of the seropositive patients showed no features of advanced HIV-related disease at the time of hospitalisation for pneumonia. *Streptococcus pneumoniae* and *Haemophilus influenzae* were the most frequently isolated organisms, a finding previously reported in patients with AIDS (Polsky et al. 1986). A recent study of IDUs in New York found that bacterial pneumonia and sepsis were important predictors of progression to AIDS and acted as a significant source of HIV-related morbidity and mortality (Selwyn et al. 1992). Although these data suggest that HIV-seropositive IDUs should be offered pneumococcal and Hib vaccination, studies have documented a variable response of HIV infected subjects to both of these vaccines (Ballett et al. 1987; Klein et al. 1989; Steinhoff et al. 1991; Unsworth et al. 1993).

By way of immunosuppression, HIV infection reflects and magnifies diseases which are endemic to a population. Since drug abuse is a risk factor for tuberculosis (Reichman et al. 1979) one may have predicted the high incidence of tuberculosis which has been reported in HIV infected IDUs (O'Donnell and Pappas 1988). In the USA, tuberculosis in HIV infected patients is seen primarily in IDUs and ethnic minorities (Theuer et al. 1990). Active tuberculosis most often results from reactivation of latent infection in patients with HIV, Selwyn et al. (1989) studied a group of IDUs on a methadone maintenance programme and found that 14% of HIV seropositive patients with a history of a positive tuberculin skin test developed tuberculosis over a 2-year period. Reports of increasing numbers of cases of multiple drug resistant tuberculosis amongst HIV-infected IDUs in New York are of particular concern (Shafer et al. 1991; Frieden et al. 1993).

Although pulmonary tuberculosis presents classically with chest symptoms, it is often extrapulmonary and disseminated in patients with HIV infection (Sunderam et al. 1986; Chaisson and Slutkin 1989) and may demonstrate marked hilar and peripheral lymphadenopathy (Aguado and Castrillo 1987). Classical apical infiltrates on chest x-ray are found in only a small minority (Pitchenik and Rubinson 1985; Sunderam et al. 1986).

Oral Symptoms

The oral complications of HIV infection do not differ from those found in non-drug using patients, however they may be compounded in the IDU by poor oral hygiene, a high prevalence of dental caries and periodontal disease (Pallasch and Joseph 1987).

Jaundice

IDUs who share injecting equipment are at high risk of acquiring viral hepatitis. Past or present hepatitis B (HB) infection has been reported in 56% to 87% of IDUs (Weller et al. 1984; Conte et al. 1987; Chamot et al. 1990, 1992; Hart et al. 1991). Although the majority develop HB core and HB surface antibodies and are therefore considered immune, there have been reports of hepatitis B reactivation in patients with HIV infection (Lazizi et al. 1988; Vento et al. 1989). The severity of HB-associated liver disease has been reported to be greater in IDUs than non-IDUs and may be related to associated hepatitis C infection or drug-induced hepatotoxicity (Housset et al. 1992).

HIV-positive IDUs show a higher prevalence of cirrhosis than HIV-negative subjects, which may be due to HIV lifting the usual inhibitory effect of delta virus on hepatitis B virus replication (Cassidy et al. 1989; Housset et al. 1992). Severe delta virus hepatitis has been reported in drug users (Lettau et al. 1987; Shattock et al. 1985) and there is evidence to suggest increased delta virus (DV) replication, delayed clearance of DV antigenaemia and loss of DV antibody in some HIV infected patients (Kreek et al. 1987; Castillo et al. 1989; Lake-Baharr et al. 1989).

Serological evidence of hepatitis C infection has been reported in up to 80% of IDUs (Esteban et al. 1989; Chamot et al. 1990, 1992) and resulting liver damage may be potentiated by HIV infection (Martin et al. 1989).

Confusion, Seizures, Other CNS Symptoms

Drug overdosage and drug withdrawal may precipitate confusion or seizures and has been particularly well documented with cocaine abuse (Myer and Earnest 1984). There is no evidence to suggest an increased rate of HIV dementia in IDUs and cognitive deficits in HIV-infected IDUs are more likely directly related to drug abuse (Egan et al. 1990; McKegney et al. 1990).

Oliguria, Polyuria, Oedema

A variety of renal syndromes affect the IDU in the absence of HIV infection. Heroin abusers may develop acute renal failure caused by rhabdomyolysis or septic glomerulonephritis (Rao et al. 1974) and intradermal injectors ("skin-poppers") are prone to chronic renal failure secondary to renal amyloidosis. Heroin-associated nephropathy describes a condition of focal and segmental glomerulosclerosis leading to nephrotic syndrome and renal insufficiency (Arruda and Kurtzman 1977) and is therefore similar to the well described AIDS-associated nephropathy (Rao et al. 1984). HIV infection, and in particular the development of AIDS, may worsen the prognosis of drug-related renal disease. Conversely, the malnutrition and recurrent sepsis related to drug abuse may adversely affect the outcome of HIV-related renal disease. It has been suggested that maintenance haemodialysis is not effective in prolonging the life of patients with AIDS-associated nephropathy and uraemia nor in patients with end-stage renal failure in whom AIDS develops during the course of maintenance dialysis (Rao et al. 1987).

Malignancies

Kaposi's sarcoma (KS) occurs less frequently in IDUs than in homosexual men with AIDS. A study from New York City reported KS as the initial AIDS diagnosis in 46% of non-drug-using homosexual or bisexual men compared to 4% of heterosexual male IDUs. Interestingly, the percentage of female IDUs with KS was higher, at 12.5% (Des Jarlais et al. 1984). More recently, Beral et al. (1990) reported KS in less than 3% of IDUs.

Both non-Hodgkin's and Hodgkin's lymphoma have been well documented in IDUs. As with other HIV-infected patients, the disease is often extranodal and generally has a poor prognosis. Solid neoplasms may also occur earlier and be more aggressive in HIV-infected IDUs than in HIV-seronegative controls (Monfardini et al. 1989; Gachupia-Garcia et al. 1992).

Sexually Transmitted Infections

The drug user is at risk for acquiring sexually transmitted diseases, usually through prostitution, which may be used as a means of funding a "drug habit" (Marshall and Hendtlass 1986; Hart et al. 1989). A recent study of almost 3000 IDUs in Baltimore reported that 60% had previously had a sexually transmitted disease (Nelson et al. 1991). In the USA a relationship has been noted between syphilis and prostitution amongst drug users (Centers for Disease Control 1988). In addition, the use of cocaine or crack has been associated with an increased incidence of syphilis, gonorrhoea and chancroid (Centers for Disease Control 1988; Whittaker et al. 1989; Rolfs et al. 1990; Farley et al. 1990). Although the majority of HIV infected patients who acquire syphilis will present with typical clinical features, there is some evidence to suggest that the clinical spectrum and natural history of syphilis may be altered by concomitant HIV infection (Berry et al. 1987; Hicks et al. 1987; Johns et al. 1987; Lukehart et al. 1988).

Investigations

The investigations performed on the injecting drug user are no different from those performed on HIV-infected patients from other risk groups. However, there are a few points which need to be considered when interpreting results.

As mentioned previously, IDUs are prone to a variety of pulmonary disorders, as a result of drug injection. Foreign particle emboli are common and may cause arteriolar and capillary obstruction resulting in a reduction of the carbon monoxide-diffusing capacity (Overland et al. 1980). Although these changes are in most cases insufficient to cause significant symptoms, and abnormalities in gas exchange during exercise tend to be mild, they should be borne in mind when interpreting lung function tests.

Concern regarding an increase in syphilis amongst IDUs has been mentioned and emphasises the need for adequate screening. However, over 10% of IDUs have false-positive syphilis serology (Cushman and Sherman 1974; Kaufman et al. 1974; Cushman et al. 1977) and therefore specific treponemal serological tests, such as the TPHA or FTA, will be required to confirm true infection.

Many injecting drug users self-medicate with a variety of drugs. Of particular importance is the use of antibiotics which may interfere with sputum and blood cultures and hence delay the diagnosis of bacterial infections. Self-medication has previously been reported as a risk factor for the development of methicillin-resistant staphylococcus aureus bacterial endocarditis (Crane et al. 1986).

As with other groups, the CD4 lymphocyte count and percentage of CD4 lymphocytes appear to be the most appropriate markers for assessing disease progression. Increased levels of $\beta 2$-microglobulin have been reported in

HIV-seronegative IDUs and probably reflect immunostimulation resulting from chronic antigenic challenge associated with continued drug injection (Flegg et al. 1991; Gorter et al. 1992).

Clinical Management

Drug users show a wide variation in psychological makeup and personality type (Cohen 1977) and although many lead chaotic lives and are somewhat unreliable, others may possess a high level of education and a variety of social assets. Generally speaking, however, the clinical management of currently injecting drug users is problematic. Out-patient care may prove difficult mainly owing to the high attendance default rates of between 30% and 50% (Welsby 1988; personal observation). This can be improved by incorporating methadone prescribing with medical care (Brettle et al. 1992). In-patient care may also require modification (Welsby 1988) and medical staff will need to improve their understanding of the principles of detoxification and appreciate the difficulties frequently encountered in its management. Advice and guidance should be sought at an early stage from a drug dependency unit if there is uncertainty among ward staff.

Tolerance is soon developed to the analgesic effect of methadone and hence drug users on methadone maintenance still experience pain and indeed may require higher and more frequent doses of analgesics (Ho and Dole 1979). Pain management in the opiate user requires skilful and sympathetic handling and may be achieved by educating staff to use appropriate doses of analgesics (Kenner and Foley 1981).

The possibility of drug interactions should be considered when prescribing for the drug user on methadone maintenance. For example, rifampicin and phenytoin may induce symptoms of opiate withdrawal by enhancing the hepatic metabolism of methadone (Kreek et al. 1976; Tong et al. 1981). Other drugs have been shown in animal models to affect the metabolism of methadone; however the relevance of these findings to human subjects is uncertain (Kreek 1983). There are conflicting clinical data on the interaction between methadone and zidovudine (Burger et al. 1993). It appears that in a subgroup of patients methadone increases plasma levels of zidovudine and may produce side effects. The exact mechanism of this interaction is unknown. All female drug users should be offered cervical cytology. Personal health often takes a low priority and many will never have had a cervical smear. This is of particular relevance to the HIV infected patient who is more than ten times as likely to develop cervical intraepithelial neoplasia than a non-infected individual (Byrne et al. 1989; LaGuardia 1993).

Although some studies have suggested that HIV infected IDUs who continue to inject at high levels (more than 45 injections per month) may show increased rates of CD4 cell loss (Des Jarlais et al. 1987; Fiegg et al. 1989) and progress more rapidly to AIDS (Crovari et al. 1988), these results have not been confirmed by more recent studies (Selwyn et al. 1992; Finnegan et al. 1993). Reports of immunological dysfunction in heroin addicts (Brown et al. 1974) and of opiate-induced depression of both T lymphocyte function and number (McDonough 1980) lend theoretical support for drug-induced immunosuppression; however, this has not been confirmed by clinical studies (McLachlan et al. 1993). Non-sterile injection irrespective of drug use, may result in increased HIV replication (Zagury et al. 1986) and reduce T-lymphocyte reactivity (Mientjes et al. 1991) but this does not appear to lead to a more rapid progression to AIDS (Rezza et al. 1990). In summary, the evidence to date does not indicate a significantly increased risk of disease progression in those IDUs who continue to inject.

Other Issues

Infection with human T-cell lymphotropic viruses (HTLV) is common in IDUs and is primarily caused by HTLV-II (Robert-Guroff et al. 1986; Giadelone et al. 1988; Cantor et al. 1989; Stevens et al. 1989; Ehm et al. 1989; Khabbaz et al. 1992; Zanetti and Galli 1992). There is no evidence to date of an increase in HTLV-related clinical disease, such as adult T-cell leukaemia or myelopathy, in these groups. However, it has been suggested that HTLV may act as a risk factor for the progression of HIV disease in IDUs (Hattori et al. 1989; Weiss et al. 1989).

There has been increasing evidence of an excess morbidity and mortality from "non-AIDS" illnesses among HIV-infected IDUs in the USA. To incorporate some of this non-AIDS morbidity, the US Centers for Disease Control (CDC) revised its surveillance definition for AIDS to include HIV-infected patients with pulmonary tuberculosis, recurrent pneumonia or CD4 cell counts $<200 \times 10^6/l$.

Conclusion

Providing long-term medical care for injecting drug users can at times prove challenging. Both drug use and drug injection lead to psychological and physical problems which, when taken in conjunction with HIV infection, lead to difficulties in diagnosis and management. Caring for HIV-infected injecting drug users requires an understanding of drug abuse and drug-related problems. Unfortunately these remain a much neglected part of both undergraduate and postgraduate medical training.

References

Aguado JM, Castrillo JM (1987) Lymphadenitis as a characteristic manifestation of disseminated tuberculosis in intravenous drug abusers infected with human immunodeficiency virus. J Infect 14: 191

Arruda JAL, Kurtzman NA (1977) Heroin addiction and renal disease. Contrib Nephrol 7: 69–78

Ballet JJ, Sulcebe G, Couderc LJ et al. (1987) Impaired anti-pneumococcal antibody response in patients with AIDS-related persistent generalised lymphadenopathy. Clin Exp Immunol 68: 479–487

Beral V, Peterman TA, Berkelman RL, Jaffe HW (1990) Kaposi's sarcoma among persons with AIDS: a sexually transmitted infection? Lancet i: 123–128

Berry CD, Hooton TM, Collier AC, Lukehart SA (1987) Neurological relapse after benzathine penicillin therapy for secondary syphilis in a patient with HIV infection. N Engl J Med 316: 1587–1589

Brettle RP, Gore SM, McNeil A (1992) Outpatient medical care of injection drug use related HIV. Int J STD AIDS 3: 96–100

Brown SM, Stimmel B, Taub RN, Kochwa S, Rosenfield RE (1974) Immunological dysfunction in heroin addicts. Arch Int Med 134: 1001–1006

Burger DM, Meenhorst PL, Koks CHW, Beijnen JH (1993) Drug interactions with zidovudine. AIDS 7: 445-451

Butz WC (1969) Pulmonary arteriole foreign body granulomata associated with angiomatoids resulting from the intravenous injection of oral medications, eg propoxyphene hydrochloride. J Forensic Sci 14: 317-326

Byrne MA, Taylor-Robinson D, Munday PE, Harris JRW (1989) The common occurrence of human papillomavirus infection and intraepithelial neoplasia in women infected by HIV. AIDS 3: 379-382

Cantor KP, Weiss SH, Goedert J, Battjes R (1989) HTLV-I/II seroprevalence and HIV/HTLV coinfection among IV drug abusers in the U.S. (abstract Th.A.P.18) In: Proceedings of the V International Conference on AIDS. Montreal, Canada

Cassidy WM, Govindarajan S, Gupta S, Valinluck B, Redeker AG (1989) Influence of HIV on chronic hepatitis B and D infection (abstract). Hepatology 10: 690

Castillo I, Bartolome J, Martinez MA, et al. (1989) Influence of HIV infection in hepatitis delta chronic carriers (abstract M.B.P.221). In: Proceedings of the V International Conference on AIDS. Montreal, Canada

Centers for Disease Control (1988) Continuing increase in infectious syphilis-United States. MMWR 37; 35-38

Centers for Disease Control (1988) Relationship of syphilis to drug use and prostitution in Conneticut and Philadelphia, Pennsylvania. MMWR 37: 755-758, 764

Chaisson RE, Slutkin G (1989) Tuberculosis and human immunodeficiency virus infection. J Infect Dis 159: 96-100

Chamot E, Hirschel B, Wintsch J, et al (1990) Loss of antibodies against hepatitis C in HIV-seropositive intravenous drug users. AIDS 4: 1275-1277

Chamot E, de Saussure Ph, Hirschel B, Deglen JJ, Perrin LH (1992) Incidence of hepatitis C, hepatitis B, and HIV infection among drug users in a methadone-maintenance programme. AIDS 6: 430-431

Cohen A (1977) A typology of drug addicts. National Drug Abuse Conference, San Francisco

Collignon PJ, Sorrell T (1987) Candidiasis in heroin abusers. J Infect Dis 155: 595

Conte D, Ferroni P, Lorini GP et al. (1987) HIV and HBV infection in intravenous drug addicts from northeastern Italy. J Med Vir 22: 299-306

Crane LR, Levine DP, Zervos MJ, Cummings G (1986) Bacteremia in narcotic addicts at the Detroit Medical Center. 1. Microbiology, epidemiology, risk factors, and empiric therapy. Rev Infect Dis 8: 364-372

Craven DE, Rixinger AI, Bisno AL, Goularte TA, McCabe WR (1986) Bacteremia caused by group G streptococci in parenteral drug abusers: epidemiological and clinical aspects. J Infect Dis 153: 988-992

Crovari P, Penco G, Valente A et al. (1988) HIV infection in two cohorts of drug addicts prospectively studied. Association of serological markers with clinical progression (abstract 4527). In: Proceedings of the IVth International Conference on AIDS. Stockholm, Sweden

Cushman P Jr, Sherman C (1974) Biologic false-positive reactions in serologic tests for syphilis in narcotic addiction. Am J Clin Path 61: 346-351

Cushman P Jr, Gupta S, Grieco MH (1977) Immunological studies in methadone maintained patients. Int J Addict 12: 241-253

Des Jarlais DC, Marmor M, Thomas P, Chamberland M, Zoll-Pazner S, Sencer DJ (1984) Kaposi's sarcoma among four different AIDSs risk groups. N Engl J Med 310: 1119

Des Jarlais DC, Friedman SR, Marmor M et al. (1987) Development of AIDS, HIV seroconversion, and co-factors for T4 cell loss in a cohort of intravenous drug users. AIDS 1: 105-111

Des Jarlais DC, Friedman SR, Choopanya K, Vanichseni S, Ward TP (1992) International epidemiology of HIV and AIDS among injecting drug users. AIDS 6: 1053-1068

Dupont B, Drouhet E (1985) Cutaneous, ocular, and osteoarticular candidiasis in heroin addicts: new clinical and therapeutic aspects in 38 patients. J Infect Dis 152: 577-591

Egan VG, Crawford JR, Brettle RP, Goodwin GM (1990) The Edinburgh cohort of HIV-positive drug users: current intellectual function is impaired, but not due to early AIDS dementia complex. AIDS 4: 651-656

Ehm-I, Pauli G, Thiele B et al. (1989) Investigations of the presence of HTLV-I infection in intravenous drug abusers and homosexuals in the Federal Republic of Germany (abstract Th.A.P.29). In: Proceedings of the V International Conference on AIDS. Montreal, Canada

Esteban JI, Viladomiu L, Gonzalez A et al. (1989) Hepatitis C virus antibodies among risk groups in Spain. Lancet ii: 294-296

Farley TA, Hadler JL, Gunn RA (1990) The syphilis epidemic in Connecticut: relationship to drug use and prostitution. Sex Transm Dis 17: 163-168

Finnegan LP, Davenny K, Hartel D (1993) Drug use in HIV-infected women. In: Johnson MA, Johnstone FD (eds) HIV infection in women. Churchill Livingstone, Edinburgh, p133-155

Flegg PJ, Jones ME, MacCallum LR et al. (1989) Continued injecting drug use as a cofactor for progression of HIV (abstact M.A.P.92). In: Proceedings of the V International Conference on AIDS. Montreal, Canada

Flegg PJ, Brettle RP, Robertson JR, Clarkson RC, Bird AG (1991) β2-microglobulin levels in drug users: the influence of risk behaviour. AIDS 5: 1021-1024

Frieden TR, Sterling MPH, Pablos-Mendez A, Kilburn JO, Cauthen GM, Dooley SW (1993) The emergence of drug resistant tuberculosis in New York City. N Engl J Med 328: 521-526

Gachupin-Garcia A, Selwyn PA, Salisbury Budner N (1992) Population-based study of malignancies and HIV infection among injecting drug users in a New York City methadone treatment programme, 1985-1991. AIDS 6: 843-848

Giadelone A, Zani M, Barillari G et al. (1988) HTLV-I and HIV infection in drug addicts in Italy. Lancet ii: 753-754

Glassroth J, Adams G, Schmoll S (1987) The impact of substance abuse on the respiratory system. Chest 91: 596-602

Gorter RW, Vranizan KM, Osmond DH, Moss AR (1992) Differences in laboratory values in HIV infection by sex, race, and risk group. AIDS 6: 1341-1347

Hahn HH, Schweid AI, Beaty HN (1969) Complications of injecting dissolved methylphenidate tablets. Arch Int Med 123: 656-659

Hart GJ, Sonnex C, Petherick A et al. (1989) Risk behaviours for HIV infection among injecting drug users attending a drug dependency unit. Br Med J 298: 1081-1083

Hart GJ, Woodward N, Johnson AM, Tighe J, Parry JV, Adler MW (1991) Prevalence of HIV, hepatitis B and associated risk behaviours in clients of a needle-exchange in central London. AIDS 5: 543-547

Hattori T, Koito A, Takatsuki K et al. (1989) Frequent infection with human T-cell lymphotropic virus type 1 in patients with AIDS, but not in carriers of human immunodeficiency virus type 1. J AIDS 2: 272-276

Helpern M, Rho Y-M (1966) Deaths from narcotism in New York City. New York J Med 66: 2391-2408

Hicks CB, Benson PM, Lupton GP, Tramont EC (1987) Seronegative secondary syphilis in a patient infected with the human immunodeficiency virus (HIV) with Kaposi sarcoma: a diagnostic dilemma. Ann Int Med 107: 492-495

Ho A, Dole VP (1979) Pain perception in drug-free and in methadone-maintained human ex-addicts. Proc Soc Exp Biol Med 162: 392-395

Hopkins GB (1972) Pulmonary angiothrombotic granulomatosis in drug offenders. JAMA 221: 909-911

Housset C, Pol S, Carnot F et al. (1992) Interactions between human immunodeficiency virus-1, hepatitis delta virus and hepatitis B virus infections in 260 chronic carriers of hepatitis B virus. Hepatology 15: 578-583

Johns DR, Tierney M, Felsenstein D (1987) Alteration of the natural history of neurosyphilis by concurrent infection with the human immunodeficiency virus. N Engl J Med 316: 1569-1572

Johnston EH, Goldbaum LR, Whelton RL (1969) Investigation of sudden death in addicts, with emphasis on the toxicological findings in thirty cases. Med Ann D C 38: 375-380

Kaufman RE, Weiss S, Moore JD, Falcone V, Wiesner PJ (1974) Biological false positive serological tests for syphilis among drug addicts. Br J Vener Dis 50: 350-353

Kenner RM, Foley KM (1981) Patterns of narcotic use in a cancer pain clinic. Ann NY Acad Sci 362: 161-72

Khabbaz RF, Onorato IM, Cannon RO et al. (1992) Seroprevalence of HTLV-I and HTLV-II among intravenous drug users and persons in clinics for sexually transmitted diseases. N Engl J Med 326: 375-80

Klein RS, Selwyn PA, Maude D, Pollard C, Freeman K, Schiffman G (1989) Response to pneumococcal vaccine among asymptomatic heterosexual partners of persons with AIDS and intravenous drug users infected with HIV. J Infect Dis 160: 826-831

Kreek MJ, Garfield JW, Gutjahr CL, Guisti M (1976) Rifampin-induced methadone withdrawal. Ann Int Med 294: 1104-1106

Kreek MJ (1983) Factors modifying the pharmacological effectiveness of methadone. In: Research on the Treatment of Narcotic Addiction, Cooper JR, Altman F Brown BS, Czechowicz D (eds). Treatment Research Monograph Series DHSS Publication no (ADM) 83-1281, pp 95-107

Kreek MJ, Des Jarlais DC, Trepo G et al. (1987) Hepatitis delta antigenemia in intravenous drug abusers with AIDS (abstract Th.P.216). In: Proceedings of the III International Conference on AIDS, Washington, DC

LaGuardia KD (1993) Other sexually transmitted disease: cervical intraepithelial neoplasia. In: Johnson MA, Johnstone FD (eds) HIV infection in women. Churchill Livingstone, Edinburgh, p 247-61

Lake-Baharr G, Bhat K, Goundarajan S (1989) HIV infection and delta hepatitis in intravenous drug addicts (abstract M.B.P.218) In: Proceedings of the V International Conference on AIDS. Montreal, Canada

Lazizi Y, Grongeot-Keros L, Delfraissy J-E et al. (1988) Reappearance of hepatitis B virus in immune patients infected with the human immunodeficiency virus. J Infect Dis 158: 666-667

Lettau LA, McCarthy JG, Smith MH et al. (1987) Outbreak of severe hepatitis due to delta and hepatitis B viruses in parenteral drug abusers and their contacts. N Engl J Med 317: 1256-1262

Lukehart SA, Hook EW III, Baker-Zander SA, Collier AC, Critchlow CW, Handsfield HH (1988) Invasion of the central nervous system by Treponema pallidum: implications for diagnoses and therapy. Ann Int Med 109: 855-862

Luttgens WF (1949) Endocarditis in "main line" opium addicts. Arch Int Med 83: 653-654

Marshall N, Hendtlass J (1986) Drugs and prostitution. J Drug Issues 16: 237-248

Martin P, Di Bisceglie AM, Kassianides C, Lisker-Melman M, Hoofnagle JH (1989) Gastroenterology 97: 1559-1561

McDonough RJ, Madden JJ, Falek A et al. (1980) Alteration of T and null lymphocyte frequencies in the peripheral blood of human opiate addicts: in vivo evidence for opiate receptor sites on T lymphocytes. J Immunol 125: 2539-2543

McKegney FP, O'Dowd MA, Feiner C, Selwyn P, Drucker E, Friedland GH (1990) A prospective comparison of neuropsychologic function in HIV-seropositive and seronegative methadone maintained patients. AIDS 4: 565-569

McLachlan C, Crofts N, Wodak A, Crowe S (1993) The effects of methadone on immune function among injecting drug users: a review. Addiction 88: 257-263

McMeeking AA, Holzman RS(1988) Group G streptococcal bacteremia and parenteral drug abusers. J Infect Dis 157: 612

Mientjes GH, Miedema F, van Ameijden EJ et al. (1991) Frequent injecting impairs lymphocyte reactivity in HIV-positive and HIV-negative drug users. AIDS 5: 35-41

MMWR (1991) Update: Acquired immunodeficiency syndrome–United States, 1981-1990. 40: 358-369

Monfardini S, Vaccher E, Pizzocara G et al. (1989) Unusual malignant tumours in 49 patients with HIV infection. AIDS 3: 449-452

Munoz-Fernandez S, Macia MA, Pantoja L et al. (1993) Osteoarticular infection in intravenous drug abusers: influence of HIV infection and differences with non drug abusers. Ann Rheum Dis 52: 570-574

Myer JA, Earnest MP (1984) Generalised seizures and cocaine abuse. Neurology 34: 675-687

Nelson KE, Vlahov D, Cohn S, Odunmbaku M, Lindsay A, Anthony JC, Hook III EW (1991) Sexually transmitted disease in a population of intravenous drug users: association with seropositivity to the human immunodeficiency virus. J Infect Dis 164: 457-463

Novick DM (1992) The medically ill substance abuser. In: Lowinson J, Ruiz P, Millman R (eds) Substance abuse: a comprehensive textbook, 2nd edn. Williams and Wilkins, Baltimore, MD, pp 657-674

O'Donnell AE, Pappas LS (1988) Pulmonary complications of intravenous drug abuse. Chest 94: 251-253

Overland ES, Nolan AJ, Hopewell PC (1980) Alteration of pulmonary function in intravenous drug abusers. Prevalence, severity, and characterization of gas exchange abnormalities. Am J Med 68: 231-237

Pallasch TJ, Joseph CE (1987) Oral manifestations of drug abuse. J Psych Drugs 19: 375-376

Pitchenik AE, Rubinson HA (1985) The radiographic appearance of tuberculosis in patients with the acquired immunodeficiency syndrome (AIDS) and pre-AIDS. Am Rev Respir Dis 131: 393-396

Podzamczer D, Guidol F (1986) Systemic candidiasis in heroin abusers. J Infect Dis 153: 1182-1183

Polsky B, Gold JWM, Whimbey E et al. (1986) Bacterial pneumonia in patients with the acquired immunodeficiency syndrome. Ann Int Med 104: 38-41

Rao TKS, Nicastri AD, Friedman EA (1974) Natural history of heroin associated nephropathy. N Engl J Med 290: 19-23

Rao TKS, Filippone EJ, Nicastri AD et al. (1984) Associated focal and segmental glomerulosclerosis in the acquired immunodeficiency syndrome. N Engl J Med 310: 669-673

Rao TKS, Friedman EA, Nicastri AD (1987) The types of renal disease in the acquired immunodeficiency syndrome. N Engl J Med 316: 1062-1068

Reichman L, Felton C, Edsall J (1979) Drug dependence, a possible new risk factor for tuberculosis disease. Arch Int Med 139: 337–339

Rezza G, Menniti-Ippolito F, Lazzarin A et al. (1990) Psychoactive drug use and AIDS. JAMA 263: 372–373

Robert-Guroff M, Weiss SH, Gibbs WN et al. (1986) Prevalence of antibodies to HTLV-I, -II, and -III in intravenous drug abusers from an AIDS endemic region. JAMA 255: 3133–3137

Rolfs RT, Goldberg M, Sharrar RG (1990) Risk factors for syphilis: cocaine use and prostitution. Am J Public Health 80: 853–857

Ruggeri P, Sathe SS, Kapila R (1988) Changing patterns of infectious endocarditis in parenteral drug abusers with human immunodeficiency virus infections (abstract 8028). In: Proceedings of the IVth International Conference on AIDS. Stockholm, Sweden

Salmaso S, Conti S, Sasse H, and the Second Multicenter Study Group on Drug Users (1991) Drug use and HIV-1 infection: report from the second Italian multicenter study. J AIDS 4: 607–613

Sapira JD (1968) The narcotic addict as a medical patient. Am J Med 45: 555–585

Selwyn PA, Feingold AR, Hartel D et al. (1988) Increased risk of bacterial pneumonia in HIV-infected intravenous drug users without AIDS. AIDS 2: 267–272

Selwyn PA, Hartel D, Lewis VA et al. (1989) A prospective study of the risk of tuberculosis among intravenous drug users with human immunodeficiency virus infection. N Engl J Med 320: 545–550

Selwyn PA, Alcabes P, Hartel D et al. (1992) Clinical manifestations and predictors of disease progression in drug users with human immunodeficiency virus infection. N Engl J Med 327: 1697–1703

Shafer RW, Chirgwin KD, Glatt AE, Dahdouh MA, Landesman SH, Suster B (1991) HIV prevalence, immunosuppression, and drug resistance in patients with tuberculosis in an area endemic for AIDS. AIDS 5: 399–406

Shattock AG, Irwin FM, Morgan BM et al. (1985) Increased severity and morbidity of acute hepatitis in drug abusers with simultaneously acquired hepatitis B and hepatitis D virus infections. Br Med J 290: 1377–1380

Siegel H (1972) Human pulmonary pathology associated with narcotic and other addictive drugs. Human Pathol 3: 55–66

Siegel H, Helpern M, Ehrenreich T (1966) The diagnosis of death from intravenous narcotism. J Forensic Sci 11: 1–16

Slim J, Boghossian J, Perez G, Johnson E (1988) Comparative analysis of bacterial endocarditis in HIV positive and HIV negative intravenous drug abusers (abstract 8027). In: Proceedings of the IVth International Conference on AIDS. Stockholm, Sweden

Steinhoff MC, Auerbach BS, Nelson KE et al. (1991) Antibody responses to Haemophilus influenzae type B vaccines in men with human immunodeficiency virus infection. N Engl J Med 325: 1837–1842

Stern W, Subbarao K (1983) Pulmonary complications of drug abuse. Semin Roentgenol 18: 183–197

Stevens R, Wethers J, Samsonoff C, Berns D (1989) Human immunodeficiency and human T-lymphotropic virus infections associated with intravenous drug use (abstract T.A.P.53). In: Proceedings of the V International Conference on AIDS. Montreal, Canada

Sunderam G, McDonald RJ, Maniatis T, Oleske J, Kapila R, Reichman LB (1986) Tuberculosis as a manifestation of the acquired immunodeficiency syndrome. JAMA 256: 362–366

Theuer CP, Hopewell PC, Elias D, Schecter GF, Rutherford GW, Chaisson RE (1990) Human immunodeficiency virus infection in tuberculosis patients. J Infect Dis 162: 8–12

Tong TG, Pond SM, Kreek MJ et al. (1981) Phenytoin induced methadone withdrawal. Ann Int Med 94: 349–351

Unsworth DJ, Rowen D, Carne CA, Sonnex C, Baglin T, Brown DL (1993) Defective IgG2 response to Pneumovax in HIV seropositive patients. Genitourin Med 69: 373–376

Vento S, di Perri G, Luzzati R et al. (1989) Clinical reactivation of hepatitis B in anti-HBS-positive patients with AIDS. Lancet i: 332–333

Weiss SH, French J, Holland B et al. (1989) HTLV-I/II coinfection is significantly associated with risk of progression to AIDS among HIV+ intravenous drug abusers (abstract Th.A.O.23). In: Proceedings of the V International Conference on AIDS. Montreal, Canada

Weller IVD, Cohn D, Sierralta A et al. (1984) Clinical, biochemical, serological, histological and ultrastructural features of liver disease in drug abusers. Gut 25: 417–423

Welsby PD (1988) Caring for intravenous drug abusers with HIV infection: some lessons from Edinburgh. Postgrad Med J 64: 575–577

Whittaker S, Calsyn D, Saxon A, Freeman G Jr (1989) Sexual behaviours of intravenous drug users (abstract W.D.P.85). In: Proceedings of the V International Conference on AIDS. Montreal, Canada

Zagury D, Bernard J, Leonard L et al. (1986) Long term cultures of HTLV-III infected T cells: a model of cytopathology of T-cell depletion in AIDS. Science 231: 850–853
Zanetti AR, Galli C (1992) Seroprevalence of HTLV-I and HTLV-II. N Engl J Med 326: 1783
Zientara M, Moore S (1970) Fatal talc embolism in a drug addict. Human Pathol 1: 324–326

10 AIDS in Africa

Adam Malin and Anton Pozniak

The Size of the Problem

In 1992, the World Health Organization estimated that more than 6 million people in sub-Saharan Africa were infected with the Human Immunodeficiency Virus (HIV) – 2.5% of the adult population. This accounted for over 60% of the estimated worldwide HIV infections (Global Programme on AIDS 1992). Admittedly, generalisations concerning the extent and distribution of HIV infection are difficult to make. Prevalence rates between countries, urban and rural areas and even within individual city localities may differ greatly. However, evidence indicates that the spread of HIV continues unabated in areas of both high and low prevalence.

HIV Prevalence

The epidemic is concentrated in large towns and cities and is highest among sexually active adults (15–45 years). More women are infected than men (female : male ratio, 1.4 : 1) and peak age prevalence occurs about 5 years earlier in women, at 20–24 years, compared with male peak prevalence at 25–29 years (Berkley et al. 1990). In the worst afflicted countries, levels of infection in urban areas have reached 12%–30% in sentinel populations such as pregnant women (Anderson et al. 1991). In Kigali, Rwanda, seroprevalence in antenatal clinics is more than 25% with an annual increase of 3%–5% (Bucyendore et al. 1993). By contrast, prevalence in rural areas (where 80% of the population live) is much lower, with rates ranging from 1%–12% (Berkley et al. 1990). However, there is evidence of a shift in burden of HIV infection from urban to rural areas.

HIV Incidence

There have been few prospective HIV seroincidence studies and assumptions are derived mainly from multiple anonymous cross-sectional serosurveys (Nkowane 1991). However, some cohort data are available. Two high-risk groups, prostitutes from Kinshasa and women with STDs from Nairobi, showed a 12% and 22% incidence per year respectively. But these data are flawed because the follow-up rate was not reported. Similarly, a cohort of post-natal women with an incidence of 3% per year had only a 37% follow-up (Nkowane 1991).

AIDS

Surveillance of AIDS cases is of limited value to assess the future trends of this pandemic, since reported AIDS cases reflect HIV infection which occurred many years previously. Significant problems also exist regarding accuracy, completeness and timing of reporting of AIDS cases. For a variety of reasons, perhaps only 20% of all adult AIDS cases that have occurred in Africa have been reported to WHO. HIV surveillance is therefore more relevant for public health planning since future numbers of all HIV-related disease will reflect the number of persons infected with HIV.

AIDS has already become the major cause of death in adults in Abidjan, Ivory Coast (De Cock et al. 1990). In Rwanda, a prospective 2-year cohort study demonstrated that HIV disease accounted for 90% of deaths among child-bearing women. The 2-year mortality among all HIV-infected women and those fulfilling the WHO criteria for AIDS at entry was 7% and 21% respectively. By contrast, women not infected with HIV had a 2-year mortality of 0.3% (Lindan et al. 1992). The survival time from diagnosis of AIDS is shorter in Africa than in the USA or Europe. In part, this is due to differing levels of medical care (Colebunders and Latif 1991).

The "African myth"

Controversy surrounds the extrapolation of reported statistics (Nicholl 1993). Proponents of the "African Myth" argue that surveillance methods are not representative, that the extent of cross-reactivity in HIV testing is unknown, and that AIDS cannot be reliably diagnosed in Africa. Moreover, some suggest that the statistics are deliberately inflated in order to avert funds towards self-interested AIDS scientists and away from other treatable tropical conditions which have been mistakenly diagnosed as AIDS. The body of evidence contradicts these charges. All recent serosurveys utilise serologic algorithms which approach a 100% specificity. Whilst the representativeness of sentinel surveillance may not perfectly reflect population rates, large cross-sectional serosurveys of clearly-defined subgroups (blood donors, pregnant women) will give a strong indication of trend (Bucyendore et al. 1993; Hunter 1993; Lindan et al. 1992). More specifically, a study in Mwanza province, Tanzania, further supported the validity of sentinel surveillance by comparing sentinel groups with the general population. If anything, antenatal clinic attenders underestimated the population prevalence, whilst blood donors were the most representative (Borgdorff 1993). The final charge contends that because AIDS is sometimes diagnosed in those without the disease, the figures are inflated. This is wholly spurious. It is just as easy to argue the alternative: AIDS is often undiagnosed as a result of inadequate diagnostic and reporting facilities – a statement which has more scientific support (Chin and Mann 1989). It is widely accepted that HIV causes AIDS and the large majority of those infected with HIV will develop the disease. Therefore, at present, sero-epidemiology offers the best means of monitoring the trend and thus health planning. It also offers a means to assess the efficacy of control programmes.

Projected rates of HIV and AIDS

WHO has developed a short-term projection model which estimates a 4% adult prevalence rate (10 million persons) and 2 million adult AIDS cases in sub-Saharan Africa by 1994 (Chin et al. 1992). For the same period, the worldwide estimate is 17 million. Sub-Saharan Africa will therefore account for 60% of the global prevalence of HIV; yet the region supports less than 9% of the world population (Hunter 1993).

Transmission Modes

Heterosexual

In contrast to the industrialised world, the majority of HIV in the African continent is acquired by heterosexual sexual intercourse (80% of total) (Heymann and Edstrom 1991). There are two peaks of high seroprevalence related to age, one is in the under-one age group and the another is in the 16–29 year old age group with peak age prevalence occurring about 5 years earlier in women (Berkley et al. 1990). The first peak reflects maternal–fetal transmission, the second peak sexual transmission – the major mode of spread of HIV in Africa.

Studies in prostitutes confirm bidirectional transmission of HIV. The male:female HIV seropositivity ratio is 1 : 1.4 (Berkley et al. 1990). This higher rate may be due to differential rates of transmission between men and women, higher rates of female sexual exposure, or longer survival in HIV infected women compared with men.

Concurrent sexually transmitted disease (STD), both ulcerative and non-ulcerative, have the strongest association with transmission of HIV. Overall, genitourinary disease (GUD) is the most important cofactor (Nsubuga ct al. 1990). However, in areas where the prevalence of GUD is low, such as Kinshasa, Zaire, non-ulcerative STD confers a higher attributable risk (Laga et al. 1993). Other risk factors include: number of sexual partners (Serwadda et al. 1992), a history of prostitution or contact with a prostitute, less condom use (Allen et al. 1992), high socioeconomic status (Allen et al. 1991), lack of male circumcision (Plummer et al. 1991) and the use of oral contraceptives (Plummer et al. 1991). Whilst concurrent STD, number of partners and condom use all appear as independent risk factors, the evidence for the others is less apparent. Some are certainly markers for sexual behaviour e.g. socioeconomic status and affordability of multiple partners. Evidence also suggests that sexual transmission of HIV is more likely among couples if the index case acquired HIV sexually rather than from transfusion of blood or blood products (Holmes and Kreiss 1988).

Blood and Blood Products

Blood transfusion and injections probably account for 10% of all AIDS cases in Africa, thus making it the third most important mode of transmission (Heymann and Edstrom 1991). The proportion of blood donors who are HIV positive is greater in Africa than in the developed world. The use of unscreened blood has led to many recipients, especially children, being infected (Gumodoka et al. 1993). However the situation is improving. Zimbabwe was the third country in the world to screen their blood and blood products for HIV and many other countries have developed comprehensive blood screening programmes.

Transmission by Injection

Intravenous drug use is not common in Africa. Even when it does occur, it contributes little to HIV seropositivity rates compared to heterosexual spread. In Zaire and the Congo, an association has been found between frequency of needle exposure (medical, not intravenous drug misuse) and HIV seropositivity in children of seronegative women (Berkley 1991). However, the controls were not matched for severity of symptoms and the number of injections may have been increased as a result of symptomatic HIV treatment.

Scarification

Medicinal blood letting, ritual and medicinal scarification, group circumcision, genital tattooing and shaving of body hair are customs that may be potential modes of HIV transmission. It is unlikely that traditional medicine plays a large role, especially as fresh razor blades, non-hollow instruments such as needles, are used by the traditional healers (Pela and Platt 1989). In a study of traditional healers in Ghana, 88% used scarification, 53% reused their instruments and only 13% attempted sterilisation. Interestingly, those who used traditional healers were less likely to be HIV positive (Berkley et al. 1989). This may be a reflection of one self-selected group having a more traditional rural lifestyle.

Traditional vaginal agents such as herbs or stones used for tightening or discharge may play some part in transmission of HIV due to their irritative and erosive effect on mucosal surfaces.

There is no evidence to suggest widespread transmission by arthropods such as mosquitoes or bed bugs. Laboratory evidence indicates that the soft tick, *Ornithodoros moubata*, could transmit HIV, but there is no epidemiological evidence to suggest that this means of transmission is at all important (Humphrey-Smith et al. 1993).

Perinatal Transmission

Up to 30% of antenatal attenders have been found to be HIV positive in Africa (Nkowane 1991) and 10%–65% of children are infected in utero (Ryder and Temmerman 1991). These rates are considerably higher than the European Collaborative study which showed a vertical transmission rate of 12.9%.

Explanations for this disparity include: (1) that pregnant/nursing women in the African studies may have been more immunocompromised (i.e. more viraemic) and thus more likely to transmit the virus either placentally or in breast milk; (2) that presence of chorioamnionitis is associated with a higher perinatal transmission rate and may be linked with STD and extent of HIV-related immune deficiency.

During the 1990s WHO estimates that AIDS will kill an additional 3 million women and children. Infant and child mortality could be 30% greater than predicted and there will be a million uninfected children who could be orphaned as a result of their parent dying from AIDS (Chin 1990).

Transmission to Medical Staff in Africa

There have been 33 reports of health care workers contracting HIV as a result of their work in the tropics, of whom four were expatriates (Veekan et al. 1991). Health care workers must do their best to follow guidelines to protect themselves against occupational exposure in spite of hazards such as lack of gloves and sharps boxes, no hand-washing facilities, inadequate training of technical procedures and busy schedules. The risk to surgeons whose patients have a high prevalence of HIV (25%–35%) has been calculated as one infection every 8 years (with a case load of 15,000 per year) (Gazzard and Wastell 1990).

Origins

There is an assumption that AIDS is an old disease in Central Africa (Sonnet et al. 1987), having been a sporadic and ill-defined entity perhaps, until the start of the present outbreak. However there is no conclusive evidence to show that HIV originated in Africa (Pela and Platt 1989). Clinical record keeping is necessarily of low priority in Africa and any clinical data are usually little supported by laboratory evidence. Clinicians working in Africa had not, prior to this epidemic, recognised the clinical presentations of HIV-related disease such as candidiasis, Kaposi's sarcoma or lymphadenopathy (Biggar 1987). It is difficult to believe that these conditions would be consistently overlooked as clinicians can now diagnose 80% of HIV positive persons on clinical grounds alone. Affluent Africans used to go to Europe for health care and reviews of their hospital records show that cases consistent with a diagnosis of AIDS have only become common since 1980 (Biggar 1986). Moreover, the cumulative frequency of cases in Africa corresponds to the same epidemic curve seen for the USA and Europe. These points, plus the fact that the HIV epidemic is still spreading through Africa, suggests that it is a new disease. Finally, if HIV had started decades ago in poorer or more rural areas, then it would have been seen in urban centres over the last 30 years because of the migratory labour system (Biggar 1986).

There is still no answer as to whether HIV is an age-old virus or a new phenomenon but there is antibody evidence that HIV or a closely related virus existed in Uganda and Zaire in the late 1950s (Saxinger et al. 1985). Although the HIV genome was identified in a UK sailor who died in 1959, there is no evidence that he ever visited Africa (Saxinger et al. 1985). HIV's origin has puzzled scientists since its discovery over a decade ago. Theories have included origins in outer space, a political plot involving biological warfare, or a harmless blood or vaccine contaminant which transformed into a lethal virus. Viruses have been known to "jump" species with disastrous consequences after modification as a vaccine and in the early days of polio vaccine production green monkey kidney culture was used and this could have been contaminated with a simian immunodeficiency virus (SIV_{AGM}). This particular virus is not sufficiently structurally close to HIV-1, however, to support the idea that it was the progenitor of HIV. Although many modes of monkey to human transmission exist and changes in genetic sequence can occur over a few decades, simian and human immunodeficiency viruses may have evolved in parallel as there is no evidence that simian viruses preceded HIV. SIV_{MAC} (from macaques) was the first SIV to be discovered. Although it causes immunosuppression in monkeys, SIV_{MAC} has only been found in laboratories, not in wild macaques. This virus shares overall sequence homology to HIV-1 of 40% and 75% to HIV-2 and has serological cross reactivity with HIV-2 but it is probably not the forerunner of HIV-2 as several of its genes are distinctly different to HIV-2. SIV_{SM} from the sooty mangabey has a close geographical and molecular relationship to HIV-2 and these viruses may well be closely related.

SIV_{CPZ} from chimpanzees has a genetic sequence similar to HIV-1 but is distinct from it and another simian virus from mandrills has recently been found (SIV_{MND}). There now appears to be four main virus groups – HIV-1 and -2, SIV_{MAC}, $SIV_{SM/AGM}$ and SIV_{MND} – which all might have evolved simultaneously from a common ancestor (Tsujimoto et al. 1989).

DNA and protein sequencing of isolates from different geographical regions indicate different subgroups of HIV-1, a homogeneous North American group and a heterogeneous African group (De Leys et al. 1990). Whether or not these strain variations/variants have produced any differences in the characteristics of the epidemic in Africa has yet to be seen.

HIV-2

In 1985, serum samples collected from a group of healthy Senegalese showed a strong antibody response to simian immunodeficiency virus (SIV) and a relatively weaker response to HIV-1 (Barin et al. 1985). The following year, Montangnier's group identified a new human immunodeficiency virus, HIV-2 (Clavel et al. 1986). Early reports based on case studies suggested that the clinical features of HIV-2 were identical to HIV-1. However, a prospective study of Senegalese prostitutes suggested that the infection was largely benign and thereby threw into question the pathogenicity of HIV-2 (Marlink et al. 1988). Subsequent studies have clearly demonstrated that HIV-2 is independently associated with symptomatic HIV and AIDS with clinical and laboratory features similar to HIV-1 (Gnaore et al. 1993; Le Guenno et al. 1991; Naucler et al. 1991; Whittle et al. 1992). A cohort study of symptomatic HIV-1 and -2 infection in the Gambia showed that CD4 counts, serum β_2-microglobulin and serum neopterin were all powerful predictors of death (Whittle et al. 1992). The same study also suggested median survival times of 6 months for HIV-1 and 13 months for HIV-2 (failed to reach significance). Questions concerning the duration of latency and the number of HIV-2 positive asymptomatic individuals progressing to disease remain unanswered. However, much circumstantial evidence suggests that HIV-2 is less virulent and disease progression is slower (Markovitz 1993).

Epidemiology of HIV-2

Transmission of HIV-2 is predominantly heterosexual with some parenteral transmission. In contrast to HIV-1, perinatal transmission is less common (<10% as compared with >30% for HIV-1 (African rates)). HIV-2 occurs in most parts of West Africa with general population seroprevalence rates ranging from as low as 0.2% in Benin to 9.5 in Guinea-Bissau (De Cock et al. 1991a). Among female prostitute populations 15%–64% are infected (Markovitz 1993). Increasing numbers of HIV-2 cases have been identified in the Americas and Europe but these infections have usually come from West Africa. Interestingly, HIV-2 is also found in southern Africa, in Angola and Mozambique – two ex-Portuguese colonies which have maintained links with Guinea-Bissau and Cape Verde. In the far West of the continent, HIV-2 is more common than HIV-1. Further East, in Cote-d'Ivoire, Burkina-Fasso and parts of Nigeria, HIV-1 predominates and dual infection with both types of HIV is common. In future, it appears that there will be a general trend in West Africa for HIV-1 to become a bigger problem than HIV-2. Observing the HIV-2 epidemic poses significant difficulties as the serological diagnosis of HIV-2 can be difficult to interpret, even with Western blotting. This will be improved by synthetic peptide-based tests (Brattegaard et al. 1993).

HIV-2 Structure and Function – Clues to Origin and Latency

Nucleotide sequence analysis shows 75% similarity to certain strains of SIV, but only 42% similarity to HIV-1. SIV_{MAC} and SIV_{SM} are two particularly closely related strains, found in macaque and sooty mangabey monkeys respectively. Indeed, so close are *pol* and *env* gene sequences in SIV_{SM} and HIV-2, that it might suggest that the 2 viruses are one and the same (Markovitz 1993).

HIV-1 and HIV-2 gene organisation and function are very similar. Both viruses include gag, pol and env genes. *vpu* and *vpx* are specific for HIV-2 and HIV-1 respectively. Under certain circumstances *vpx* is believed to be important in replication. Other differences between HIV-1 and HIV-2 include different requirements for the induction of replication. NF-κB, the dominant cellular protein involved in stimulating the HIV-1 enhancer in activated T cells, also plays a role in HIV-2 induction. However, other purine rich cellular protein binding sites (PuB_1 and PuB_2), which are found upstream from the NF-κB receptor site, are also required. Potential disruption in this region might explain the difference in pathogenesis (Markovitz 1993).

The Natural History of HIV Infection in Africa

The majority of HIV infected persons in Africa are asymptomatic but, unlike the developed world, there are few data on rates of progression to AIDS. Surrogate markers or combinations of variables such as β_2-microglobulin, presence of p24 antigen, monitoring p24 antibodies together with careful clinical observation have been suggested as having the highest predictive value in marking progression to AIDS in HIV asymptomatic patients in Africa (Katzenstein et al. 1990).

The progression rates to ARC in asymptomatics were 20.4 cases per 100 person-years in one study and occurred in 117/285 (41%) in one cohort at presentation (Katzenstein et al. 1990). The progression rates to AIDS in asymptomatics was shown to be 2.3 cases per 100 person years (Mann et al. 1986). The annual mortality from AIDS is not known although it appears that the majority of deaths occur within the first year of the diagnosis of AIDS being made. Large cohorts are being followed and the results, unlike those in the developed world, will not often be affected by the use of antiviral therapy.

The acute HIV seroconversion syndrome may be missed as fever is common in Africa and is often treated as malaria and any rash may be easily overlooked in black skins. Persistent generalised lymphadenopathy (PGL) is one of the commonest earliest presentations occurring in up to 47% of patients followed over 2 years. In one cohort PGL was present in 88% (234/265) (Katzenstein et al. 1990). The glands should fulfil the CDC criteria of being at least 1 cm in size, occur in 2 extra-inguinal sites and be present for at least 3 months duration. However some workers in Africa doubt the validity of this rigid definition and have modified it. The commonest histological appearance of PGL is of benign hyperplasia and in one study this was seen in 97%, the other 3% of nodes were tuberculous. The nodes can become large, painful and sometimes asymmetrical, the pain often responding to non-steroidal anti-inflammatory drugs. A biopsy should be performed in any symptomatic patient or anyone whose nodes become large, painful or asymmetrical in order to exclude tuberculosis, Kaposi's sarcoma or lymphoma.

WHO Case Clinical Definition for AIDS

For the purpose of surveillance, the CDC AIDS case definition was inapplicable in Africa because of inadequate facilities for serodiagnosis of HIV and diagnosis of AIDS indicator diseases. Therefore, in 1985 in Bangui, Central African Republic, the WHO developed a clinical case definition for AIDS to be used in parts of Africa where HIV testing was not used or impractical. It depended on two major and at least one minor criteria being diagnosed in the absence of other causes of immunosuppression such as cancer or malnutrition. Major criteria are weight loss >10%; chronic diarrhoea >1 month; and prolonged fever >1 month, constant or intermittent. Minor criteria are persistent cough >1 month; recurrent herpes zoster; oropharyngeal candida; chronic progressive or disseminated herpes simplex; persistent generalised lymphadenopathy; generalised pruritic dermatitis.

Development of cryptococcal disease or the epidemic form of Kaposi's sarcoma would alone meet the case definition.

The case definition's use in Kinshasa had a specificity of 90% and a sensitivity of 59% with a 74% positive predictive value (Colebunders et al. 1987). Even at its best, the definition lacks sensitivity, has only moderate positive prediction and fails to include useful discriminatory clinical features common to AIDS in Africa such as neurological disease (De Cock et al. 1991c).

A modified case definition used in Abidjan prescribed the need for (1) any CDC case definition or (2) a positive HIV test plus either "slim disease" (see their definition), multi-organ, disseminated or extrapulmonary TB, KS, or neurological features interfering with independent daily life and not explainable by a non-HIV cause (De Cock et al. 1991c). This definition improved the predictive value by excluding those HIV-negative individuals with diseases resulting in cough, fever or wasting (for example, TB or malignancy). Sensitivity was also enhanced by including HIV-positive patients with localised KS and neurological disease (for example cryptococcus or AIDS-dementia complex). In Nairobi, an increased rate of life-threatening bacterial infections was identified in HIV-positive patients, many of whom failed to meet any of the definitions of AIDS (Gilks et al. 1990a). Gilks argues that in Africa serious HIV disease should be identified for surveillance purposes and not AIDS (Gilks 1991).

Whilst proponents of the earlier, WHO/Bangui case definition continue to argue for its use given that HIV testing is still limited in many parts of Africa others feel that the political climate is such that a more rigorous definition is required to justify continued funding (Nicholl 1993). When the natural history of HIV infection in Africa is established, monitoring of HIV seroincidence and prevalence will offer the most useful surveillance tool (Gilks et al. 1990a)

Gastrointestinal Disease

Diarrhoea and Slim

Chronic diarrhoea and severe weight loss is so common and recognisable, with an overall frequency of 30%–80%, that it is known locally as "Slim" (Conlin et al. 1990; Serwadda et al. 1985; Sewankambo et al. 1987). The diarrhoea may be intermittent with asymptomatic periods followed by diarrhoeal episodes. Stools are usually liquid or semi-solid and blood and mucous is not usually found. Infective causes have been found in 30%–80% of cases depending on the extent of the investigation and clinical presentation. If those patients with unexplained chronic diarrhoea are then more extensively investigated occult infection may be found in 50% (Dryden and Shanson 1988). Obviously in Africa there is limited resource for sophisticated investigation.

Mycobacterial gut infection is contributing to the diarrhoea in the developed world but seems to play no role in Africa where *Cryptosporidium* was found in 10%–21% and Isospora in 7% in studies from Zaire and Uganda (Sewankambo et al. 1987). *Enterocytozoon bieneusi* and other species of microsporidia are important causes of diarrhoea in HIV infected people (Orenstein et al. 1990). Gastrointestinal infection with *Blastocystis hominis* was more frequent in HIV-infected Tanzanian children when compared with an HIV-negative chronic diarrhoea group (Cegielski et al. 1993).

A specific HIV enteropathy has been described with abnormal villus and crypt architecture and is probably due to T cell dysfunction but this appearance seems to be independent of whether the patient has diarrhoea or not (Greenson et al. 1991). Treatment for diarrhoea in Africa is usually symptomatic and supportive as extensive investigation beyond microscopy and culture is not widely available and anti-diarrhoeals or antibiotics are given empirically. Helminth infestation is found to a comparable degree in both HIV positive and HIV negative persons although one study has shown that a large proportion of HIV positive children with chronic diarrhoea had intestinal parasites which might have been responsible for their symptoms (Cegielski et al. 1993).

Salmonella infections, especially *S. typhimurium*, occur more often in HIV positive persons and are more likely to be bacteraemic and recurrent in spite of appropriate therapy.

In one cross-sectional survey of adults acutely admitted to hospital in Nairobi, pneumococcal and *Salmonella typhimurium*, bacteraemia accounted for almost one quarter of HIV related acute medical admissions and the mortality from these episodes of bacteraemia was higher in the HIV positives than in HIV negatives (Gilks et al. 1990a). The *S. typhimurium* bacteraemia was often resistant to therapy with resulting prolonged bacteraemia and recurrence.

Other diseases can affect the gut such as Kaposi's sarcoma and cytomegalovirus but have not been directly implicated in the pathogenesis of "Slim".

A study of skeletal muscle biopsy in slim disease demonstrated that muscle fibre atrophy was non-specific, and could not be distinguished from wasting related to dual infection with TB and HIV or HIV plus chronic diarrhoea and/or prolonged fever. Furthermore, the latter syndrome failed to reach the CDC case definition of HIV wasting syndrome in 5 of 10 patients (Mhiri et al. 1992).

Candida

Oral candida is a sensitive clinical marker of immunosuppression and is common in African HIV patients. Extension into the oesophagus results in odynophagia; usually a clinical diagnosis. Topical therapy may be given but the results are often unsatisfactory and oral long-term systemic agents are required. Ketoconazole is not available in all countries. Expense, resistant strains arising from long-term use and toxicity are all factors in limiting its use. Even fewer countries can afford the newer azole compounds such as fluconazole and itraconazole. Gentian violet appears to be a cheap and effective anti-candidal drug and more useful than topical nystatin and short course ketoconazole. Its use as first line treatment for oral thrush will continue in many parts of Africa.

Pulmonary Disease

Tuberculosis (TB)

Tuberculosis (TB) has become the most important manifestation of HIV infection in Africa (De Cock et al. 1992). The rise in tuberculosis cases represents the major threat to public health as, unlike other opportunistic infections, TB can spread to the HIV negative population. TB probably accounts for 7% of all deaths in the developing world and for 26% of preventable adult deaths (Murray et al. 1990).

The prevalence of HIV infection among TB patients is high. In several African studies 20%–67% of TB cases are HIV positive compared with 10%–20% of controls (De Cock et al. 1992). A cohort study in Abidjan calculated that 35% of TB cases could be attributed to HIV infection (De Cock et al. 1991b) and in an autopsy study, 36% of all HIV positive deaths were due to disseminated, multibacillary TB (De Cock et al. 1992). These facts are not surprising considering the high HIV seroprevalence in Africa, coupled with an estimated annual risk of TB infection of 1.5%–2.5% (Murray et al. 1990) and a TB prevalence rate (harbouring infection without disease) of greater than 50% in adults (Slutkin et al. 1988).

Clinical TB in HIV probably arises from reactivation of latent infection but there appears to be an increased risk of person-to-person spread if an HIV-positive person is exposed to a sputum positive index case (Di Perri et al. 1989). There is no evidence, however, that persons with HIV and TB are more infectious. The interaction between the two diseases is such that with decreasing immunity and abnormal immunological surveillance, latent TB becomes active in persons with HIV. However not only does TB itself lower CD4 counts, but immune stimulation by tuberculosis could theoretically switch on HIV replication and increase the rate of immunosuppression. Evidence to support this theory includes the fact that the development of TB is a recognised risk factor for the development of AIDS (Sunderam et al. 1986). If this is the case, then early prevention and diagnosis of TB in HIV-positive persons would be even more important.

One strategy to decrease the risk of reactivation of TB would be to give HIV-positive persons isoniazid chemoprophylaxis. In one study from Zambia, 6 months of isoniazid appeared to be efficacious as chemoprophylaxis in HIV-infected patients but the optimum duration and protection has not been determined. Practically, the funding and organisation of providing chemoprophylaxis to all HIV-positive patients in Africa would be an impossible task; in addition, drug-resistant TB could develop if supervision of chemoprophylaxis were poor.

Patterns of clinical presentation correlate with the host immune status and these are reflected in the microbiology and histopathological appearances. The spectrum ranges from "paucibacillary" TB, usually pulmonary or lymphadenopathic disease, associated with relatively high CD4 counts, giant and epithelioid cells and caseating granulomas to a non-reactive, disseminated "multibacillary" disease with low CD4 counts, a granular necrotic appearance and reduced macrophages. This spectrum is analogous to leprosy (De Cock et al. 1992). Pulmonary disease is still commonest in HIV-positive persons with TB but the proportion of extrapulmonary or disseminated TB has increased (Pitchenik et al. 1987; Sunderam et al. 1986). TB cases infected with either HIV-1 or -2 differ significantly from seronegatives in having AIDS-related features such as wasting, chronic diarrhoea, oral candidiasis and generalised lymphadenopathy (Gnaore et al. 1993).

The chest radiograph may be atypical although classical upper zone involvement, a primary-like picture in an adult, or two or more thoracic structures involved are suggestive of underlying immunosuppression. The tendency not to form cavities because of poor immune responses is thought to be the reason why patients are often sputum negative but culture positive (Pitchenik et al. 1987). Up to 50% of patients are anergic. Paradoxically, this fact may support the diagnosis of HIV once a diagnosis of TB has been established. Tuberculous lymphadenitis may be diagnosed by wide needle aspiration with a sensitivity of 96% (Bem et al. 1993).

The American Thoracic Society recommend that treatment of TB in HIV should be continued for 6 months after cultures become negative and that treatment for extrapulmonary TB should continue for 9 months. These recommendations are not based on any data. They also suggest that treatment should continue for 18 months if regimens do not contain isoniazid or rifampicin. These guidelines cannot be followed by most developing countries where TB culture is not routine, and excellent compliance difficult to achieve.

In much of Africa various drug regimes are used, based on research done in East Africa. Two common regimes are isoniazid, pyrazinamide, streptomycin and thiacetazone for 2 months followed by a continuation phase of isoniazid and thiacetazone to complete a year of total treatment. An alternative for sputum positive cases is to add rifampicin for the first 2 months and maintain the same continuation phase but for 6 months only.

There are potential hazards of administering streptomycin as injections carry a risk of transmitting HIV. For this reason the International Union against Tuberculosis and Lung Disease have suggested that streptomycin no longer be used.

Hypersensitivity drug reactions occur more commonly with streptomycin and even more so with thiacetazone. Serious reactions such as epidermal necrolysis and Stevens-Johnson syndrome are more common with thiacetazone in HIV positives compared with HIV negative persons (Nunn et al. 1991).

Although overall cure rates for TB are similar in HIV positive compared with HIV negative persons, overall mortality is much higher in the HIV positive group because of death from non-tuberculous disease (Chaisson and Slutkin 1989; De Cock et al. 1990). WHO still recommends the use of BCG in all neonates, children and adults except in suspected or symptomatic HIV infection. Whether BCG actually provides protection in HIV positive persons is conjecture.

BCG appears to be safe although anecdotal reports of dissemination and severe reactions to its use have been noted in HIV positive persons even occurring many years after vaccination (Armbruster et al. 1990). These are probably not of major significance overall. It has also been suggested that infants who do not react to BCG may be HIV positive.

It is estimated that 1.5×10^6 people are dually infected with TB and HIV in subSaharan Africa and this number is rapidly increasing. TB is already a major burden on African government health services. Many countries are seriously attempting to develop new strategies for coping with this marriage of old and new epidemics but the recent vision of a tuberculous-free world is fading away.

Mycobacterium Avium Infection

Resources are limited in the developing world and precise identification of different mycobacterial species may not always be feasible. Although *Mycobacterium avium* is common in the environment in Africa, very little *M. avium* has been documented. The diagnosis of *M. avium* is time consuming and not often technologically available in Africa. Many studies have failed to identify *M. avium* (De Cock et al. 1991b; Gilks et al. 1990a).

Pneumococcal Disease

High rates of pneumococcal bacteraemia have been reported in patients with HIV (Gilks et al. 1990b). Epidemiological data strongly suggest that acute bacterial pneumonia is an important cause of death in some high risk groups, even though acute bacterial pneumonia is not part of AIDS surveillance. Acute pneumococcal pneumonia is a common illness in Africa and appears to be on the increase due to an association with HIV (Gilks et al. 1990b). In Rwanda, in children less than 2 years old, bacteraemia was significantly more common in those who were HIV positive. Similar findings have been found in San Francisco where the rate of pneumococcal bacteraemia is 100 fold greater in AIDS patients than the rate reported in patients before the HIV epidemic arose (Redd et al. 1990). Interestingly, more than half of all the episodes of pneumococcal bacteraemia are occurring in HIV infected patients without AIDS. This tendency to develop pneumococcal disease may reflect deficiency of IgG2 which has been noted in AIDS patients.

Pneumocystis Carinii Pneumonia (PCP)

Fifty six percent of all AIDS patients present with pneumocystis carinii pneumonia (PCP) in America and Europe and there have been over 60,000 cases of PCP in the USA since 1981. However, it is debatable whether PCP is an important opportunistic infection in Africa, although it has been well documented in Africans with AIDS living in Europe. In similar experiments to those performed by Walzer, Griffin and Lucas did not detect PCP infection in their immunosuppressed mice in Kenya and speculated that climatic and geographic factors could be important in the transmission of PCP (Griffin and Lucas 1982).

Before AIDS, PCP was occasionally found in Africa in immunosuppressed patients in Nigeria, the Congo and the Republic of South Africa. Although thought to be uncommon, PCP has occurred in HIV positive patients with pneumonia in several African countries. Of 78 seropositive autopsies in Abidjan, PCP was found in 9% (Abouya et al. 1992). Among patients with HIV and clinical or radiological pneumonia, 22% were found to have PCP in one study from Zimbabwe (McLeod et al. 1989), the clinical picture being similar to patients in the developed world. The numbers studied were small and selected and may have overemphasised the importance of PCP.

In Zambia, 4 of 27 AIDS patients with clinical pneumonia of unknown aetiology were found to have probable trophozoites of *Pneumocystis*, although no cysts were present in their sputum and no definite diagnosis of PCP was made (Elvin et al. 1989).

The reason for the global variation in prevalence of PCP may be due to lack of diagnostic skills, facilities and techniques (such as induced sputum or "Diff-quick" staining). Genetic or environmental differences remain speculative. It may well be, and there are some supportive data, that other infections, especially TB, infect HIV patients earlier in their immune suppression and that patients die from these initial or subsequent infections before their CD4 count drops below 200 cells/mm^3 and so are at high risk of developing PCP (Elvin et al. 1989).

There have been so few cases of PCP reported in Africa that the database regarding therapy, complications and relapse is inadequate to draw any firm conclusions. But, in Zimbabwe, treatment for PCP with high dose oral cotrimoxazole was due to the lack of availability and the cost of intravenous preparations. Clindamycin and primaquine in combination could be given to those who reacted to co-trimoxazole as these drugs are more often easily available in

Africa. Prophylaxis with dapsone or co-trimoxazole was then encouraged after a first episode of PCP. Pentamidine was unavailable for both treatment and prophylaxis.

Fungal Infections

Disseminated histoplasmosis can occur in HIV positive persons (Graybill 1988) usually from reactivation of quiescent infection. It can resemble TB or Pneumocystis carinii pneumonia (PCP), although hypoxia is not a feature. *Histoplasma spp.* can be isolated from any site especially sputum, lymph nodes, marrow or spleen. Infection with *H. duboisii*, the African variety of *Histoplasma*, appears to be rare. Whether it is because *H. duboisii* acts differently from *H. capsulatum* or because it is found in remote areas where HIV prevalence is low is not known.

Aspergillosis is unusual in AIDS patients and when it occurs it does so in two distinct forms: invasive or obstructive bronchial aspergillosis (Denning et al. 1991). It infects patients with severe immunosuppression or neutropenia and responds poorly to treatment. As yet there have been no reports of these forms of aspergillosis from Africa where, even if diagnosed, the scope for treatment would be limited.

Tumours

Kaposi's Sarcoma (KS)

Kaposi's sarcoma (pronounced Kop-osh-ee) was initially recognised in 1872 in elderly males of Mediterranean or Ashkanazic Jewish origin. Epidemiologically, KS can be classified into (i) classical, (ii) African, (iii) immunosuppression-associated such as organ-transplant recipients and (iv) AIDS-related (Peterman et al. 1993). Whilst there is considerable overlap, these categories do give an indication of natural history. For example, when an immunosuppressive agent is stopped, as in the case of a transplant recipient, the KS may regress and sometimes disappear entirely.

Classical KS is considered an indolent cutaneous disease of old men, but even in the original paper, Kaposi alluded to the fact that the disease has the propensity to involve extracutaneous sites. The African form of KS was recognised in the 1950s and appeared to occur in well defined geographical areas of Central Africa, accounting for about 10% of all malignancies in the Congo, Kenya and Tanzania. Both the classical and African form of KS have a strong male predominance (15 : 1 in Kaposi's original description). This ratio has gradually diminished with time and may be the result of an increasing agent or co-factor in women (Wahman et al. 1991). In African children the sex ratio was only 3 : 1 and the tumour is rapidly progressive and fatal. The association with immunosuppression was first noted in renal transplant recipients in the 1970s (Wahman et al. 1991). In 1980, an unusual aggressive form of KS was reported in male homosexuals from the USA. This new aggressive form of KS was also recognised in Zambia and found to be related to HIV seropositivity. Its incidence still appears to be increasing and it accounts for about 90% of all the KS seen in Africa.

Clues as to the aetiology of KS have been summarised recently (Peterman et al. 1993; Wahman et al. 1991). The frequency of AIDS-related KS is highest amongst New York and Californian homosexual men and lowest amongst recipients of clotting factors. Rates are also relatively high for Africans and blood transfusion recipients and relatively lower for injecting-drug users. Rates of KS in sexual partners of the above groups tend to reflect the rate of the group belonging to sexual contact. These epidemiological factors strongly implicate a sexually-transmitted infectious KS agent. Faeco-oral transmission has also been suggested, but not demonstrated, in all studies. The fact that blood transfusion is a higher risk factor than factor VIII concentrate may reflect that the putative agent is highly cell-associated or destroyed by the preparation process (Peterman et al. 1993).

As opposed to the localised nodular endemic disease which may also involve local lymph nodes, the epidemic HIV-related type commonly presents with multifocal lesions, red to purple plaques or papules which can progress to nodules or form ulcerating lesions. The cutaneous lesions tend to be smaller in this HIV-related type compared with the classical endemic form and tend to involve the mouth, head, neck and upper trunk more commonly whereas 75% of the endemic form occurs only on the legs. The mucous membranes, mouth, anus, lymph nodes, gastrointestinal tract and lungs are also more often involved and woody oedema of the limbs is also commonly seen in Africa.

At autopsy, HIV related KS lesions have been noted in virtually every organ including the brain (Gill et al. 1990). Pulmonary involvement is relatively common and may present with cough and fever, haemoptysis and infiltrates seen on the chest film. This presentation is often clinically misdiagnosed as tuberculosis in Africa and occasionally as PCP.

There is no uniformly accepted staging system for KS and it is felt that tumour regression and survival after treatment are related to the degree of immune deficiency and not to tumour bulk or site. Clinically, KS has been divided into four types: nodular, florid, infiltrative and lymphadenopathic. All types can be found in AIDS-related KS and they do not give an indication of prognosis.

Many patients are treated in Africa and although the quality of life has improved and major symptoms alleviated, there is no proof that any treatment prolongs life (Volberding et al. 1989). These treatments have usually been limited to chemotherapy or local or systemic radiotherapy which is easy, cheap, and well tolerated once the infrastructure to use it has been organised. Chemotherapy with vincristine, vinblastine, doxorubicin, bleomycin, and VP16 as single or combination agents is also used but these treatments have a palliative role to play and run the risk of further increasing immune suppression. The cost of the drugs, medical care and side effects are an additional burden to patient and health care systems which may not be affordable or desirable, and the use of high dose interferons and zidovudine is beyond the economic capabilities of many African countries.

Other Tumours

Squamous cell tumours of the skin, mouth, epiglottis, lung, anorectum, conjunctiva, cervix and many other sites have already been reported in HIV. Malignancies may be on the increase in HIV-positive children. Although studies from America have demonstrated an increase in high grade non-Hodgkin's lymphoma in HIV (Beral et al. 1991), no clear association has been seen in Africa. Burkitt's lymphoma has a strong association with HIV and occurs 1000 times more commonly in AIDS patients in the USA (Mbidde et al. 1990) but this association has yet to be extensively studied in Africa.

Skin Diseases

Leprosy

There are no convincing data for any association between leprosy and HIV. Although an association was suggested there has been no evidence for this in Malawi (Meeran 1989), in Ethiopia (Tekle-Haimanot et al. 1991) or in Guinea-Bissau with HIV-2 (Ferro et al. 1990). This may reflect the slow rate of disease progression and differences may become apparent with further observation. Fleming believes that there is accelerated progress of both HIV and leprosy diseases in dually-infected patients (Fleming 1990). It might be expected that if an interaction were to take place, there would be a down-grading from tuberculoid-type disease (paucibacillary with well-formed granulomas) to lepromatous cases (multi-bacillary with no granulomas).

Fungal Infections

Fungal infections figure prominently among the opportunistic infections that are so characteristic of AIDS. Mucocutaneous candidiasis, cryptococcosis and histoplasmosis depend on compromised, cell-mediated immunity and are common problems in HIV positive patients, whereas disseminated candida or aspergillosis depend on bloodstream invasion due to profound neutropenia and are not found as often (Mandal 1989).

It is difficult to assess whether HIV is associated with a greater incidence of superficial mycosis, as most reports come from institute-based series with no comparable control groups of immunocompetent persons. Seborrhoeic dermatitis was previously rare in Africans but it is now common in patients with HIV infection. Although seborrhoeic dermatitis may be related to the uninhibited growth of *Pityrosporum* or related fungi, one detailed dermatopathological study from Europe found little to support this theory (Soeprono et al. 1986).

Other infections such as blastomycosis and mucormycosis (Cuadrado et al. 1988) occur rarely in HIV but as the epidemic evolves, some of the lesser known fungal diseases may well assume prominence.

Herpes Zoster

The incidence of herpes zoster in HIV positive individuals is about seven times greater than that of the general population, and the incidence of HIV seropositivity in members of high risk groups who present with zoster is 92% (Colebunders et al. 1988). The positive predictive value of a history of shingles for HIV positivity is 90%. The progression by such HIV positive individuals to AIDS is at the rate of about 1% per month after presentation (Melbye et al. 1986). Zoster often occurs as the first manifestation of progressive HIV infection preceding candida and oral leucoplakia by an average of 1.5 years (Colebunders et al. 1988). The clinical presentation may be typical with radicular pain or dermatomal eruption (Gulick et al. 1991), but two or more dermatomes and dissemination are common and the morbidity and mortality are increased and clinical relapse common. Spontaneous healing occurs but the rate of post-herpetic neuralgia is undefined in Africa.

Treatment with acyclovir, especially high dose intravenous therapy, is too costly and impracticable for Africa.

Generalised Prurigo

Other skin diseases related to HIV such as molluscum contagiosum and cutaneous cryptococcosis occur in Africans and are described in detail elsewhere. One of the most specific in Africans is an itchy widespread nodular prurigo (Liautaud et al. 1989) which occurred in 21% of HIV infected patients in Zaire.

Hair Changes

In advanced HIV infection, the normally curly hair of Africans tends to become straight and silky and the changes in the hair resemble those seen in protein-calorie malnutrition. Moreover, the eyelashes become long and black lines can be seen on the nails (Pozniak, personal observation).

Sexually Transmitted Diseases

Sexual Behaviour – Traditional and Modern

Attitudes vary widely among different ethnic groups and among regions in subSaharan Africa. However, the majority of traditional African tribes used to expect virginity in the females at first marriage. Many cultures imposed sanctions against promiscuity, whilst others would accept premarital non-penetrative sex (Prual et al. 1991). If premarital sexual intercourse did occur, the woman's kin would be concerned that pregnancy, not loss of virginity, would spoil a marriage. Consequently the level of premarital births was usually below 5% of the total number of annual births. Male chastity was not praised and male premarital experience was often limited to rare contact with prostitutes. Men tended to marry later than women because of dowry problems, polygamy levels, labour migration and land shortage. Men could only be accused of adultery if they had sex with another man's wife. For married women, all other men were taboo (Prual et al. 1991). Punishment for adultery was strict and severe, but long periods of sexual abstinence post-partum (from 40 days to over a year) was a major reason for men seeking sex elsewhere, traditionally with other wives.

Economic pressure encouraged married men to separate from their families and migrate from the rural areas to cities, thus creating a group of unattached men. This urbanisation reduced social control and began the move away from the traditional codes of marriage. In many cities in eastern and southern Africa men usually outnumber women and a core group of prostitutes and bar girls offer an alternative male sexual outlet. In subSaharan Africa, the concept of prostitution must be understood broadly. Sexual permissiveness for urban women changed with the emergence of a more sophisticated sexual structure allowing mistresses, lovers and concubines. Moreover, women in regular but poorly paid employment now sold sex to supplement their income. This core group of sex workers together with their clients have been termed "high frequency transmitters" (Moses et al. 1991). Up to 80% of male STD patients in these areas reported that prostitutes were the source of their infection, in contrast with <20% in Europe and North America (Laga et al. 1991).

Prior to the advent of HIV, sexually transmitted diseases (STDs) were a major health care problem in Africa. In 1972, very high rates of STDs were reported among Rwandan male university students. Incidence rates of gonorrhoea and syphilis were 30% and 9% respectively over a 9-month period (Laga et al. 1991). Pelvic inflammatory disease is the commonest cause of gynaecological admission in Africa. This is associated with a high rate of ectopic pregnancy and mortality (due to poor critical care facilities). Further obstetric problems include prematurity, stillbirth and infertility. The high rate of STDs also contributes to infant morbidity including congenital syphilis, ophthalmia neonatorum and chlamydia pneumonia. Treatment is often inappropriate or inadequate and has resulted in widespread antibiotic resistance for both gonorrhoea and chancroid. To compound all of these problems, HIV, itself an STD, has severely aggravated the situation.

Interrelationship between HIV and STDs

The relationship between HIV and STDs is complex. Three means of interaction are possible. (1) The presence of an STD in either the HIV positive or negative partner can enhance transmission (Laga et al. 1991). (2) HIV disease may affect STDs by increasing the frequency, altering the natural history, diagnosis and response to treatment. Thus, an STD may act as a marker of HIV-related immunosuppression. (3) STDs may accelerate progression of HIV infection.

Given that HIV is itself an STD, an association between HIV and other STDs may merely be the consequence of high risk behaviour. Furthermore, an increase in an STD may be subsequent to HIV induced-immunodeficiency as seen with an increase in herpes attacks. These methodological problems are answered, at least in part, by prospective cohort studies identifying a temporal relationship between STDs and subsequent HIV seroconversion.

Both genital ulcer disease (GUD) and non-ulcerative STD increase the transmission of HIV (Laga et al. 1993; Plummer et al. 1991). The increase in infectiousness is biologically plausible. STDs increase the pool of T lymphocytes and macrophages which are the HIV-susceptible or of HIV-infected cells found in genital secretions. Moreover, STDs cause a breakdown in the epithelial barrier, either macroscopically, in GUD, or as micro-ulcerations in the genital mucosa of non-ulcerative STD. Ulcers bleed easily and HIV has been found in biopsies of the ulcer base. The dense lymphocytic infiltrate around these ulcers is a primary target for HIV infection. An increased viral shedding from the ulcer would increase the infectivity of the index case. Any ulcer would also provide an easy portal of entry for HIV infection.

Genital Ulcer Disease (GUD)

Of all STDs, GUD and HIV infection have the strongest association. The most convincing evidence that GUD enhances HIV transmission comes from prospective studies of clients and prostitutes from Nairobi. Relative risk (RR), adjusted after multivariate analysis (confounders included sexual activity and condom use), demonstrated an independent relationship between GUD and subsequent HIV seroconversion in male partners (RR 4.7) (Cameron et al. 1989) and in female prostitutes (RR 3.3) (Plummer et al. 1991).

Chancroid (*H. ducreyi*)

Chancroid is the commonest cause of GUD in Africa and in one study accounted for 85% of genital ulcers in STD clinic attenders and prostitutes in Nairobi (Nsanze 1981). HIV positivity causes both an increase in incidence and persistence of chancroid ulceration in spite of standard antibiotic treatment. This lack of responsiveness has been used as a predictor for HIV status. Transmission of HIV to wives of HIV positive men is much more likely if the man has had a history of genital ulcer (Latif et al. 1989).

Syphilis

Although a positive TPHA result is associated with HIV positivity in Nairobi prostitutes and a cohort of homosexual men, the same was not found in Kinshasa or in Nairobi male STD attenders (Simonsen et al. 1988). It is likely that primary syphilis does increase transmission of HIV, but evidence is less good than for the other STDs.

The impact of HIV on syphilis is unclear, and assumptions about natural history and serology have been based on a number of studies which have lacked an HIV negative patient comparison group. These studies have suggested that co-infection with HIV may result in atypical clinical presentation, false-negative or false-positive serological tests and more frequent progression (or latent reactivation) to neurosyphilis (Hook 1989).

A small study, which included an HIV negative control group, offered some evidence of the failure of benzathine penicillin in the treatment of early syphilis in patients with HIV co-infection (Lukehart et al. 1988). However, more frequent progression to neurosyphilis was not supported by other studies (McMillan et al. 1990). Procaine penicillin cured syphilis and prevented the occurrence of late manifestations in spite of infection with HIV. Furthermore, patients who had prior therapy for syphilis with benzathine penicillin might go on to develop neurosyphilis whether or not they had HIV infection (Berry et al. 1987). Secondary syphilis is usually associated with a high RPR titre, even in HIV positives, but some patients may have no positive syphilis serology. Limited data indicate that a new treponemal infection in an HIV-infected individual may not result in the development of cardiolipin or specific antibodies. Also, fewer treponemal antigens are found by immunoblotting than are usually present in secondary syphilis.

Suggested guidelines for HIV positive patients are that any patient previously treated for syphilis should have serological testing. Those whose sera show a rise in cardiolipin or treponemal antibody titres should have their CSF examined and treated appropriately without delay (McMillan et al. 1990).

In some parts of Africa where antibody titres are not available it may be that the most practical course of action is to treat all suspected cases with procaine penicillin and accept that some patients are overtreated.

Herpes Simplex Virus 2 (HSV-2)

A prospective cohort study of homosexual men in the USA has demonstrated a strong association between HSV-2 seroconversion and subsequent HIV seroconversion (RR 4.4) (Holmberg et al. 1988). Chronic, frequent, severe episodes of HSV-2 occur in HIV positive persons. In a cohort study of female HIV positive and negative prostitutes in Zaire, GUD (mainly HSV-2) was three times more common in those who were HIV positive. Although the disease responds to treatment, there is usually a need for continuing suppressive therapy. Acyclovir is expensive and the prolonged treatment required is not available throughout Africa. Herpes is therefore usually treated symptomatically with local applications of gentian violet and oral analgesia.

Non-ulcerative STDs

Chlamydia Infection, Gonorrhoea and Trichomoniasis

Chlamydia infection was independently associated with HIV seroconversion in a prospective cohort study of a 124 female Nairobi prostitutes (Plummer et al. 1991). In Zaire, 431 HIV-negative prostitutes were enrolled into a 2-year cohort study. Multivariate analysis demonstrated increased HIV-seroconversion for gonorrhoea, chlamydial infection and trichomoniasis. Adjusted odds ratios 4.8, 3.6, and 1.9 respectively having controlled for number of partners and condom use (Laga et al. 1993). Whilst GUDs were more frequent in cases than controls, they were much less common than other non-ulcerative STDs. This was reflected in the low attributable risk of 4% (compared with 44, 22, and 18% for gonorrhoea, chlamydia and trichomoniasis respectively).

There is no evidence that HIV alters the presentation, clinical course or treatment of lower tract non-ulcerative STD. But some evidence exists to suggest a higher incidence of gonococcal PID.

Human Papilloma Virus (HPV)

There appears to be no association between HPV (wart virus infection) and HIV transmission (Kent et al. 1987). However, HIV has a marked impact on genital warts. This results in severe, prolonged and recurrent disease (McMillan and Bishop 1989) sometimes requiring surgical removal because of size. It is worrying that HIV appears to act as an important cofactor for the development of anogenital dysplasia. It remains to be seen if cervical and anal cancer will emerge as complications of HIV.

Circumcision

Lack of circumcision was noted as an independent risk factor for HIV transmission in men attending an STD clinic in Nairobi (Cameron et al. 1989). This has been confirmed by others and the observation has been extended to demonstrate higher HIV seropositivity among women whose husbands are uncircumcised. This has been explained in terms of: an increase in balanitis, a larger surface area for contact with HIV, increased trauma and trapping of virus (vaginal, cervical secretions) under the foreskin after intercourse (Hunter 1993).

One way of trying to curb HIV epidemic is by controlling STDs (Laga et al. 1991). Some countries such as Zimbabwe, which reported 1 million STDs in 1989, now have national STD programmes which aim to prevent HIV transmission. These are funded by international agencies as well as local resources and are integrated into HIV prevention campaigns.

Intervention, Counselling and Condoms

Intervention studies are required in order to evaluate health education, condom use and STD control. Two such studies have demonstrated that encouraging condom use produces a reduction in HIV (Allen et al. 1992; Moses et al. 1991). In Rwanda, both HIV and gonorrhoea rates went down in a cohort of 1548 urban women who were shown a video about AIDS, counselled and tested for HIV and given free condoms (Allen et al. 1992). In an STD/HIV control programme in Nairobi sex-workers, condoms were promoted and STDs diagnosed and treated. The authors estimated that 6000 to 10,000 cases of HIV infection were prevented per year with a cost of approximately 8-12 US$ for each case prevented (Moses et al. 1991).

Rheumatological Problems

Among patients presenting with acute septic and non-septic arthritis in Rwanda, 72% were found to be HIV positive, and in tropical Africa there appears to be an increase in reactive arthritis of the Reiters-type in HIV positive patients. The bulk of evidence in the developed world does point toward a real association between reactive arthritis and HIV positivity (Kaye 1989) but some work from the USA has found no correlation in homosexual men.

Septic arthritis with opportunistic organisms (Rogers et al. 1988) and recurrence of acute rheumatic fever are both associated with HIV positivity. However, data are still needed from Africa regarding the importance of these problems and the arthropathy associated with HIV infection has not been well documented.

Neurological Disease

There is a great need for more information about the role of HIV and neurological morbidity and mortality in Africa as there is little documented about neurological disease compared with the developed world. Early case reports, of Africans treated in Europe, described cerebral toxoplasmosis or cryptococcal meningitis (Clumeck et al. 1984). In one study from Tanzania 10.5% of 200 patients with HIV had an obvious focal neurological disorder such as cranial nerve palsies, hemiparesis, or paraparesis. Of the rest 72% had less obvious neurological disorders including dementia (54%), retinopathy (23%), areflexia (21%), pyramidal tract signs (19%) and tremor and incoordination (Howlett et al. 1989).

Guillain–Barre syndrome (Howlett et al. 1989), facial palsy (Belec et al. 1989), painful peripheral neuropathy and psychiatric syndromes appear to be increasing in Africa and many patients with severe immunosuppression appear demented. There is a strong association between endemic tropical spastic paraparesis and HTLV-1 but no association with HIV has yet been demonstrated. There is little known about the epidemiology of cytomegalovirus disease in Africa but anecdotal cases have been seen. Due to the lack of technology, many neurological conditions are treated empirically after diseases such as pyogenic meningitis, TB meningitis and neurosyphilis have been excluded by lumbar puncture.

Cryptococcus

No hard data on the frequency of cryptococcal infection are available from Africa but it appears that the incidence is increasing (Laroche et al. 1992) and is higher than the 3.2% of patients with HIV reported to the Public Health Laboratory service in the USA. Although visceral and cutaneous cryptococcus occurs, meningeal infection is commonest and in one African study, cryptococcal meningitis occurred in 8% of HIV positive patients admitted with a fever. There was a sevenfold increase in cryptococcal meningitis in 1978–1984 compared with 1973–1977, due to the interaction with HIV. Unfortunately for the clinician working in low technology areas, signs and symptoms of meningitis may be lacking and cerebrospinal fluid (CSF) changes less marked in HIV positive patients. Cryptococcal antigens in the blood and CSF are useful investigations but expensive and technology-dependent. However India ink staining of CSF is simple and needs only a microscope and a good supply of ink.

Epidemiologically, *Cryptococcus neoformans var neoformans* appears to be the commonest serogroup infecting AIDS patients even in Africa where *C. neoformans var gatti* is endemic. Treatment is costly and requires either intravenous amphotericin or oral fluconazole. Relapses from reservoirs in the prostate can occur, requiring long-term maintenance therapy. Many African countries do not treat cryptococcal infection as the treatment is too expensive.

Toxoplasmosis

Infection of humans by the protozoan *Toxoplasma gondii* is common, but relatively few immunocompetent persons develop toxoplasmosis. It is probably the most important cause of focal brain lesions in AIDS patients in the developed world. The incidence of toxoplasma encephalitis, which results from a recrudescence of latent infection, is directly related to the seroprevalence rate in a given risk group and so depends on both the risk associated with developing AIDS and the geographical variations in the seroprevalence of toxoplasma infection. This rate varies from 5%–40% of patients with AIDS. It is thought to be commoner in patients from Africa than in those from Europe or the USA (Sonnet et al. 1987) but the true incidence of CNS toxoplasmosis causing focal abscess or diffuse meningoencephalitis is not known. Unfortunately, diagnosis depends not only on the clinical situation but also on serum toxoplasma tests, a CT scan and, occasionally, brain biopsy. In most of Africa, none of these tests can be routinely performed because of lack of resources. The picture is also confused in Africa by the common occurrence of pyogenic abscess, tuberculous meningitis and meningovascular syphilis, which produce similar syndromes to toxoplasmosis.

In Africa empirical treatment with pyrimethamine and sulphonamides could be used as a diagnostic and therapeutic tool, as almost all patients with toxoplasmosis will have responded clinically by day 10–14. Unfortunately, late initiation of specific treatment and failure to consider the diagnosis of toxoplasmosis is associated with a poor prognosis. Patients who have recovered should embark upon lifelong prophylaxis which, arguably, needs more clinical certainty in making an initial diagnosis than a clinical assessment and an empirical trial of treatment.

Paediatric Problems

WHO estimated, by 1991 approximately 180,000 AIDS cases in children aged 0–4 years in subSaharan Africa. In 10 Central and East African countries, HIV and AIDS will cause between one quarter and half a million child deaths annually by the year 2000 (Preble 1990). The United Nations estimate that, without AIDS, the under-five mortality rate in these countries would be $132/10^5$, but with AIDS it will rise to between 159 and $189/10^5$. In this decade, HIV/AIDS will kill a total of between 1.5 and 2.9 million women of reproductive age in this region, producing 3.1–5.5 million AIDS orphans. This means that 6%–11% of the population under 15 will be orphans. In 1991, in four districts of Uganda, the total number of orphans was between 0.6 and 1.2×10^6. Supportive treatment is all that can be offered at present, and prevention policies are of paramount importance.

HIV can be transmitted vertically from mother to child in utero and via breast milk. However, breast feeding should be actively encouraged because, in the developing world, the benefits considerably outweigh any risk of HIV transmission. Other sources of transmission include blood transfusion and the re-use of needles without adequate sterilisation. A large study of HIV infection and severe malnutrition in Burkina Faso demonstrated 77% mother-to-child transmission, 13% resulting from transfusions and 10% from multiple injections (Prazuck et al. 1993). The clinical picture in African children is varied and as complex as in adults (Ryder et al. 1989). The incubation period for African paediatric AIDS appears to be similar to that observed in the USA with two distinct populations, one with a short incubation period and another with a longer one. Thus, the risk of developing AIDS in <18 month old children is greater than >18 months (Commenges et al. 1992).

The clinical picture includes: failure to thrive, diarrhoea, persistent cough, hepatosplenomegaly, recurrent bacterial infections – especially of the middle ear and lung, and chronic eczematous skin rash. The epidemic form of Kaposi's sarcoma is also being seen (Bouquety et al. 1989). The persistent cough is often due to lymphocytic interstitial pneumonitis and is usually misdiagnosed as miliary TB.

WHO proposed a provisional clinical case definition of AIDS in children (World Health Organization 1986) but it appears to lack sensitivity and positive predictive value when compared to HIV serology alone (Jonckheer et al. 1988).

AIDS Case Definition for African Children

The definition of AIDS in African children requires two major and two minor criteria in the absence of known causes of immune suppression. The major criteria are weight loss or abnormal slow growth; chronic diarrhoea for more than one month; and prolonged fever for more than one month. The minor criteria are generalised lymphadenopathy; oropharyngeal candida; repeated common infections (otitis, pharyngitis etc); persistent cough; generalised dermatitis; and confirmed maternal HIV infection.

Other Tropical Problems

Malaria

As both HIV and malaria are endemic in subSaharan Africa, there is concern that the immunosuppression caused by HIV might increase both the risk and severity of *Plasmodium falciparum* infection and decrease the response to antimalarial treatment. Evidence is conflicting but there appears no direct interaction of clinical importance between HIV and *P. falciparum* (Lucas 1990). Oral quinine appears to be efficacious in the treatment of non-severe falciparum malaria, whatever the HIV status. However, malaria may cause severe anaemia requiring blood transfusion and this may lead to HIV infection if the donated blood is unscreened.

One study has shown a significantly higher number of malaria positive thick films per person months among patients with recent HIV infection. This may be due to the fact that all these people had transfusion-related HIV and so presented themselves for medical attention as soon as they developed a fever (Colebunders et al. 1990). The overall mortality in this group was higher than in HIV negative controls but the number dying from malaria was not known. More research into this interaction is needed, so that malaria control programmes can respond appropriately.

Visceral Leishmaniasis

Visceral leishmaniasis is endemic in Sudan and Kenya and sporadic cases occur in Central and Southern Africa. A study from Spain has shown that in HIV positive patients there is often an absence of Leishmania antibodies (Montalban et al. 1990). These patients also follow a chronic relapsing course and it is unknown whether a real cure ever takes place after treatment (Peters et al. 1990). This relapsing disease may be a predictive marker for the development of AIDS due to other causes. One mechanism by which this type of chronic infection takes place is that in HIV patients lymphokine production is suppressed, especially the production of interferon gamma. Therefore, there is an inability of monocytes to phagocytose *L. donovani*. Drug costs prohibit the use of the recognised drugs such as pentamidine, stibogluconate and amphotericin.

Schistosomiasis

As yet, there are no data as to whether HIV worsens co-infection with clinical schistosomiasis. But in theory the clinical picture may be changed as the immunological response causing fibrosis may be diminished in HIV positive persons. There appears to be a surface protein on schistosomes, important for infection by the schistosome, which is very similar to virion infective factor, a regulatory protein produced by HIV when it replicates and enables the virus to infect cells. Various theories for the presence of this factor are that this protein may have evolved in parallel from a common origin in both HIV and schistosomes, or that schistosomes may have assimilated the gene from a retrovirus such as HIV-1, or the virus may have "picked up" the gene from a schistosome. It is, therefore, theoretically possible that in areas endemic for schistosomiasis, people may have some immunological ability to recognise HIV. Whether this ability reduces or exacerbates HIV infection is not known.

Hepatitis B Virus Infection

Hepatitis B infection is a major health problem in Africa. Theoretically two major interactions with HIV could occur. Firstly, reactivation of hepatitis B virus (HBV) followed by a subsequent increase in the already large numbers of hepatocellular carcinoma and, secondly, an increased susceptibility of new cases of HBV to develop a highly infectious HB_sAg positive state. There have been concerns about the efficacy of the HBV vaccine in patients who are HIV positive and this information is important to African countries who have invested in mass immunisation campaigns.

Tropical Pyomyositis

Pyomyositis is endemic in Africa and has been described in 7 patients in Europe and North America. Seven further HIV-associated cases have been reported from the Central African Republic (CAR) (Belec et al. 1991). However further epidemiological studies are needed to see whether this association is a real one as the seroprevalence of HIV in the CAR has increased fivefold in the at-risk population over the past 5 years.

The Future

Approximately 6 million persons are infected with HIV in subSaharan Africa, which accounts for half the world's HIV positive people and almost 1 African in 40 (Berkley 1992). By 1995, the Harvard Institute of International Development estimates the annual economic loss from AIDS deaths in one African country will be 350 million US$ and by the year 2000, Africa is destined to have 30% of the world's poor. Although AIDS is incurable, the many associated manifestations of HIV infection are treatable. Unfortunately, the manpower and economic wealth needed to deliver a standard of health care comparable to the developed world is unavailable and unobtainable in much of Africa. Treatments for HIV with antiviral agents cannot be afforded by most African states where the GNP/per capita is 100-650 US$ a year. AIDS control programmes would be failing if only the rich received drugs and vaccines and it is interesting to note that the combined expenditure on AIDS by the states of New York and California in 1 year was greater than that for the entire developing world.

Various compounds developed in Africa, such as low dose oral interferon or Kemron, have incited exaggerated claims as HIV cures. Vaccine trials in the developed world and Africa are under way. However, despite a decade of intensive research, there appears to be little hope in the near future. Even with an effective vaccine, practical problems are posed, such as who should be vaccinated and who will pay for it.

We cannot wait for an effective vaccine or drug. Strategies of risk reduction are required and must be directed at education, particularly condom use and treatment of STDs. Education of both the sexually active and pubertal population, preferably through peer pressure, need to convince communities to change sexual habits and practices. Encouraging the use of condoms appears to have a direct impact on reducing HIV transmission. For example, intervention studies have resulted in reduction of both STDs and HIV in sex workers in Kenya (Moses et al. 1991) and urban Rwandan women (Allen et al. 1992). It remains to be seen if these interventions are feasible across the subcontinent. There must be an effective programme for widespread treatment of STDs. Diagnosis and management can be simplified by utilising a syndromic approach, but adequate supply of effective drugs is essential. Countries such as Zimbabwe and Uganda are developing their own affordable and practicable guidelines of care. All aspects of HIV control are co-ordinated within national AIDS programmes (Goodgame 1990). Counselling networks, hospice and community care have all found an active role to play in the management of HIV.

The committed personnel who are working in all aspects of HIV throughout Africa need help, both economically and politically, for their work to succeed. If there is no control of STD and little change in sexual behaviour, the projected figures for the HIV epidemic in Africa may materialise and the continent may be lost to both poverty and disease.

References

Abouya YL, Beaumel A, Lucas S et al. (1992) Pneumocystis carinii pneumonia. An uncommon cause of death in African patients with acquired immunodeficiency syndrome. Am Rev Respir Dis 145: 617-620

Allen S, Lindan C, Serufilira A et al. (1991) Human immunodeficiency virus infection in urban Rwanda. Demographic and behavioral correlates in a representative sample of childbearing women. JAMA 266: 1657-1663

Allen S, Serufilira A, Bogaerts J et al. (1992) Confidential HIV testing and condom promotion in Africa. JAMA 268: 3338-3343

Anderson RM, May RM, Boily MC, Garnett GP, Rowley JT (1991) The spread of HIV-1 in Africa: sexual contact patterns and the predicted demographic impact of AIDS. Nature 352: 581-589

Armbruster C, Junker W, Vetter N, Jaksch G (1990) Disseminated bacille Calmette-Guerin infection in an AIDS patient 30 years after BCG vaccination. J Infect Dis 162: 1216

Barin F, M'Boup S, Denis F et al. (1985) Serological evidence for virus related to simian T-lymphotropic retrovirus III in residents of west Africa. Lancet ii: 1387-1389.

Belec L, Gherardi R, Georges AJ et al. (1989) Peripheral facial paralysis and HIV infection report of four African cases and review of the literature. J Neurol 236: 411-414

Belec L, Di Costanzo B, Georges AJ, Gherardi R (1991) HIV infection in African patients with tropical pyomyositis. AIDS 5: 234

Bem C, Patil PS, Elliott AM, Namaambo KM, Bharucha H, Porter JDH (1993) The value of wide-needle aspiration in the diagnosis of tuberculous lymphadenitis in Africa. AIDS 7: 1221-1225

Beral V, Peteman T, Berkelman R, Jaffe H (1991) AIDS-associated non-Hodgkins lymphoma. Lancet 337: 805-809

Berkley S (1991) Parenteral transmission of HIV in Africa. AIDS 5 (suppl 1): S87-S92

Berkley SF (1992) HIV in Africa: what is the future? Ann Intern Med 116: 339-341

Berkley SF, Widy-Wirski R, Okware SI et al. (1989) Risk factors associated with HIV in Uganda. J Infect Dis 160: 22-30

Berkley S, Naamara W, Okware S et al. (1990) AIDS and HIV infection in Uganda: are more women infected than men? AIDS 4: 1237-1242

Berry CD, Hooton TM, Collier AC, Lukehart SA (1987) Neurologic relapse after benzathine penicillin therapy for secondary syphilis in a patient with HIV infection. N Engl J Med 316: 1587-1589

Biggar RJ (1986) The clinical features of HIV infection in Africa. Br Med J 293: 1453-1454

Borgdorff M (1993) Sentinel surveillance for HIV-1 infection: how representative are blood donors, outpatients with fever, anaemia, or sexually transmitted diseases, and antenatal clinic attenders in Mwanza Region, Tanzania? AIDS 7: 567-572

Bouquety JC, Siopathis MR, Ravisse PR, Lagarde N, Georges-Courbot MC, Georges AJ (1989) Lymphocutaneous Kaposi's sarcoma in an African pediatric AIDS case. Am J Tropic Med Hyg 40: 323-325

Brattegaard K, Kouadio J, Adom ML, Doorly R, George JR, De Cock KM (1993) Rapid and simple screening and supplemental testing for HIV-1 and HIV-2 infections in West Africa. AIDS 7: 883-885

Bucyendore A, Van de Perre P, Karita E, Nziyumvira A, Sow I, Fox E (1993) Estimating the seroincidence of HIV-1 in the general adult population in Kigali, Rwanda. AIDS 7: 275-277

Cameron DW, Simonsen JN, D'Costa LJ et al. (1989) Female to male transmission of human immunodeficiency virus type 1: risk factors for seroconversion in men. Lancet ii: 403-407

Cegielski JP, Msengi AE, Dukes CS et al. (1993) Intestinal parasites and HIV infection in Tanzanian children with chronic diarrhea. AIDS 7: 213-221

Chaisson RE, Slutkin G (1989) Tuberculosis and human immunodeficiency virus infection. J Infect Dis 159: 96-100

Chin J (1990) Current and future dimensions of the HIV/AIDS pandemic in women and children. Lancet 336: 221-224

Chin J, Mann J (1989) Global surveillance and forecasting of AIDS. Bull World Health Organ 67: 1-7

Chin J, Remenyi MA, Morrison F, Bulatao R (1992) The global epidemiology of the HIV/AIDS pandemic. World Health Stat Q 45: 220-227

Clavel F, Guetard D, Brun-Vezinet F et al. (1986) Isolation of a new human retrovirus from West African patients with AIDS. Science 233: 343-346

Clumeck N, Jonnet J, Taelman H, Mascart Lemone F, De Bruyere M (1984) Acquired immunodeficiency syndrome in African patients. N Engl J Med 310: 492-97

Colebunders RL, Latif AS (1991) Natural history and clinical presentation of HIV-1 infection in adults. AIDS 5 (suppl 1): S103-S112

Colebunders R, Mann JM, Francis H et al. (1987) Evaluation of a clinical case-definition of acquired immunodeficiency syndrome in Africa. Lancet i: 492-494.

Colebunders R, Mann JM, Francis H et al. (1988) Herpes zoster in African patients: a clinical predictor of human immunodeficiency virus infections. J Infect Dis 157: 314-318

Colebunders R, Bahwe Y, Nekwei W et al. (1990) Incidence of malaria and efficacy of oral quinine in patients recently infected with human immunodeficiency virus in Kinshasa, Zaire. J Infect 21: 167-173

Commenges D, Alioum A, Lepage P, Van de Perre P, Msellati P, Dabis F (1992) Estimating the incubation period of paediatric AIDS in Rwanda. AIDS 6: 1515-1520

Conlin CP, Pinching AJ, Perera CU, et al. (1990) HIV-related enteropathy in Zambia: a clinical, microbiological, and histological study. Am J Trop Med Hyg 42: 83-87

Cuadrado LM, Guerrero A, Garcia Asenjo JA, Martin F, Palau E, Garcia Urra D (1988) Cerebral mucormycosis in two cases of acquired immunodeficiency syndrome. Arch Neurol 45: 109-111

De Cock KM, Barrere B, Diaby L et al. (1990) AIDS-the leading cause of adult death in the West African city of Abidjan, Ivory Coast. Science 249: 793-796

De Cock KM, Brun-Vezinet F, Soro B (1991a) HIV-1 and HIV-2 infections and AIDS in West Africa. AIDS 5 (suppl 1): S21-S28

De Cock KM, Gnaore EAG, Braun MM et al. (1991b) Risk of tuberculosis in patients with HIV-I and HIV-II infections in Abidjan, Ivory Coast. Br Med J 302: 496-499

De Cock KM, Selik RM, Soro B, Gayle H, Colebunders RL (1991c) For debate. AIDS surveillance in Africa: a reappraisal of case definitions. Br Med J 303: 1185-1188

De Cock KM, Soro B, Coulibaly IM, Lucas SB (1992) Tuberculosis and HIV infection in sub-Saharan Africa. JAMA 268: 1581-1587

De Leys R, Vanderborght B, Haesevelde MV et al. (1990) Isolation and partial characterization of an unusual human immunodeficiency retrovirus from two persons of West-Central African origin. J Virol 64: 1207-1216

Denning DW, Follansbee SE, Scolaro M, Norris S, Edelstein H, Stevens DA (1991) Pulmonary aspergillosis in the Acquired Immunodeficiency Syndrome. N Engl J Med 324: 654-662

Di Perri G, Danzi MC, De Checchi G et al. (1989) Nosocomial epidemic of active tuberculosis among HIV-infected patients. Lancet ii: 1502-1504

Dryden MS, Shanson DC (1988) The microbial causes of diarrhoea in patients infected with the human immunodeficiency virus. J Infect 17: 107-114

Elvin KM, Lumbwe CM, Luo NP, Bjorkman A, Kallenius G, Linder E (1989) Pneumocystis carinii is not a major cause of pneumonia in HIV infected patients in Lusaka Zambia. Trans R Soc Trop Med Hyg 83: 553-555

Ferro A, Boschetto A, Simoes O (1990) HIV1-2 seroreactivity evaluation in a group of patients with Hansen disease in Guinea Bissau. Vth International Conference on AIDS in Africa, Zaire. Abstract: W.P.E.7

Fleming AF (1990) Opportunistic infections in AIDS in developed and developing countries. Trans R Soc Trop Med Hyg 84: 1-6

Gazzard BG, Wastell C (1990) HIV and surgeons. Br Med J 301: 1003-1004

Gilks CF (1991) What use is a clinical case definition for AIDS in Africa? Br Med J 303: 1189-1190

Gilks CF, Brindler RJ, Otieno LS et al. (1990a) Extrapulmonary and disseminated tuberculosis in HIV-1 seropositive patients presenting to the acute medical services in Nairobi. AIDS 4: 981-985

Gilks CF, Brindler RJ, Otieno LS et al. (1990b) Life-threatening bacteraemia in HIV-1 seropositive adults admitted to hospital in Nairobi, Kenya. Lancet 336: 545-549

Gill PS, Naidu YM, Salahuddin SZ (1990) Recent advances in AIDS-related Kaposi's sarcoma. Current Opin Oncol 2: 1161-1166

Global Programme on AIDS WHO (1992) Current and future dimensions of the HIV/AIDS pandemic. World Health Organisation: Geneva

Gnaore E, Sassan-Morokro M, Kassim S et al. (1993) A comparison of clinical features in tuberculosis associated with infection with human immunodeficiency viruses 1 and 2. Trans R Soc Trop Med Hyg 87: 57-59

Goodgame RW (1990) AIDS in Uganda-Clinical and social features. N Engl J Med 323: 383-389

Graybill JR (1988) Histoplasmosis and AIDS. J Infect Dis 158: 623-626

Greenson JK, Belitsos PC, Yardley JH, Bartlett JG (1991) AIDS Enteropathy: occult enteric infections and duodenal mucosal alterations in chronic diarrhea. Ann Intern Med 114: 366-372

Griffin L, Lucas SB (1982) Does Pneumocystis carinii exist in Kenya? Trans R Soc Trop Med Hyg 76: 198-199

Gulick RM, Heath-Chiozzi M, Crumpacker CS (1991) Varicella-zoster virus disease in patients with human immunodeficiency virus infection. Arch Dermatol 126: 1086-1088

Gumodoka B, Vos J, Kigadye FC, van Asten H, Dolmans WMV, Borgdorff MW (1993) Blood transfusion practices in Mwanza region, Tanzania. AIDS 7: 387-392

Heymann DL, Edstrom K 1991) Strategies in AIDS prevention and control in sub-Saharan Africa. AIDS 5 (suppl 1): S197-S208

Holmberg, SD, Stewart JA et al. (1988) Prior herpes simplex virus type 2 as a risk factor for HIV infection. JAMA 259: 1048–1050

Holmes KK, Kreiss J (1988) Heterosexual transmission of human immunodeficiency virus: overview of a neglected aspect of the AIDS epidemic. J Acq Immuno Defic Synd 1: 602–610

Hook EW (1989) Syphilis and HIV infection. J Infect Dis 160: 530–534

Howlett WP, Nkya WM, Mmuni KA, Missalek WR (1989) Neurological disorders in AIDS and HIV disease in the northern zone of Tanzania. AIDS 3: 289–296

Humphrey-Smith I, Donker G, Turzo A, Chastel C, Schmidt-Mayerova H (1993) Evaluation of mechanical transmission of HIV by the African soft tick, Ornithodoros moubata. AIDS 7: 341–347

Hunter DJ (1993) AIDS in sub-Saharan Africa: the epidemiology of heterosexual transmission and the prospects for prevention. Epidemiology 4: 63–72

Jonckheer T, Levy J, Ninane J, Alimenti A, Francois A (1988) AIDS case definitions for African children. Lancet ii: 690–691

Katzenstein DA, Latif AS, Grace SA et al. (1990) Clinical and laboratory characteristics of HIV-1 infection in Zimbabwe. J Acquir Immune Defic Syndr 3: 701–707

Kaye BR (1989) Rheumatological manifestations of infection with human immunodeficiency virus (HIV). Ann Intern Med 111: 158–167

Kent C, Samuel M, Winkelstein WJ (1987) The role of anal/genital warts in HIV infection. JAMA 258: 3385–3386

Laga M, Manoka A, Kivuvu M et al. (1993) Non-ulcerative sexually transmitted diseases as risk factors for HIV-1 transmission in women: results from a cohort study. AIDS 7: 95–102

Laga M, Nzila N, Goeman J (1991) The interrelationship of sexually transmitted diseases and HIV infection: implications for the control of both epidemics in Africa. AIDS 5 (suppl 1): S55–S63

Laroche R, Dupont B, Touze JE et al. (1992) Cryptococcal meningitis associated with acquired immunodeficiency syndrome (AIDS) in African patients: treatment with fluconazole. J Med Vet Mycol 30: 71–78

Latif AS, Katzenstein DA, Bassett MT, Houston S, Emmanuel JC, Marowa E (1989) Genital ulcers and transmission of HIV among couples in Zimbabwe. AIDS 3: 519–523

Le Guenno BM, Barabe P, Griffet PA et al. (1991) HIV-2 and HIV-1 AIDS cases in Senegal: clinical patterns and immunological perturbations. J Acquir Immune Defic Syndr 4: 421–427

Liautaud B, Pape JW, DeHovitz JA et al. (1989) Pruritic skin lesions: a common initial presentation of acquired immunodeficiency syndrome. Arch Dermatol 125: 629–632

Lindan CP, Allen S, Serufilira A et al. (1992) Predictors of mortality among HIV-infected women in Kigali, Rwanda. Ann Intern Med 116: 320–328

Lucas SB (1990) Missing infections in AIDS. Trans R Soc Trop Med & Hygiene 84 (suppl 1): 34–38

Lukehart SA, Hook EW, Baker-Zander SA, Collier AC, Critchlow CW, Handsfield HH (1988) Invasion of the central nervous system by *Treponema pallidum*: implications for diagnosis and treatment. Ann Intern Med 109: 855–862

Mandal B (1989) AIDS and fungal infections. J Infect 19: 199–205

Mann JM, Bila K, Colebunders RL et al. (1986) Natural history of HIV infection in Zaire. Lancet ii: 707–709

Markovitz DM (1993) Infection with the human immunodeficiency virus type 2. Ann Intern Med 118: 211–218

Marlink RG, Ricard D, M'Boup S et al. (1988) Clinical, hematologic, and immunologic cross-sectional evaluation of individuals exposed to human immunodeficiency virus type-2 (HIV-2). AIDS Res Hum Retroviruses 4: 137–148

Mbidde E, Banura C, Kazura J, Desmomd-Hellman S, Kizito A, Hellman N (1990) Non-Hodgkin's lymphoma (NHL) and HIV infection in Uganda. Vth International Conference on AIDS in Africa, Zaire abstract: F.P.B.1

McLeod DT, Neill P, Robertson VJ (1989) Pulmonary diseases in patients infected with the human immunodeficiency virus in Zimbabwe, Central Africa. Trans R Soc Trop Med Hyg 83: 694–697

McMillan A, Bishop PE (1989) Clinical course of anogenital warts in men infected with human immunodeficiency virus. Genitourin Med 65: 225–228

McMillan A, Young H, Peutherer JF (1990) Influence of human immunodeficiency virus infection on treponemal serology, in patients who have been treated for syphilis. J Infect 21: 95–103

Meeran K (1989) Prevalence of HIV infection among patients with leprosy and tuberculosis in rural Zambia. Br Med J 298: 364–365

Melbye M, Njelesani EK, Bayley A et al. (1986) Evidence for heterosexual transmission and clinical manifestations of human immunodeficiency virus infection and related conditions in Lusaka, Zambia. Lancet ii: 1113–1115

Mhiri C, Belec L, Di Costanzo B, Georges A, Gherardi R (1992) The slim disease in African patients with AIDS. Trans R Soc Trop Med Hyg 86: 303-306

Montalban C, Calleja JL, Erice A et al. (1990) Visceral leishmaniasis in patients infected with human immunodeficiency virus. J Infect 21: 261-270

Moses S, Plummer FA, Ngugi EN, Nagelkerke NJ, Anzala AO, Ndinya Achola JO (1991) Controlling HIV in Africa: effectiveness and cost of an intervention in a high-frequency STD transmitter core group. AIDS 5: 407-411

Murray CJ, Styblo K, Rouillon A (1990) Tuberculosis in developing countries: burden, intervention and cost. Bull Int Union Tuberc Lung Dis 65: 6-24

Naucler A, Albino P, Da Silva AP, Andreasson PA, Andersson S, Biberfeld G (1991) HIV-2 infection in hospitalized patients in Bissau, Guinea-Bissau. AIDS 5: 301-304

Nicholl A (1993) The AIDS epidemic in Africa: monster not myth. Br Med J 306: 938-939

Nkowane BM (1991) Prevalence and incidence of HIV infection in Africa: a review of data published in 1990. 5 (suppl 1): S7-S15

Nsanze H FMDLe (1981) Genital ulcers in Kenya: Clinical and laboratory study. Br J Vener Dis 57: 378-381

Nsubuga P, Mugerwas R, Nsibambi J, Sewankambo N, Katabira E, Berkley S (1990) The association of genital ulcer disease and HIV infection at a dermatology-STD clinic in Uganda. J Acquir Immune Defic Syndr 3: 1002-1005

Nunn P, Kibuga D, Gathua S et al. (1991) Cutaneous hypersensitivity reactions due to thiacetazone in HIV-1 seropositive patients treated for tuberculosis. Lancet 337: 627-630

Orenstein JM, Chiang J, Steinberg W, Smith PD, Rotterdam H, Kotler DP (1990) Intestinal microsporidiosis as a cause of diarrhea in human immunodeficiency virus-infected patients: a report of 20 cases. Hum Pathol 21: 475-481

Pela AO, Platt JJ (1989) AIDS in Africa: emerging trends. Soc Sci Med 28: 1-8

Peterman TA, Jaffe HW, Beral V (1993) Epidemiologic clues to the etiology of Kaposi's sarcoma. AIDS 7: 605-611

Peters BS, Fish D, Golden R, Evans DA, Bryceson AD, Pinching AJ (1990) Visceral Leishmaniasis in HIV infection and AIDS. Clinical features and response to treatment. Q J Med 77: 1101-1111

Pitchenik AE, Burr J, Suarez M, Fertel D, Gonzalez G, Moas C (1987) Human T-Cell lymphotropic virus-III (HTLV-III) seropositivity and related disease among 71 consecutive patients in whom tuberculosis was diagnosed. A prospective study. Am Rev Respir Dis 135: 875-879

Plummer FA, Simonsen JN, Cameron DW et al. (1991) Co-factors in male-female transmission of human immunodeficiency virus type 1. J Infect Dis 163: 233-239

Prazuck T, Tall F, Nacro B et al. (1993) HIV infection and severe malnutrition: a clinical and epidemiological study in Burkina Faso. AIDS 7: 103-108

Preble EA (1990) Impact of HIV/AIDS on African children. Soc Sci Med 31: 671-680

Prual A, Chacko S, Koch Weser D (1991) Sexual behaviour, AIDS and poverty in Sub-Saharan Africa [editorial]. Int J STD AIDS 2: 1-9

Redd SC, Rutherford GW, Sande MA et al. (1990) The role of human immunodeficiency virus infection in pneumococcal bacteremia in San Francisco residents. J Infect Dis 162: 1012-1017

Rogers PL, Walker RE, Lane HC et al. (1988) Disseminated mycobacterium haemophilum infection in two patients with the acquired immune deficiency syndrome. Am J Med 84: 640-642

Ryder RW, Temmerman M (1991) The effect of HIV-1 infection during pregnancy and the perinatal period on maternal and child health in Africa. AIDS 5 (suppl 1): S75-S85

Ryder RW, Nsa W, Hassig S (1989) Perinatal transmission of the human immunodeficiency virus type 1 to infants of seropositive women in Zaire. N Engl J Med 320: 1637-42

Saxinger WC, Levine PH, Dean A (1985) Evidence for exposure to HTLV-III in Uganda before 1973. Science 22: 1036-1037

Serwadda D, Mugerwa RD, Sewankambo NK (1985) Slim disease a new disease in Uganda and its association with HTLV-III infection. Lancet ii: 849-52

Serwadda D, Wawer MJ, Musgrave SD, Sewankambo NK, Kaplan JE, Gray RH (1992) HIV risk factors in three geographic strata of rural Rakai District, Uganda. AIDS 6: 983-989

Sewankambo N, Mugerwa RD, Goodgame R, et al. (1987) Enteropathic AIDS in Uganda. An endoscopic, histological and microbiological study. AIDS 1: 9-13

Simonsen JN, Cameron DW, Gakinya MN, et al. (1988) Human immunodeficiency virus infection among men with sexually transmitted diseases: Experience from a centre in Africa. N Engl J Med 319: 274-278

Slutkin G, Leowski J, Mann J (1988) Tuberculosis and AIDS. The effects of the AIDS epidemic on the tuberculosis problem and tuberculosis programmes. Bull Int Union Tuberc Lung Dis 63: 21-24

Soeprono F, Schinella RA, Cockerell CJ, Comite SJ (1986) Seborrhoeic-like dermatitis of acquired immunodeficiency syndrome. A clinico-pathological study. J Am Acad Dermatol 14: 242–248

Sonnet J, Michaux J, Zech F (1987) Early AIDS cases originating from Zaire and Burundi (1962–1976). Scand J Infect Dis 19: 511–517

Sunderam G, McDonald RJ, Maniatis T (1986) Tuberculosis as a manifestation of the acquired immunodeficiency syndrome (AIDS). JAMA 256: 362–366

Tekle-Haimanot R, Frommel D, Tadesse T, Verdier M, Abebe M, Denis F (1991) A survey of HTLV-1 and HIV in Ethiopian leprosy patients. AIDS 5: 108–110

Tsujimoto H, Hasegawa A, Maki N (1989) Sequence of a novel simian immunodeficiency virus from a wild-caught African mandrill. Nature 341: 539–541

Veekan H, Verbeek J, Houweling H, Cobelens F (1991) Occupational HIV infection and health care workers in the tropics. Trop Doct 21: 28–31

Volberding PA, Cusick PS, Feigal DW (1989) Effect of chemotherapy for HIV-associated Kaposi's sarcoma on longterm survival. Am Soc Clin Oncol 11

Wahman A, Melnick SL, Rhame FS, Potter JD (1991) The epidemiology of classic, African, and immunosuppressed Kaposi's sarcoma. Epidemiol Rev 13: 178–199

Whittle H, Egboga A, Todd J et al. (1992) Clinical and laboratory predictors of survival in Gambian patients with symptomatic HIV-1 or HIV-2 infection. AIDS 6: 685–689

World Health Organization (1986) Acquired immunodeficiency syndrome (AIDS). Weekly Epidemiol Rec 61: 69–73

Index

Abdominal pain 91, 101
Acalculous cholecystitis 103
Acyclovir 11, 97, 98, 102
Adrenals, insufficiency 9
AIDS wasting syndrome 104
AIDS-related complex (ARC) 123
Albendazole 98, 108
Amikacin 76
Amoebiasis 170
Amphotericin B 12, 97, 98, 102, 133, 137
Amphotericin lozenges 98
Anaemia 194–195
Anorectal disease
 differential diagnosis 93, 110
 symptoms 92
Antiretroviral therapy 13–14
Anxiety 20, 26, 32–33, 51, 61, 122
 symptoms 32–33, 55
 treatment 32–33
Aphthous ulcers 99
Arthritis 8, 245
 septic 245
Aspergillosis 238
Atavaquone 70
Atopic dermatitis 163, 176
 treatment 178

Bacillary angiomatosis 167, 176
 treatment 179
Basal cell carcinoma 172
Beck Depression Inventory (BDI) 27, 54
Beta 2 microglobulin 10–11
Blastocystis homininis 233
Bone marrow 195–198
 suppression 74
Brain biopsy 130
Breathlessness 60–61, 214
Broncho-alveolar lavage (BAL) 67–69
Bronchoscopy 67–69
Bullous impetigo 166
Burkitt's lymphoma 203, 240

Candidiasis 98, 108, 181, 213
 GI tract 108

 oesophageal 89, 98, 100, 234
 oral 6–7, 12, 86, 97, 169, 172, 174, 182, 234, 240
Carcinoma 139
 cervical 15
Cauda equina syndrome 120
CD4 counts 12
Cellulitis 166
Cephalosporins 102
Cerebrospinal fluid 124, 125, 137
Cerebrovascular disease 143
Chancroid (*H. ducreyi*) 243
Chest x-ray 63
 Kaposi's Sarcoma 61–63
 mycobacterial 61–63
 Pneumocystis carinii 61, 63
Chlamydia trachomatis 15, 93, 244
Ciprofloxacin 102
Clarithromycin 76
Classification 3, 14
Clindamycin 70, 71, 237
Clinical psychologists 20–22
Clinical psychology
 assessment 26–29
 indications for referral 22
 levels 21
 treatment 30–31
Coccidiodomycosis 170
Colony stimulating factors 199
Compulsions 33–34
Computed tomography
 cranial 123, 126, 129
 pulmonary 64
Constitutional disease 14
Constitutional symptoms (malaise, weight loss, anorexia) 14, 62, 91, 104–106, 214
Continuous positive airways pressure (CPAP) 72
Cotrimoxazole 102
 Isospora belli 98
 PCP treatment 69–70, 237
 primary prophylaxis of PCP 12, 13
 side effects 69, 198
Cough 61, 214
Counselling
 children 41–42
 death and dying 38–39

Index

definition 20
haemophilia 40–41
HIV antibody testing 23–26, 51
Cryptococcus neoformans 117, 136, 170, 181, 241, 246
 cerebrospinal fluid 125
 presentation 119, 120, 136
 serology 125
 treatment 133, 137
Cryptosporidium 93, 98, 104, 107, 233
Cytomegalovirus (CMV) 93, 109, 177
 neurological 120
  encephalitis 138
  peripheral neuropathy 138
  polyradiculopathy 129, 134, 138
 cutaneous 168, 176
 gastrointestinal 93, 95, 98, 100
 oesophageal 89
 oropharyngeal 88
 pneumonitis 63, 73
 polyradiculopathy 138
 retinitis 9, 121, 134, 138–139
Cytosine arabinoside 143

Dapsone
 primary prophylaxis of PCP 12, 13
 treatment of PCP 71
Delta virus 216
Delusions 123
Demodex 178
Demodex mites 170, 176
 treatment 180
Demodicidosis 181
Dental caries 215
Depression 20, 26, 53, 122
 symptoms 33, 50–51, 52
 treatment 33, 54–55
Dermatophytes 169, 177, 181
Diarrhoea 91–92, 104, 106–111, 232, 233–234
 pathogen negative 93
 radiological investigation 94–95
 treatment 99, 109
Didanosine (ddI) 13
Dideoxycytosine (ddC) 13
Ditiocarb sodium (imuthiol) 14
Drug eruptions 166
DTPA (99m-3Tc) 66

EEG 123, 131
Eflornithine (DFMO) 71
Electromyography (EMG) 131
Endocarditis, infective 214, 217
Endoscopic retrograde cholangiopancreatology 95
Endoscopy 95–96
 sterilization of equipment 96
Entamoeba histolytica 107
Enterocytozoon bienusi 94, 108, 233
Eosinophilic folliculitis 164, 176
 treatment 179

Epstein-Barr virus (EBV) 90, 142, 203
ERCP, *see* Endoscopic retrograde cholangiopancreatology
Erythropoietin 199
Ethambutol 76

Fluconazole 12, 97, 98, 102, 133, 137
5-Flucytosine 133, 137
Folliculitis 166
 treatment 179
Foscarnet (phosphonoformate)
 GI tract 98
 pneumonitis 74
 retinitis 134, 138
 side effects 74, 98
Fungal infections 240
Fungal organism 69

Gallium-67, in the lung 65
Ganciclovir 102
Gancyclovir (DHPG) 134
 for CNS disease 138
 for GI disease 98
 for pneumonitis 74
 for retinitis 138
 side effects 74
Gastrointestinal bleeding 91, 101
Gay bowel syndrome 107
Giardia lamblia 99, 108
Gingivitis 6, 215
 treatment 12
Granuloma annulare 65

Haemophilia, psychological problems 40–41
Haemoptysis 62
Hair 172, 241
Hairy leukoplakia (OHL) 7, 86, 87, 173
 treatment 182
Hallucinations 123
Headache, differential diagnosis 118
Hepatitis 101
 A 101
 B 15, 101, 215, 249
 C 101, 102, 215, 216
 D 101, 102, 216
Herpes simplex (HSV-1) 174, 177, 180
 ano-genital 5, 86, 88, 93, 110
 cutaneous 167–168
 drug resistance 12
 encephalitis 117
 myelitis 120
 oesophageal 90, 100
 oral 12, 97, 98
 prophylaxis 11
Herpes simplex virus 2 (HSV-2) 244
Herpes zoster (HZV) 5, 240–241
 cutaneous (treatment) 11, 168, 180
Histoplasma 178
Histoplasmosis 170, 173, 176, 181, 238

HLA-B27 8
Hodgkin's Disease 197, 207
Human immunodeficiency virus (HIV)
  in Africa 225-250
  Centre for Disease Control Classification (CDC I-IV) 1-5
  encephalopathy 117, 143, 151
  interrelationship with sexually transmitted disease 242-243
  laboratory assessment 9-11
  meningitis 145-146
  muscle disease 121
  ongoing 230-231
  peripheral neuropathy 146-149
  prevention by behavioural change 23, 37-38, 42
  seroconversion illness 1, 162-163, 173, 191
  vacuolar myelopathy 146
  WHO case clinical definition 232-233, 248
Human immunodeficiency virus-2 (HIV-2) 230-231
Human papilloma virus (HPV) 110, 168, 244-245

IDA ^{99m}Tc scans 96
Inflammatory dermatoses 163-166, 176
Inosine pranobex 14
Intravenous drug users
  behaviour patterns 24, 36-37, 43, 216, 217
  clinical management 218-219
Isoniazid 235, 236
  prophylaxis 13
  treatment 75, 102
Isospora belli 98, 108
Itraconazole 97, 98

Jaundice 91, 101, 215-216
JC virus 125, 138

Kaposi's sarcoma 93, 171, 197
  in Africa 238-239
  GI tract 92-93, 95, 109, 110-111
    treatment 110-111
  in injecting drug users 216
  oral 6, 88, 173, 178
    treatment 181-182
  pulmonary 61-63, 69, 77-78
    treatment 77
Ketoconazole 12, 97, 98, 102

Leishmaniasis 248-249
Leprosy 167, 240, 246
Lumbar puncture 123, 124, 125, 126
Lung function tests
  injecting drug users 214
  Kaposi's Sarcoma 65
  Pneumocystis carinii 65
  smokers 65

Lupus anticoagulant 200
Lymph nodes, enlarged 214
Lymphadenopathy
  differential diagnosis 6
  injecting drug users 214
  persistent generalised (PGL) 5
Lymphomas 8, 203
  B cell 78
  bone marrow 197
  Burkitt-like 197
  cerebral 117, 126, 142-143, 206
  GI tract 92-93, 109
  pulmonary 78
Lymphopenia 192

Magnetic resonance imaging (MRI)
  cerebral 123, 126, 129
  spinal 129
Malabsorption 104
Malaria 248
Mechanical ventilation 72
Mental status 122-123
Metronidazole 99
Miconazole 12
Microsporidium 94, 98, 108
Molluscum contagiosum 5, 169, 174, 177, 241
  treatment 180
Mononeuritis multiplex 120, 147
Mood 120
  assessment 54-55
Mood disorder 123
Mouth 182
Mucositis, severe 88
Muscle biopsy 130-131
Mycobacteria 6, 8, 61, 63, 74-76, 93, 197
  atypical 76, 101, 104, 107, 180, 197, 236
  GI tract 101, 103-104, 107
  pulmonary
  skin 166-167
  treatment 76
  tuberculosis 8, 75-76, 103, 167, 180, 215, 234-236
    cerebral 141-142
    chest x-ray appearance 63, 235
    primary prophylaxis 13, 235
    skin 166
    treatment 76, 141
Myelography 129
Myopathy 120, 121, 149-151

Naevi 171
Nails 172, 241
Nausea 99
  treatment 98
Nebulisers
  for pentamadine treatment 70
  ultrasonic (for induced sputum) 67
Neisseria gonorrhoeae 15, 16, 93, 217, 244
Neopterin 11
Nerve conduction studies (NCS) 131

Neuropathy 120, 121
  autonomic 9
  demyelinating 120, 146–147
  distal symmetrical 120, 147–149
  drug induced 120
  sensory 124
Neurophysiology 131, 148
Neuropsychological problems 35–36, 49, 52–53, 56, 122, 123
  AIDS dementia complex (HIV-1 associated cognitive/motor complex) HACC 35, 52, 151, 216
  definition 52
  diagnosis 152
  pathology 152–153, 154–155
  treatment 36, 153–154
Neutropenia 192
Non-Hodgkin's lymphoma 202–207, 217, 239
  cerebral 143
  clinical features 204
  management 204
  presentation 204
  treatment 205–206
Nuclear medicine
  gastrointestinal 96
  pulmonary 65–66
Nystatin 12, 97, 98

Obsessions 33–34
Oesophageal disease 100–101
Open lung biopsy 69
Oximetry 64
Oxygen, assessment 64

p24 antigen 11
Papilloma virus, human 93
Paromomycin 98
Pentamidine
  GI tract 102
  primary prophylaxis 12
  side effects 70
  treatment of PCP 70
    IV/IM 70
    nebulised 70
Periodontal disease 215
Personality change 123
Pityriasis rosea 165
Pityrosporum 176, 240
Pneumocystis carinii pneumonia (PCP)
  continuous positive airways pressure (CPAP) 72
  corticosteroids 71
  examination findings 62
  incidence 60, 206, 214, 237
  induced sputum 67
  lung function tests 65, 217
  mechanical ventilation 72
  nuclear medicine 65–66
  oximetry 64, 217
  presentation 60–62, 170
  prophylaxis
    indications 12, 206
    primary 12
    secondary 72
  radiology 62–64
  serodiagnosis 66
  treatment 69–72
Pneumonia
  bacterial 61–64, 76–77, 214, 236
  fungal 77
  Pneumocystis carinii (see under *Pneumocystis carinii*)
Pneumonitis
  lymphocytic interstitial 61, 63, 69, 78
  non-specific interstitial 61, 63, 69
Primaquine 70, 71, 237
Progressive multifocal leukoencephalopathy (PML) 117, 137–138
  presentation 119, 120, 137–138
  radiology 129
  treatment 137–138, 138
Protein S deficiency 200
Protozoa, GI tract 107–108
Prurigo 241
Pruritus (generalised) 165, 166
Psoriasis 5, 163–164, 176
  treatment 179
Psychiatry, assessment 55–56
Psychosis 49, 51–52
Psychotherapy
  categories 20
  definition 20
  treatment 30–31
Pyogenic bacterial 63
Pyomyositis, tropical 249
Pyrazinamide 75, 236
Pyrexia 213–214
Pyrimethamine 102, 133

Reiter's Syndrome 164
Renal syndromes, in injecting drug users 216
Rifabutin 76
Rifampicin 75102

Salmonella 93, 104, 106, 234
Scabies 171, 176, 178
  treatment 181
Scalded skin syndrome 166
Schistosomiasis 249
Sclerosing cholangitis 95, 103
Seborrhoeic dermatitis 5, 163, 176
  treatment 11, 178
Seizures 122
Seroconversion 175–176
Sexual problems 34
Sexually-transmitted disease 4, 14–16
  in Africa 241–245
  in injecting drug users 217
  screening tests 15
  treatment 15

Shingles 11
Simian immunodeficiency virus (SIV) 230
Skin 5, 162–185
  bacteria 166–167
  biopsy 175
  in children 174
  drug reactions 165–166
  in haemophiliacs 174–175
  scrapings 175
  swabs 175
  viruses 167–169
Slim disease 104, 233, 234
Somatosensory evoked potentials (SEPs) 131
Spielberger State-Trait Anxiety Inventory
    (STAI) 27, 55
Sporotrichosis 170
Sputum, induced 67
Staphylococcal folliculitis 179
Staphylococcus aureus 174
Streptomycin 236
Suicide 53–54
Sulphadiazine 133
Syphilis 15, 16, 93, 126, 139–141, 167, 177, 217, 243–244
  treatment 140

T-lymphocyte subsets (CD4, CD8) 10, 12, 13, 191, 217, 237
Thalidomide 182
Therapy 33
Thiacetazone 236
Thrombocytopenia 192–194, 200
  treatment 202
Thrombotic thrombocytopenic purpura 200

Toxic megacolon 106
Toxoplasma gondii 117, 132–136, 246–247
  presentation 119, 120, 132
  prophylaxis, primary 13
  radiology 120, 132
  serology 124–125
  treatment 132–133, 136
Transbronchial Biopsy (TBB) 67–69
Treponema pallidum 93
Trichomonas vaginalis 15, 16, 244
Trimethoprim 71
Trimetrexate 71

Ulceration
  oesophageal 100
  oral 6, 88, 98, 172
    management of 12
    treatment 182

Vacuolar myelopathy 120
Visual problems 121–122

Walking difficulty, differential diagnosis 120
Worried well 39–40

Yaws 167

Zidovudine (AZT) 13, 14, 138, 153
  anaemia 194, 198
  myopathy 151